**Proceedings of the Centennial Symposium
Manhattan Eye, Ear and Throat Hospital**

VOLUME ONE # OPHTHALMOLOGY

Proceedings of the Centennial Symposium
Manhattan Eye, Ear and Throat Hospital

VOLUME ONE OPHTHALMOLOGY

Edited by

ARNOLD I. TURTZ, M.D.

Attending Surgeon and Chief, Cataract Service II,
Manhattan Eye, Ear and Throat Hospital; Clinical
Professor of Ophthalmology, New York Medical College,
New York, N. Y.

With 247 illustrations

Saint Louis

The C. V. Mosby Company

1969

To

Manhattan Eye, Ear and Throat Hospital
on this hallmark occasion,
as it commences its second century of service.

Copyright © 1969 by
The C. V. Mosby Company

All rights reserved. No part of this book may be
reproduced in any manner without written permission
of the publisher.

Printed in the United States of America

Standard Book Number 8016-5138-7

Library of Congress Catalog Card Number 78-91798

Distributed in Great Britain by Henry Kimpton, London

Contributors

Peter H. Ballen, M.D.

Attending Surgeon, Mercy Hospital, Rockville Centre; Clinical Assistant Professor, State University of New York, Downstate Medical Center, Brooklyn, New York

José I. Barraquer, M.D.

Chief, Ophthalmology, Marly Clinic; President, Instituto Barraquer de America, Bogota, Colombia

M. A. Bedford, F.R.C.S.

Consultant Eye Surgeon, St. Bartholomew's Hospital; Senior Lecturer, Department of Clinical Ophthalmology, Moorfields Eye Hospital, London, England

John G. Bellows, M.D.

Surgeon, St. Joseph Hospital; Associate Professor, Northwestern University; Professor of Ophthalmology, Cook County Graduate School of Medicine, Chicago, Illinois

Irving Berlin, M.D.

Attending Anesthesiologist, Manhattan Eye, Ear and Throat Hospital, New York, New York

C. D. Binkhorst, M.D.

Surgeon, Ophthalmology, Flamish-Zeeland, Holland

Goodwin M. Breinin, M.D.

Director of Eye Service, New York University Hospital; Daniel B. Kirby Professor and Chairman, Department of Ophthalmology, New York University Medical Center, New York, New York

Nathaniel R. Bronson II, M.D.

Associate Attending Surgeon, Manhattan Eye, Ear and Throat Hospital; Attending Surgeon, Southampton Hospital, Southampton, New York

Harold W. Brown, M.D.

Attending Surgeon, Manhattan Eye, Ear and Throat Hospital, New York, New York

Stuart I. Brown, M.D.

Assistant Attending Surgeon and Director, Cornea Research Laboratory, and Assistant Professor of Surgery, New York Hospital, New York, New York

Alston Callahan, M.D.

Surgeon, Carraway Methodist Hospital, University Hospital; President, The Eye Foundation Hospital, Birmingham, Alabama

Ramon Castroviejo, M.D.

Chief, Department of Ophthalmology, St. Vincent's Hospital and Medical Center; Professor, Clinical Ophthalmology, New York University Postgraduate Medical School; Clinical Professor in Ophthalmology, Mt. Sinai School of Medicine of the City University of New York, New York

Robert S. Coles, M.D.

Associate Attending Surgeon, Mt. Sinai Hospital; Director Uveitis Clinic, Bellevue Hospital; Associate Clinical Professor, New York University, New York, New York

Frank H. Constantine, M.D.

Surgeon-Director, Manhattan Eye, Ear and Throat Hospital; Professor of Ophthalmology, New York University Medical Center, New York, New York

John Marquis Converse, M.D.

Surgeon-Director, Plastic Surgery Department, Manhattan Eye, Ear and Throat Hospital; Lawrence D. Bell Professor of Plastic Surgery, New York University School of Medicine, New York, New York

Brian J. Curtin, M.D.

Attending Surgeon and Chief, Myopia Clinic, Manhattan, Eye, Ear and Throat Hospital; Assistant Professor of Clinical Ophthalmology, New York University College of Medicine, New York, New York

Andrew de Roetth, Jr., M.D.

Assistant Attending Ophthalmologist, Presbyterian Hospital; Assistant Professor of Clinical Ophthalmology, Columbia University College of Physicians and Surgeons, New York, New York

Arthur Gerard DeVoe, M.D.

Director, Institute of Ophthalmology, Presbyterian Hospital; Professor and Chairman, Department of Ophthalmology, College of Physicians and Surgeons, Columbia University, New York, New York

Edward A. Dunlap, M.D.

Clinical Professor of Surgery, Cornell University Medical School, New York, New York

Sidney A. Fox, M.D.

Consultant Ophthalmologist, Goldwater Memorial Hospital, Bronx Veterans' Hospital; Clinical Professor of Ophthalmology, New York University School of Medicine, New York, New York

Professor Jules François

Director, Ophthalmological Clinic, University of Ghent, Ghent, Belgium

Miles A. Galin, M.D.

Attending Ophthalmologist, Flower and Fifth Avenue Hospitals; Professor and Chairman, Department of Ophthalmology, New York Medical College, New York, New York

Antonio R. Gasset, M.D.

Resident in Ophthalmology, University of Florida College of Medicine, Gainesville, Florida

Marc H. Gobin, M.D.

Surgeon, Ophthalmology, Antwerp, Holland

Dan M. Gordon, M.D.

Associate Attending Surgeon, New York Hospital; Associate Professor (Surgery), Cornell University Medical College, New York, New York

George Gorin, M.D.

Attending Surgeon, Manhattan Eye, Ear and Throat Hospital; Assistant Clinical Professor of Ophthalmology, Albert Einstein Medical School, New York, New York

Herbert L. Gould, M.D.

Assistant Attending Surgeon and Director, Scleral Lens Clinic, Manhattan Eye, Ear and Throat Hospital; Visiting Lecturer in Surgery, State University of New York, Downstate Medical Center, Brooklyn, New York

Raymond Harrison, M.D.

Attending Surgeon and Chief, Glaucoma Clinic, Manhattan Eye, Ear and Throat Hospital, New York, New York

Wendell L. Hughes, M.D.

Consulting Ophthalmologist, Hempstead General Hospital; Assistant Professor, New York University School of Medicine, New York, New York

Herbert M. Katzin, M.D.

Attending Surgeon, Manhattan Eye, Ear and Throat Hospital, New York, New York

Herbert E. Kaufman, M.D.

Professor and Chairman, Department of Ophthalmology, College of Medicine, University of Florida, Gainesville, Florida

Charles D. Kelman, M.D.

Attending Surgeon, Manhattan Eye, Ear and Throat Hospital; Assistant Clinical Professor of Ophthalmology, New York Medical School, New York, New York

Samuel J. Kimura, M.D.

Francis I. Proctor Foundation for Research in Ophthalmology and Department of Ophthalmology, University of California San Francisco Medical Center, San Francisco, California

Philip Knapp, M.D.

Attending Surgeon, Institute of Ophthalmology, Presbyterian Hospital; Associate Professor, Clinical Ophthalmology, Columbia University College of Physicians and Surgeons, New York, New York

Professor Tadeusz Krwawicz

Director, Ophthalmological Clinic and Professor and Chairman, Ophthalmology, Medical Academy, Lublin, Poland

Paul A. M. Leonard, M.D.

Surgeon, Ophthalmology, Flamish-Zeeland, Holland

Irving H. Leopold, M.D.

Director, Department of Ophthalmology, Mt. Sinai Hospital; Chairman and Professor, Department of Ophthalmology, Mt. Sinai School of Medicine, New York, New York

Harvey Lincoff, M.D.

Assistant Clinical Professor, Ophthalmology, Cornell Medical Center, New York, New York

Professor Maurice H. Luntz

Chief Ophthalmologist, Johannesburg Teaching Hospitals; Professor of Ophthalmology, University of Witwatersrand, Johannesburg, South Africa

Seamus Lynch, M.D.

Director, Anesthesiology, Manhattan Eye, Ear and Throat Hospital, New York, New York

Miguel Martinez, M.D.

Co-Director, Wilmer Surgical Research Laboratory, The Wilmer Institute, The Johns Hopkins Hospital, Baltimore, Maryland

A. Edward Maumenee, M.D.

Professor of Ophthalmology, The Wilmer Institute of Ophthalmology, The Johns Hopkins University School of Medicine and Hospital, Baltimore, Maryland

P. Robb McDonald, M.D.

Ophthalmologist in Chief, Lankenau Hospital; Chief, Retina Service, Wills Eye Hospital; Professor of Ophthalmology, Jefferson Medical College; Lecturer in Ophthalmology, Graduate School of Medicine, University of Pennsylvania, Philadelphia, Pennsylvania

†John McLean, M.D.

Professor and Chairman, Department of Ophthalmology, Cornell Medical Center, New York, New York

Margaret Fealy Obear, M.D.

Assistant Attending Surgeon, Manhattan Eye, Ear and Throat Hospital, New York, New York

Edward Okun, M.D.

Surgeon, McMillan Hospital; Assistant Professor, Clinical Ophthalmology, Washington University, St. Louis, Missouri

Marshall M. Parks, M.D.

Chairman, Eye Department, Children's Hospital; Senior Attending Surgeon, Washington Hospital Center, Washington, D. C.

David Paton, M.D.

Consultant in Ophthalmology, Ft. Howard Veterans Hospital; Associate Professor of Ophthalmology, The Wilmer Institute; Co-Director, Wilmer Surgical Research Laboratory, Baltimore, Maryland

R. Townley Paton, M.D.

Consultant-Ophthalmology, Huntington Hospital, Southampton Hospital; Vice President, Manhattan Eye, Ear and Throat Hospital, New York, New York

Adolph Posner, M.D.

Attending Surgeon, Manhattan Eye, Ear and Throat Hospital, New York, New York

Edward W. Purnell, M.D.

Associate Ophthalmologist, University Hospitals; Assistant Professor, Ophthalmology, Case-Western Reserve School of Medicine, Cleveland, Ohio

Algernon B. Reese, M.D.

Consulting Ophthalmologist, Manhattan Eye, Ear and Throat Hospital, New York, New York

Frederick Ridley, F.R.C.S.

Senior Surgeon and Director, Contact Lens Department, Moorfields Eye Hospital; Lecturer in Ophthalmology, University of London, London, England

---

†Deceased.

Richard Robbins, M.D.

Department of Ophthalmology, New York Medical College, New York, New York

Cyril Sanger, M.D.

Anesthesiologist, Manhattan Eye, Ear and Throat Hospital, New York, New York

Walter S. Schachat, M.D.

Attending Surgeon, Manhattan Eye, Ear and Throat Hospital, New York, New York

Harold G. Scheie, M.D.

William F. Norris and George E. de Schweinitz Professor of Ophthalmology and Chairman of the Department, University of Pennsylvania School of Medicine, Philadelphia, Pennsylvania

Abraham Schlossman, M.D.

Attending Surgeon, Manhattan Eye, Ear and Throat Hospital, New York; Clinical Associate Professor of Ophthalmology, State University of New York, Downstate Medical Center, Brooklyn, New York

Donald M. Shafer, M.D.

Acting Chairman, Department of Ophthalmology, New York Hospital—Cornell Medical Center; Secretary, Board of Surgeon Directors, Manhattan Eye, Ear and Throat Hospital, New York, New York

Byron Smith, M.D.

Director, Ophthalmic Plastic Surgery and Chairman, Department of Ophthalmology, Manhattan Eye, Ear and Throat Hospital, New York, New York

David B. Soll, M.D.

Director, Department of Ophthalmology, Frankford Hospital; Associate, Department of Ophthalmology, University of Pennsylvania, Philadelphia, Pennsylvania

R. David Sudarsky, M.D.

Associate Attending Surgeon, Manhattan Eye, Ear and Throat Hospital, New York, New York

H. Saul Sugar, M.D.

Chief of Ophthalmology, Sinai Hospital of Detroit; Clinical Professor, Wayne State University School of Medicine, Detroit, Michigan

Richard R. Tenzel, M.D.

Surgeon, Jackson Memorial Hospital, North Miami Beach; Clinical Assistant Professor, University of Miami School of Medicine; Chief, Ophthalmic Plastic Surgery Service, Bascomb Palmer Eye Institute, Miami, Florida

Frederick H. Theodore, M.D.

Attending Ophthalmic Surgeon and Director, External Disease and Infections Clinic, Manhattan Eye, Ear and Throat Hospital; Attending Surgeon, Mt. Sinai Hospital; Associate Clinical Professor of Ophthalmology, New York University, New York, New York

Richard C. Troutman, M.D.

Professor and Head, Division of Ophthalmology, Department of Surgery, State University of New York, Downstate Medical Center, Brooklyn; Surgeon-Director, Manhattan Eye, Ear and Throat Hospital, New York, New York

Arnold I. Turtz, M.D.

Attending Surgeon and Chief, Cataract Service II, Manhattan Eye, Ear and Throat Hospital; Clinical Professor of Ophthalmology, New York Medical College, New York, New York

Professor Rudolf Witmer

Chairman and Head, University Eye Clinic, Zurich; Chief, Outpatient Department, University Eye Clinic, Bern, Switzerland

Gerald L. Wolf, M.D.

Attending Anesthesiologist, Manhattan Eye, Ear and Throat Hospital, New York, New York

Lorenz E. Zimmerman, M.D.

Chief, Division B—General and Special Pathology and Chief, Ophthalmic Pathology Branch, Armed Forces Institute of Pathology, Walter Reed Army Medical Center, Washington, D. C.; Lecturer, Department of Ophthalmology, Johns Hopkins University School of Medicine, Baltimore, Maryland; Associate in Pathology, George Washington University School of Medicine, Washington, D. C.

Judah Zizmor, M.D.

Roentgenologist, Manhattan Eye, Ear and Throat Hospital, New York, New York

Preface

The idea for the Centennial Symposium gained definition in October, 1966, with the appointment by the Board of Directors and Board of Surgeon Directors of Manhattan Eye, Ear and Throat Hospital of Drs. William F. Robbett and Arnold I. Turtz as co-chairmen. Having drawn up a tentative outline for the symposium, complete with a preliminary program, the co-chairmen presented the project in December, 1966, to the Irene Heinz Given and John La Porte Given Foundation for its financial support. With the granting of that assistance, the plans rapidly took on shape and substance.

The Centennial Symposium was, of course, designed to be the first major event in honor of Manhattan Eye, Ear and Throat Hospital's centennial anniversary. It was believed that an international medical symposium presenting the tremendous changes that have occurred in the fields of ophthalmology, otolaryngology, and plastic surgery would be exceedingly valuable and a truly fitting occasion to celebrate the Hospital's 100 years of dedicated service to medical science and humanity.

Thus, in preparing for this meeting, current medical topics of high interest were selected and speakers were invited from all parts of the United States and a number of foreign countries. The co-chairmen expended a great deal of thought in the selection of topics and honored guests who would present their views on these subjects. It is believed that the concepts of diagnosis and therapy that these specialists discussed reflect the best thinking on these topics today.

The Centennial Symposium was held at the Hotel Pierre, New York City, June 3 to 7, 1968, and was attended by a capacity audience of 668 physicians from all parts of the United States and 22 foreign countries. Some of the modern trends and ideas presented during the ophthalmology, otolaryngology, and plastic surgery sessions were deliberately selected for their controversial nature. It is hoped that by the resulting free exchange of different opinions the symposium proved to be of great educational value.

In addition to the distinguished medical program that the Centennial Symposium offered, there were comparable social events to add to the centennial celebration.

The twofold purpose of the symposium was thus accomplished: a commemorative event was held in honor of Manhattan Eye, Ear and Throat Hospital's centennial anniversary and an outstanding medical conference was presented.

Arnold I. Turtz, M.D.

Contents

Section III   Pediatric ophthalmologic problems
Presiding Chairman: **Algernon B. Reese**

Section IV   Ophthalmic plastic surgery
Presiding Chairman: **Byron Smith**

Section V **New techniques in ophthalmology**
Presiding Chairman: **Goodwin M. Breinin**

Section VI **Complications in ocular surgery**
Presiding Chairman: **Arnold I. Turtz**

NEW CONCEPTS IN OCULAR THERAPY

Presiding Chairman: **R. Townley Paton**

Chapter 1

Trends in ocular therapy

Irving H. Leopold

Development of adrenergic agents

The concept that excitation might be transferred from a nerve ending to an effector organ by release of a chemical substance was developed over a century ago. Elliott, in 1905, suggested that an epinephrine-like compound was the substance released at sympathetic nerve endings.[1] Nearly half a century passed before it was established that the epinephrine-like substance was norepinephrine.[2]

Considerable increase in information concerning the action of drugs in the adrenergic nervous system has appeared in the last decade. This increase has been brought about by new pharmacologic agents, electron microscopic studies, improved histochemical techniques, and microchemical analysis. The identification of various metabolic products of the catecholamines and the discovery of drugs which alter their formation, storage, release, metabolism, transport, and physiologic activity have resulted in a rapid advance in the knowledge of the physiology, biochemistry, and pharmacology of the adrenergic system.

The receptor concept of drug-effector interaction is a useful device in pharmacologic investigations. The adrenergic receptor is the part of certain effector cells that allows them to detect and respond to epinephrine and related compounds. This adrenergic receptor concept was conceived by Sir Henry Dale. He noted that ergot alkaloids blocked only some effects of epinephrine. Barger and Dale (1910) noted two separate sets of responses to catecholamines.[3, 4] (The term catecholamine usually refers to primary or secondary 3, 4 dehydroxyphenyl-ethanolamines with substitutes in the 1-carbon of methyl or ethyl and in the nitrogen of methyl or isopropyl.) The differentiation between alpha and beta receptors is based on the observation that only two sets of structure activity relationships seemed to exist within a small group of related catecholamines.

Adrenergic alpha receptor is believed to be associated with vasoconstriction, contraction of the iris dilator musculature, retraction of the third eyelid, contraction of splenic smooth muscles, relaxation of intestinal muscles, and myometrial contraction.

The beta receptor is associated with vasodilatation, relaxation of the smooth muscles of bronchi, intestines, and uterus, and the adrenergic-positive cardiac inotropic and chronotropic effects.

Specific stimulators or agonists for alpha receptors are phenylephrine and norepinephrine; isoproterenol is specific for beta receptors; and epinephrine stimulates both alpha and beta receptors.

Pharmacologically the beta receptor blocking agents are substances that specifically block catecholamine-evoked responses stated to be associated with beta receptors, but do not block adrenergic responses associated with alpha receptors. Alpha receptor blocking agents are substances that specifically block catecholamine-evoked responses stated to be associated with alpha receptors, but do not block those associated with beta receptors.

An adrenergic alpha receptor blocking agent would specifically block responses to norepinephrine and phenylephrine, block part of the responses to epinephrine, and have no effect on responses to isoproterenol.

Adrenergic beta receptor blocking agents specifically block the responses to isoproterenol, block part of the responses to epinephrine, and have no effect on the responses to norepinephrine and phenylephrine.

Ophthalmologic use of adrenergic agents

Many adrenergic compounds have been tried for ophthalmologic purposes. Studies in ophthalmology have included trials of agents that:

1. Act on alpha adrenergic receptors (phenylephrine, norepinephrine, epinephrine)
2. Act on beta adrenergic receptors (isoproterenol, epinephrine)
3. Block alpha adrenergic receptors (phentolamine)
4. Block beta adrenergic receptors (propranolol)
5. Inhibit monamine oxidase (pargyline)
6. Inhibit catechol-o methyl transferase (pyrogallol, quercetin)
7. Interfere with uptake of catecholamine in nerve tissue (protriptyline)
8. Interfere with storage of catecholamine in nerve tissue (reserpine, guanethidine)
9. Deplete stores of catecholamine from nerve tissue (tyramine, reserpine, guanethidine)

These agents produce varying degrees of pupillary changes, vessel caliber alterations, and intraocular pressure fluctuations. No one of these adrenergic agents has supplanted epinephrine for the reduction of intraocular pressure.

Epinephrine topically applied is believed to lower intraocular pressure by reducing aqueous humor formation and improving the facility of aqueous humor outflow.

Guanethidine has been shown to reduce intraocular pressure following systemic and local administration. It appears to reduce inflow essentially with only a minor effect on the outflow mechanism. This compound has also been employed to reduce the lid retraction associated with hyperthyroidism.

Protriptyline (Vivactil [Merck]) is an antidepressant drug that is thought to suppress the mechanism for pumping catecholamine across the membrane back into nervous tissue for storage. It is not a monamine oxidase inhibitor. Langham studied this compound experimentally for ocular effects and was impressed with its ability to lower intraocular pressure.[5] However, in our studies with 0.01%, 0.025%, and 0.05% solutions in human eyes with previously untreated ocular hypertension, protriptyline has failed to produce a significant drop in intraocular pressure. Therapy has been continued with each concentration for 14 to 21 days. Higher concentrations of protriptyline in the range of 0.2% solution have been noted to produce corneal opacification. Perhaps closely allied derivatives of this compound may prove more effective with less local toxicity.

Propranolol is the first beta adrenergic receptor blocking agent available in the United States for general use. At present its use is limited in the U. S. to pheochromocytomas, cardiac arrhythmias, and idiopathic hypertropic subaortic stenosis. It has been used topically in England to reduce the lid retraction associated with thyroid gland dysfunction, but has not been studied seriously regarding its effect on aqueous humor dynamics.[6, 7]

Management of glaucoma

Over the years the use of topical agents for the management of glaucoma has demonstrated a number of previously unknown side effects. Within recent years interest has been shown in the possibility of systemic side effects, as well as those in ocular tissues. Both adrenergic and cholinergic compounds can produce various undesired actions. It has been stressed that patients should not be embarrassed by the use of miotics or adrenergic compounds simply to treat ocular hypertension. Therapy for glaucoma should be commenced only when one can be certain of the presence of the disease and particularly of a progressive course.[8]

The latest member of the cholinergic compounds to be used in glaucoma therapy is aceclydine. This compound in 1% concentration appears to be the equivalent of 2% pilocarpine. It is slightly irritating initially in its present formulation and appears to lose some of its potency in a matter of months when in 1% concentration at room temperature.

Prophylaxis of intraocular infections

Antibiotics have been used extensively—probably excessively—for prophylaxis or prevention of infection. Their administration for this purpose is indicated and effective only in specific instances. In general surgery and medicine, the rapidly accumulating evidence illustrates clearly the inadvisability of indiscriminate use of antibiotics for prophylaxis. However, the problem of postoperative ocular infections is an example of an area in which evidence appears to point to a favorable effect of prophylaxis.

In general surgery mild postoperative infections are not uncommon, but serious infections are rare. However, all infections associated with intraocular surgery are serious and are often disastrous. Therefore, all studies directed toward reduction of the frequency and severity of intraocular infection are important.

All institutions strive to develop and attain an aseptic technique. This includes preparation of the patient, the operating room theater, instruments, and team. Loopholes in technique may be penetrated by an opportunistic organism and induce a vision-threatening infection.

Prophylactic antibiotics have been recommended as an additional defense against infection. Antibiotics can be administered topically, subconjunctivally, or systemically for this purpose. There is some evidence that prophylactic antibiotics reduce, but do not eliminate, secondary postoperative infection. Topical and subconjunctival antibiotics are thought to reduce the likelihood of systemic toxicity. However, subconjunctivally adminis-

tered antibiotics in large doses often produce significant plasma levels. The one injection technique is less likely to be systemically toxic than repeated subconjunctival or systemic doses.

If the surgeon decides to include a subconjunctival antibiotic injection in his routine for intraocular surgery, it is important that he use a drug that will inhibit or destroy the organisms most likely to induce the infection. The drug must also be given in a dosage that will provide an effective concentration in the ocular tissue and fluids.

The organisms encountered in most infections have been *Staphylococcus aureus*, resistant *Staphylococcus aureus*, *pyocyaneus*, *Bacillus proteus*, and *E. coli*. Other organisms, including fungi, are found less frequently.

Studies of the penetration of antibiotics into the ocular tissues and fluids have been made by many investigators over the past 25 years.[10-13] Recently Drs. McPherson, Presley, and Crawford analyzed the penetration in animal and human eyes of subconjunctivally administered penicillin, streptomycin, ampicillin, and chloramphenicol, and have suggested from their studies that ampicillin and penicillin G provide excellent penetration with the doses they employed.[14] They have recommended ampicillin because of its penetrating activity and because it has a broader antibacterial spectrum than penicillin.

Chloramphenicol failed to provide adequate levels in their experiments, but the fact that they used chloramphenicol succinate may possibly explain the absence of evidence of chloramphenicol in aqueous humor by this technique. Chloramphenicol succinate is inactive unless hydrolyzed in the body. If a culture is tested for inhibition by chloramphenicol, there will be inhibition if the chloramphenicol powder is used. However, if chloramphenicol succinate is employed, there will be no inhibition in vitro. Perhaps the subconjunctival injection studies did not provide sufficient time for the hydrolysis necessary for activation. In previous studies in which subconjunctival injections of chloramphenicol were shown to penetrate, the succinate was not used.

There are many factors that must be considered in comparing data by various investigators using a bioassay technique to analyze penetration of antibiotics. For example, it is important to know the concentration of the standard control antibiotic which is predetermined against the control organisms used in the assays. It is also important to note that different preparations of the same general drug can show dissimilar penetration characteristics.

Penetration is important; however, it is also essential to select antibiotics that will overcome the likely invading organism. Polymyxin, colistin, and neomycin are effective against many strains of *B. pyocyaneus,* and all have been shown to penetrate after subconjunctival injection.[15, 16] Many of the semisynthetic penicillins, such as methicillin and ampicillin, are effective against the resistant staphylococcus.[17, 18] Vancomycin is an effective drug for resistant staphylococcus, and studies in our laboratory have demonstrated excellent penetration. However, at present it would seem advisable to reserve this drug for therapy of active infection rather than for prophylaxis.

The cephalosporin agents, such as cephalothin (Keflin) and cephaloridine (Loridine), also penetrate satisfactorily and have a wide spectrum according to recent investigations.

Preoperative cultures. Preoperative cultures can be helpful, but negative preoperative cultures do not assure freedom from postoperative infections. Eyes have been successfully operated upon without complication in the presence of a pathogenic organism in the preoperative culture. Infection has also developed in the presence of a cul-de-sac yielding negative preoperative cultures. The use of daily instillations of a bacteriostatic or bacteriocidal agent prior to surgery will rarely do harm but, of course, it does not give blanket protection. Cultures taken at the time of surgery can be informative and can be used as a guide to subsequent therapy if infection caused by an organism present in the cul-de-sac should appear postoperatively.

Preparation for cul-de-sac decontamination. Many preparations are available to reduce the bacterial flora in the cul-de-sac. These include neomycin, bacitracin, polymyxin, chloramphenicol, sulfonamides, detergents, quaternary ammonium compounds, and various combinations of these drugs. There are disadvantages for each, however, such as hypersensitivity, a limited antibacterial spectrum, and systemic toxicity.

Subconjunctival antibiotics. Evidence has appeared supporting the beneficial aspects of antibiotics administered subconjunctivally during the operative procedure. Such agents, when properly selected and administered in a safe but effective dosage, can provide some protection against the development of infection. Similarly, well-chosen systemically administered agents in proper dosage can be helpful. The subconjunctival route has the advantage of reduced exposure of the entire body to the adverse effects of the antibiotic. Subconjunctival administration produces significant blood levels of the antibiotic and the drug is given only once. Systemically administered drugs, however, must be given repeatedly to be effective; they may not provide as large a concentration of the drug in the ocular fluids at any one time as the subconjunctivally administered drugs. However, a proper time sequence and minimal dosage can be worked out for the desired agent if the surgeon prefers the systemic route for any patient.

Selection of specific antibiotic. Drugs that suppress microbial multiplication must be differentiated from drugs capable of killing microorganisms. Almost all antibiotics have both bacteriostatic and bacteriocidal activity, but achievable therapeutic blood levels of the antibiotics commonly referred to as "broad spectrum" are principally bacteriostatic.

The distinction between these types of antimicrobial agents is important since killing of the microorganisms by the drug can eradicate infection independent of mechanisms of host resistance, whereas suppression of the infection may not eliminate the disease if host defense proves incomplete or inadequate.

REFERENCES

1. Elliott, T. R.: The action of adrenalin, J. Physiol. (London) **32**:401, 1905.
2. Von Euler, U. S.: Noradrenaline, Springfield, Ill., 1956, Charles C Thomas, Publisher, p. 383.
3. Barger, G., and Dale, H. H.: Chemical structure and sympathomimetic action of amines, J. Physiol. (London) **41**:19, 1910.
4. Moran, N. C., and Perkins, M. E.: Adrenergic blockade of the mammalian heart by a dichloro analogue of isoproterenol, J. Pharmacol. Exp. Therap. **125**:223, 1958.
5. Langham, M. E.: The role of adrenergic receptors in the regulation of intraocular pressure. In Paterson, G., Miller, S. J. H., and Paterson, G. D., editors: Drug mechanisms in glaucoma, London, 1966, J. & A. Churchill Ltd.
6. Lee, W. Y., Morimoto, P. K., Bronsky, D., and Waldstein, S. S.: Studies of thyroid and sympathetic nervous system interrelationships. I. The blepharoptosis of myxedema, J. Clin. Endoc. **21**:1402, 1961.
7. Sneddon, J. M., and Turner, P.: Adrenergic blockade and the eye signs of thyrotoxicosis, Lancet **2**:525, 1966.
8. Leopold, I. H.: Glaucoma masque, Amer. J. Ophthal. **67**:176, 1967.
9. Lieberman, T. W., and Leopold, I. H.: The use of aceclydine; pharmacology laboratory report, New Brunswick, N. J., 1965, Smith, Miller and Patch, Inc.
10. Leopold, I. H.: Surgery of ocular trauma, Arch. Ophthal. **48**:738, 1952.
11. Von Sallmann, L., Meyer, K., and Grand, J.: Experimental study on penicillin treatment of exogenous infection of vitreous, Arch. Ophthal. **32**:179, 1944.
12. Sorsby, A., and Ungar, J.: Preliminary note on the treatment of hypopyon ulcer, Brit. J. Ophthal. **32**:878, 1948.
13. Leopold, I. H.: Antibiotics and antifungal agents; problems and management of ocular infections, Invest. Ophthal. **3**:504, 1964.
14. McPherson, S. D., Presley, G. D., and Crawford, J. R.: Antibiotics in post-operative infection, Trans. Amer. Ophth. Soc. (in press).
15. Pryor, J. G., Apt, L., and Leopold, I. H.: Intraocular penetration of colistin, Arch. Ophthal. **67**:612, 1962.
16. Vogel, A. W., Nichols, A., and Leopold, I. H.: Neomycin; ocular tissue tolerance and penetration when locally applied in the rabbit eye, Amer. J. Ophthal. **34**:1357, 1951.
17. Green, W. R., and Leopold, I. H.: Intraocular penetration of methicillin, Amer. J. Ophthal. **60**:800, 1965.
18. Kurose, Y., Levy, P. M., and Leopold, I. H.: Intraocular penetration of ampicillin. II. Clinical experiment, Arch. Ophthal. **73**:366, 1965.

Chapter 2

Flush-fitting contact lenses

Frederick Ridley

Principles and methods of fitting

Use of scleral lenses. If the cornea is diseased the eye will not tolerate a corneal contact lens. Either the patient will experience pain and tearing, or the epithelium will strip and the cornea will ulcerate, or both. A large contact lens must be used in such conditions. In our experience in London about 70% of therapeutic cases need scleral lenses; the remaining 30% are largely aphakics and high myopes.

Reason for taking impression. The globe, including the cornea, is of irregular asymmetric form; even in the healthy eye this may be conspicuous. When the variations derived from gross refractive errors (especially astigmatism), disease conditions such as keratoconus and corneal ulceration and its sequelae, and corneal grafting and surgical procedures of all kinds are added to the form irregularities, it is evident that if there is to be a universal approach to the fitting of a large contact lens, it must be based upon an accurate impression of the front of the eye.

Impression technique

The future may produce improved techniques for copying all the variations in form of the globe but, at the present time, an alginate molding material supported by a tray that conforms roughly to the shape and size of the eye, is generally agreed to be best. Personally, I prefer an injection molding technique, and I prefer Ophthalmic Zelex and a range of molding trays so that I can choose one which will allow roughly 1 mm.

of material all over the front of the eye. The viscosity of the material will cause an indentation of the globe if the film between the eye and the tray is too thin at any point. For this reason the tray should be freely perforated using quite large holes so that no localized pressure can develop. When the injection is completed the upper and lower lids should be lifted away from the tray to liberate any pressure generated in the fornices. The material should flow freely through the holes covering the front of the tray, which, when it is removed, should be embedded in the material. Spraying the inside of the tray lightly with Hold* secures adhesion of the alginate to the Perspex shell and, to a large extent, eliminates the tendency for the material to be pulled away from the tray on removal.

Production technique

Dental stone model. A good impression will give a stone cast that will show the minutest details of the cornea and conjunctival surface. The model should be marked carefully for vertical and horizontal, and these marks should be carried forward to the flush-fitting shell so that its orientation in the eye can be determined precisely.

Making the plastic shell. The best material to date for making the plastic shell is polymethyl methacrylate—ideally Imperial Chemical Industries' CQ (Clinical Quality)—which is guaranteed to be fully polymerized and to contain no additives possibly

---

*Wm. Getz Corp., Chicago, Ill.

harmful to the tissues or liable to elicit an allergic response. (The importance of choosing the right material and processing it properly is fully dealt with in "Safety Requirements for Contact Lens Materials."[1]) To adapt a sheet of Perspex to a stone model it is essential that:

1. The material be pure
2. The material be heated to not more than 160° C.
3. The material be pressed onto the model uniformly, preferably with the vacuum elimination of any air or steam that might be trapped between the stone and Perspex

It is possible to get away with a good deal of ill-treatment of this material. Thus it is often heated in a naked flame as opposed to using a thermostatically controlled heating device. It is sometimes softened by monomer, which it readily absorbs and which leaks out and is irritating to the eye. I think these practices are wrong. It is our duty to take every precaution to protect the patient from injury or even discomfort, and the technical problem is a simple one.

When the sheet of Perspex has been pulled or pressed down onto the model and allowed to cool, its elastic memory will cause it to spring very slightly away from the model in a uniform manner. This fortuitous circumstance is, nonetheless, important. If the technique employed secures a perfect fit it may be necessary to use a separator of known and uniform thickness between the stone model and the Perspex sheet to secure the desired looseness of fit.

Fitting the shell. The orientation of the flush-fitting shell is best determined by marking it in production. When it is put into the eye with a little dilute fluorescein it should lie in exactly this orientation. If it does not do so it should be turned into its true position and any high spots marked and eliminated by grinding and repolishing. It should now fall into position accurately and if it does not do so, a new mold should be taken. Unless the shell is an accurate reproduction

and is in its proper position we are wasting our time.

A flush-fitting shell is one which shows a uniform fluorescein picture over the whole area in contact with the eye, including the cornea. This is the basic contact lens. The shell can be tested by inserting fluorescein; the fluid exchange under such a lens is very free and reaches every point under the shell in approximately 20 seconds. Medicaments can be applied and are fully effective without removing the shell. Such shells are very comfortable and can be worn in many cases indefinitely. One of our patients wore such a shell without taking it out for more than 3 months. The shell was comfortable and caused no congestion. Another patient, a man of 58 whose eye was injured in a boiler explosion, has worn a flush-fitting lens day and night for 9 years, removing it only once or twice a week, with no untoward effects. These shells permit medication and examination at all times with a minimum of disturbance. By definition they do not have good optical properties. An optic cannot be put on the back surface of such a shell opposite to the cornea without creating a loose area and introducing all the difficulties inherent in normal contact lens fitting. However, an optic can be put on the front and, if necessary, with the aid of astigmatic spectacles, an eye so fitted will usually attain one line less than is possible with a back curve. The image, however, is imperfect.

Mode of action and clinical effects of optical front curve

A flush-fitting shell with an optical front curve and a spectacle lens to correct any astigmatism can give useful vision and can be worn for long periods with great comfort.

Such a flush-fitting shell or lens is a splint. It immobilizes and supports the ocular tissues and gives them clinical rest. It protects damaged or diseased tissues from injury caused by exposure or by being rubbed by a lid which may itself be diseased or injured. It protects the eye from drying, supports the conjunctiva of the globe and lids, prevents symblepharon, and affords a mechanical barrier to irritation of the globe and cornea by ingrowing lashes, inturning lids, or rough tarsal plates. By removing irritability of the eye, such a shell abolishes epiphora and promotes a rapid return to a normal lysozyme titer in the tears with consequent recovery from infection. Discharge ceases and the conjunctiva and lid become normal. Dramatic clinical improvement is often observed, sometimes within a few days. Scarring may be inevitable. Support, rest, protection, useful vision, and the clinician's ability to examine the eye at any time and to apply whatever medication is desirable are the advantages available from using a flush-fitting shell or lens.

The disadvantage of such a lens is its indifferent optical property. If worn substantially day and night indefinitely there is some evidence that corneal vascularization is liable to occur; however, this is not excessive considering the conditions for which these shells are used.

Changing a flush-fitting shell into a normal contact lens

The fitting of a flush-fitting shell does not preclude turning it into a normal scleral or haptic lens by grinding an optical surface on the inside as well as on the outside. However, it must be remembered that a pool of fluid is created between the lens and the cornea, which is locked in by a close fitting shell. Such an area invariably develops a negative pressure, and leads to edema and veiling unless it is relieved by putting it into communication with the atmosphere. This may be achieved by drilling a hole in the appropriate place just inside the limbus or by grinding out a gutter leading from the precorneal pool of tears to the lens edge.

A flush-fitting shell may be thought of as a device to attain a clinical objective, as a first step toward the fitting of a normal haptic lens, or both. When such a lens is fitted to a diseased eye it must be observed regularly and modified as necessary

because the edematous eye tissues will shrink as they heal.

Clinical and surgical applications
Protection

Burns and chemical injuries. When the corneas and conjunctivas have been burned by heat or chemicals, a flush-fitting shell fitted within a few days of injury has prevented a symblepharon and has led to a surprising degree of preservation of clarity of the cornea. Such shells are often worn with great comfort day and night for several weeks. Any medicament applied to the conjunctival sac when such a shell is in position immediately passes under the shell and reaches every part of the eye surface.

Ulceration of the cornea. Very broadly, it may be said that a flush-fitting contact shell gives the same result as a tarsorrhaphy for ulceration of the cornea, and it also enables the patient to retain the use of the eye. Cases of acne rosacea, recurrent dendritic ulceration and disciform keratitis, mustard gas keratitis, ulceration associated with a deep corneal crater, and corneal grafts that either ulcerate or are deteriorating have responded well to this approach.

Pemphigus. Apart from improved visual acuity, the contribution contact lenses and shells can make in pemphigus is to hold the fornices open, preventing contraction and adhesion in the subacute stage. They cannot be worn in the acute stage of the disease. When the disease is quiescent, lenses should be fitted if possible and are usually worn very well; continuous wearing is not unusual. Under these conditions it is probable that visual acuity need not deteriorate over the years at all. If the eyes have any natural tear secretion this may be adequate when evaporation is prevented by the contact lens. If the eye is dry, instillation of drops of 2% sodium bicarbonate, 0.6% Ringer saline, methylcellulose, or artificial tears may be necessary, but this is a simple thing to do. Once all-day wear is established, any discharge ceases, the cornea often clears steadily over several months, vascularization subsides, the eye becomes quiet, and the fornices re-form to a considerable extent by reexpansion of the contracted conjunctiva now permanently wetted. If the case relapses the patient should be refitted as soon as possible after the acute phase subsides. Several patients with old trachoma, in whom a similar problem is seen, have been fitted. As examples, a patient has been back at work with 20/80 vision in each eye for 6 years who, during the previous 6 years, was on the blind register. Another patient still has 20/60 vision after 24 years of wearing a contact lens.

Elderly people with active lesions and wet eyes are difficult to fit and tend to do badly. They often have good visual acuity and so derive no immediate reward from contact lenses. Patients in the quiescent stage following these diseases in early life—and usually with dry eyes and corneal involvement—do very well. Apart from increased visual acuity, freedom from discharge and complete comfort are achieved at once.

Bullous keratitis. Cases of bullous keratitis have been reported in which flush-fitting shells have given relief, but the effect is palliative.

Special applications. In nerve V paralysis, in lid deformities involving exposure of the globe, or irritation by inturning lashes or by scarred lids (as in trachoma and in nerve VII palsy) contact shells give permanent comfort and protection.

Splints

Symblepharon. Provided the adhesions are not too extensive and dense scar tissue is not excessive, symblepharon may be treated by dividing the adhesions, preferably close to the globe, and taking an impression on the table while the patient is under the anesthetic. This impression should be as large as possible, extending out into the fornices. Within 3 hours a flush-fitting shell copying exactly the contour of the soft tissues is prepared and inserted. Such a shell is worn day and night and at the end of 10 days or so

the fornices will be found to have epithelialized. The epithelium grows freely over the polished surface of the acrylic; this seems to be greatly facilitated by the fact that there are no dead spaces under the lens. This approach avoids the need to use either mucous membrane or split-skin grafts with their attendant disadvantages. Caustic alkali injuries with extensive adhesions and a great deal of dense scar tissue have not responded satisfactorily to the use of the flush-fitting shell.

Cataract surgery. In 30 cataract operations a flush-fitting scleral shell was used as a splint and no corneoscleral stitches were used. The previously fitted shell was inserted at the end of the operation. The procedure was uneventful and uniformly successful. The eye so protected is probably quite safe, since any pressure or movement tends to close the wound, not to open it. This can hardly be a routine procedure, but it established the feasibility of the approach.[2, 3]

Lamellar grafts. A flush-fitting shell prepared and fitted before surgery forms a perfect splint to support a lamellar graft without the use of stitches. This is of particular importance when grafting is undertaken in a degenerate cornea, which may be either so thin that stitches cannot safely be inserted or of such poor quality that they cut out.[2, 3]

Penetrating grafts. Penetrating grafts have been done with a flush-fitting shell as a splint, but the impossibility of injecting air into the anterior chamber at the end of the operation after the shell has been inserted has led to its discontinuance.[2, 3]

Contact shells to carry radioactive material

Melanosis conjunctivae. Whenever it is required to apply radioactive material to treat the surface of the eye or the internal aspect of the lids, a shell may be produced in which the radioactive material may be localized accurately and surrounded by the required thickness of Perspex to protect the tissues from burning. This has been applied in both tantalum (gamma ray) and strontium foil (beta ray) applicators. The approach gives protection to the eye and control of the radiation dose with effective localization to the affected area.[4]

Cosmetic uses

Masking of deformed or ugly eyes. A clear shell with a black pupil built in may be used to occlude a white cataractous lens. Such a shell that incorporates an iris and pupil may be used to occlude an iridectomy with an opaque lens behind it.

An artificial eye in the form of a rather thick contact lens may be used to mask an ugly eye. It is better not to operate upon a divergent eye that has adequate movement, since such an eye is more stable than the same eye would be postoperatively. The lens is fitted over the diverging eye and is de-centered when converted into an artificial eye shell; the natural eye continues in its position of divergence, but the artificial eye is in the normal position. Movement is good and the result has proved stable. This approach is important if the useless eye has a sensitive cornea. A clear shell is made and fitted and, when this is worn satisfactorily, is converted into an artificial eye.

Wider application

Throughout the world there must be several million people (particularly with old trachoma) who have nebulae, ulceration, in-turning lashes, or chronic conjunctivitis with discharge who are partially blind and very miserable. Much of this could be remedied, almost overnight, by the fitting of these simple shells and, in the course of time, the cornea would clear and vision would improve considerably in most cases. For such partially sighted patients optimum vision can

usually be obtained with added spectacles for distance and reading. A front curve can be put onto these shells at minimum expense giving still further advantage. In the world of physical misery and disability there is hardly any other condition in which so little effort and expense could achieve so much. An approach to this problem might well be made by the World Health Organization.

Conclusion

A great deal of work has been done with flush-fitting shells and lenses here in America and there is, I think, very satisfactory agreement as to suitable cases and the kind of result that may be expected. In clinical management and treatment and in ophthalmic surgery the flush-fitting shell or lens may make an important contribution.

REFERENCES

1. Estevez, J. M. J., and Ridley, F.: Safety requirements for contact lens material and their manipulation and use, Amer. J. Ophthal. **62:** 132, 1966.
2. Ridley, F.: The contact lens in investigation and treatment, Trans. Ophthal. Soc. U. K. **74:** 377, 1954.
3. Ridley, F.: General application of contact lenses in surgical conditions, Il Curso Internacional de Oftalmologia, Instituto Barraquer, Barcelona, 1958.
4. Ridley, F.: Applications for irradiation of the conjunctival sac, Trans. Ophthal. Soc. U. K. **78:**171, 1958.

ADDITIONAL READINGS

Ridley, F.: Contact lenses. In Rycroft, B. W., editor: Corneal grafts, London, 1955, Butterworth & Co. Ltd.
Ridley, F.: Aphakia and binocular vision; Keratoconus—etiology, pathology, and treatment with contact lenses. In Girard, L., editor: Corneal and scleral contact lenses; Proceedings of the International Congress, St. Louis, 1967, The C. V. Mosby Co.
Ridley, F.: Therapeutic uses of scleral contact lenses, Int. Ophthal. Clin. **2:**687, Oct. 1962.

Chapter 3

Therapy for the edematous cornea (Fuchs' dystrophy and aphakic bullous keratopathy)

Stuart I. Brown

Corneal transplant

Early in the course of Fuchs' endothelial dystrophy, vision may be improved by partial dehydration of the epithelium with the use of hypertonic solutions, such as 5% sodium chloride; this is especially useful immediately after awakening. However, when the edema becomes advanced and vision is consistently reduced, the definitive treatment is a corneal transplant. This is also the treatment for irreversible postoperative bullous keratopathy. Stocker was the first to indicate that keratoplasty can be successful with Fuchs' dystrophy,[1] but it remained for Max Fine, in 1964, to demonstrate that corneal transplantation has a favorable prognosis in the treatment of both Fuchs' dystrophy and aphakic bullous keratopathy.[2] Fine's report also negated the popular concept that in order for a corneal transplant to be successful with Fuchs' dystrophy, the graft must be large enough to include the endothelial pathology. Many recent studies have given an anatomic basis for not needing large grafts. Pioneered by Helen Chi, this work proved that the essential endothelial cell layer of a corneal transplant can survive indefinitely, and consequently the transplant should act as an island of healthy tissue in the host bed.[3]

Another popular concept is that the prognosis for a transparent corneal graft is worsened if the epithelial edema is allowed to progress to the limbus. Evidence against this comes from the results of corneal transplantation in our last fourteen patients with limbus-to-limbus bullous keratopathy. Six of these patients had either fibrous downgrowth, absent anterior chamber, or vitreous adhesions. Eight were aphakic, and five had their cataractous lenses removed at the time of corneal surgery. We were fortunate to obtain transparent grafts never larger than $7\frac{1}{2}$ mm. in diameter in all but one of these patients (Figs. 3-1 and 3-2). Therefore, I think it is safe to conclude that the transplanted cornea can be healthy and can function independently, even though it is surrounded by diseased edematous tissue.

One form of aphakic bullous keratopathy which deserves extra mention is central vitreous touch after cataract extraction. This complication does not always result in corneal edema; however, these patients, especially those with pre-existing endothelial pathology, should be watched carefully for signs of early stromal edema. If edema is seen, I attempt to relieve the touch by aspirating liquid vitreous through the pars plana; through the same incision, a curved

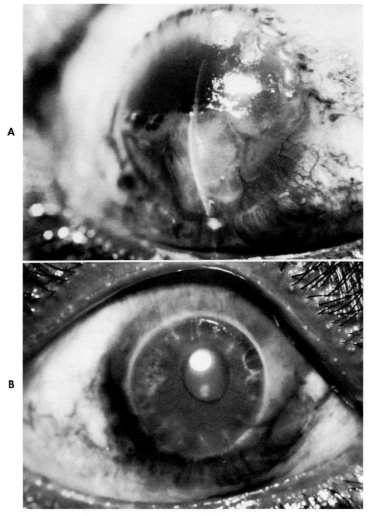

Fig. 3-1. A, Preoperative view of a 55-year-old male. Blunt trauma to eye resulted in total corneal edema. **B,** Postoperative view. Partial penetrating keratoplasty of 7.5 mm. Ten months after surgery, the corrected vision was 20/20.

needle is inserted behind the iris into the anterior chamber to fill it with air. This is best accomplished with the magnification of the surgical microscope.

When the vitreous is attached to the cornea, as indicated by the observation of attachment lines on the posterior cornea, the chance for the successful surgical release of the attachment is practically nil, and release frequently results in a distorted anterior chamber. The treatment for corneal edema from vitreous touch is corneal transplantation. The most important part of the procedure is the removal of all of the vitreous from the anterior chamber after the host corneal button is excised. This is best accomplished by wiping the surface of the iris with a cellulose sponge and excising any vitreous that has been picked up. After the iris has been completely freed of vitreous, the sponge is used to pick up and excise a small quantity of vitreous through the pupil-

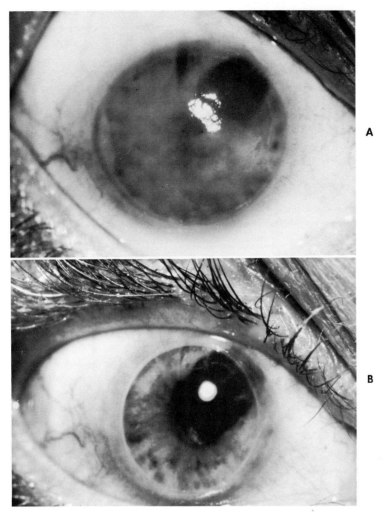

Fig. 3-2. A, Preoperative view of a 58-year-old female patient. Corneal edema and scarring to limbus. A previous iridectomy was performed for angle-closure glaucoma. **B,** Postoperative view after combined 7.5 mm. penetrating keratoplasty and cataract extraction. One year postoperatively the corrected vision was 20/50.

lary aperture. This should leave the area free of vitreous, whereupon the graft can be sutured to the host.

Corneal prosthetics—silicone implants

It is my feeling that indications for corneal prosthetics have become quite narrowed over the last 5 years. The reason for this is that many of the disease states previously thought to present difficulties can now be easily and successfully treated by corneal transplanta-

tion. This recent improvement in prognosis, which therefore expands the scope of corneal grafting, is most certainly due to the combination of (1) microsurgery, using finer and less irritating sutures, which allows for superior wound approximation, immediate ambulation, and also, for a safer use of corticosteroids; (2) greater experience with vitreous aspiration and excision in aphakic eyes; and (3) the realization that routine sized grafts (7 to 8 mm.) suffice, regardless of the host pathology. Consequently, I feel that the indications for corneal prosthetics must be repeated unsuccessful corneal grafts *which the surgeon feels certain were done to his satisfaction.* For these few patients, I use silicone corneal implants, which function as water barriers.[4, 5]

Design. The design of the silicone implants was based on the theory that a water-impermeable intralamellar membrane would act as a barrier to a fluid movement across the cornea, which would then allow evaporation to partially dehydrate the stroma in front of the membrane. This theory was eventually proved by Brown and Dohlman,[4] and quantitated by Brown and Mishima, who showed that evaporation increased the tonicity of the tears directly over the implant, and that this increased tonicity then pulled water from the cornea in front of the water barrier.[6] The grafts in front of these water-impermeable membranes would be kept free from edema and, therefore, blood vessels. The first of these was the buried silicone implant, which has been used in various centers in the United States to treat more than one hundred patients. In the fifty patients with whom I have been involved, the follow-up is almost 6 years.

Complications. Because this implant is not exposed, the complications are few. To date in our series, we still have not had a case of infection, and I have seen only 4 cases of impending extrusion. However, one common complication is that in about 30% of the patients a *fibrous membrane* grows behind the cylinder, reducing vision. We have been able to treat these successfully by sweeping the membranes away with a Zeigler knife. In addition to the retroimplant membrane, other problems with the silicone implant are superficial corneal ulceration during the early postoperative course (which will be mentioned later) and the modest visual results. Although the best visual acuity has been 20/40 after 5 years, vision is generally 20/60 to 20/80, and usually becomes worse in bright light. Recently, Dr. Michael

W. Dunn and I have developed a technique to coat the implant with a black silicone in the hope of increasing visual efficiency.[7] This combination was found to be tolerated in rabbits and has been in place for 18 months in one patient who has a visual acuity of 20/70 in a bright room.

In an attempt to further improve on the visual system of the buried corneal implant and to obviate the retroimplant membranes, a technique was devised whereby the water barrier was moved to the back of the cornea, which, in effect, created an artificial endothelium.[5] Essentially, the procedure entails the suturing of a silicone membrane to the back of a corneal graft with 10-0 Perlon sutures. These barrier membranes can be attached to a routinely trephined fresh or preserved corneal graft, or, as Dohlman and Ahmad have recently innovated, to a mushroom-shaped preserved graft.[9] As our experience is increasing with the artificial endothelium procedure, the incidence of improved vision has increased from 30 to 60% with the best visual acuity being 20/40 plus after a follow-up period of almost 3 years. The main complications with the artificial endothelium procedure are central corneal ulcers and a plastic iritis.

Central corneal ulcers seem to be inherent in barrier procedures, and the cause for this is being studied in our laboratory at the present time. Recently, Drs. Weller and Wassermann, and I have found a significant concentration of a collagenolytic enzyme in the ulcers in front of intralamellar membranes, in addition to the ulcers and perforations of the alkali-burned cornea. We have been able to prevent the ulcers of the alkali-burned corneas by the use of enzyme inhibitors and are investigating the possibility of the prevention of the ulcers in front of water barriers in the same way.[8]

The last complication is a *plastic iritis,* which I have seen in three patients and which occurs during the first 3 weeks postoperatively. This condition responds dramatically to systemic corticosteroids, but always leads to a prolonged postoperative course with breakdown and slow healing of the central epithelium of the graft.

Although we are constantly improving on all aspects of this technique, there are still many problems that need to be solved. They involve the suitability of the barrier material, the method of its attachment, and, of course, the epithelial ulcers.

Modifications of technique. Modifications of the existing water barrier techniques are presently under investigation in our laboratory. A particularly promising innovation is spot welding the membrane to the graft with microquantities of a diluted silicone adhesive. This method is suitable for preserved corneas; it is simple and requires no elaborate instrumentation. Another area of study that seems promising is the use of a new material in the field of alloplastics. This is a transparent collagen that has been pretreated to remove its immunogenic properties; it has been found by Dunn and colleagues to be well tolerated by the animal cornea.[10] One of the areas we are presently investigating is its use as a water barrier. When used as a barrier, this unique transparent collagen can be biologically cemented to the back of a corneal graft. That is, we can cross link, at a molecular level, the collagen of the barrier to the collagen lamellae of the corneal graft without using foreign cements. Preliminary studies of this technique in the laboratory animal are encouraging, and we hope to have our results ready for presentation in a short time.

It must be emphasized that although water barrier procedures are spectacular when successful, the indications for their use at this point in their development are rare, and I believe are becoming even more rare. As knowledge of corneal physiology and immunology increases and as the technique of microinstrumentation continues to improve, there will be increasingly fewer corneal conditions that cannot be treated successfully by corneal transplantation.

REFERENCES

1. Stocker, F. W.: Successful corneal graft in a case of endothelial and epithelial dystrophy, Amer. J. Ophthal. **35**:349, 1952.
2. Fine, M.: Therapeutic keratoplasty in Fuchs' dystrophy, Amer. J. Ophthal. **57**:371, 1964.
3. Chi, H. H., Teng, C. C., and Katzin, H. M.: Fate of the endothelial cells in corneal homografts, Amer. J. Ophthal. **59**:186, 1965.
4. Brown, S. I., and Dohlman, C. H.: A buried corneal implant serving as a barrier to fluid, Arch. Ophthal. **73**:635, 1965.
5. Dohlman, C. H., Brown, S. I., and Martola, E. L.: Artificial corneal endothelium, Arch. Ophthal. **75**:454, 1966.
6. Brown, S. I., and Mishima, S.: The effect of intralamellar water impermeable membrane on corneal hydration, Arch. Ophthal. **76**:702, 1966.
7. Brown, S. I., and Dunn, M.: Unpublished results, 1967.
8. Brown, S. I., Weller, C. A., and Wassermann, H. E.: Collagenolytic activity in alkali burned corneas, Arch. Ophthal. **81**:370, 1969.
9. Holmberg, A., Dohlman, C. H., and Ahmad, B.: Machining donor material for keratoplasty, Amer. J. Ophthal. **66**:341, 1968.
10. Dunn, M., Nishihara, T., Stenzel, K., Branwood, A. W., and Rubin, A. L.: Collagen-derived membrane; corneal implantation, Science **1**:157, 1967.

Chapter 4

Ocular tumor management

Moderator:
Frank H. Constantine

Panelists:
Lorenz E. Zimmerman
Algernon B. Reese
Harvey Lincoff
Jules François
Michael Bedford

Pathologic considerations in iris tumors

Lorenz E. Zimmerman

Not too many years ago, tumors of the iris were rather routinely treated by enucleation. In any large ophthalmic pathology laboratory collection, which contains cases dating back more than a decade, many specimens can be found such as the ones shown in Fig. 4-1, in which iris tumors have been treated by enucleation of the eye. Subsequently, iridectomy became the standard operation for tumors confined to the iris, and tumors that involved the chamber angle were routinely handled by enucleation of the eye; therefore another large group of iris tumors present in any pathology collection would include specimens such as the one shown in Fig. 4-2. In Fig. 4-2 the tumor of the iris has encroached upon the chamber angle and has invaded the adjacent ciliary body. Such tumors were long considered inoperable from the standpoint of excisional surgery. In more recent years, there have been cases in which the first step was iridectomy to establish a histopathologic diagnosis rather than to proceed directly with enucleation. If postoperative gonioscopic examination showed evidence

that the tumor had infiltrated the adjacent ciliary body, the eye would generally be enucleated (Fig. 4-3).

Then came the advent of more courageous excisional surgery, such as that proposed by Professor Müller and his associates[2] in Bonn, and by Mr. Stallard[3] in London, for resection of tumors involving the ciliary body.* Recently ophthalmic surgeons in the United States have also reported encouraging results with these new eye-saving operations.[4-7] The specimen shown in Fig. 4-4 is from one of Professor Müller's original iridocyclectomies; he has done a neat job of removing the iris and ciliary body well posterior to the tumor. Ever since I first heard about these new operations, I have championed this type of excisional surgery for tumors involving the periphery of the iris and adjacent ciliary body.[8, 9] However, many other ophthalmic pathologists are not quite so happy about this. As a matter of fact, at the recent meeting of the Verhoeff Society in Washington,† there was a good bit of heated discussion about the wisdom of doing this type of excisional therapy for tumors of the iris and ciliary body. Because of that discussion, I would like to indicate why I believe this type of therapy has a place and why I am in favor of iridocyclectomy for these tumors.

In 1967 Burch and Maumenee wrote a paper advocating the use of iridocyclectomy

---

*Since the presentation of this paper, Dr. A. B. Reese and his associates have reviewed their surgical experience with tumors of the iris and ciliary body.[4] In their paper they point out that some efforts were made to excise tumors of the ciliary body long before the more recent surge of interest in cyclectomy.
†April 22-23, 1968.

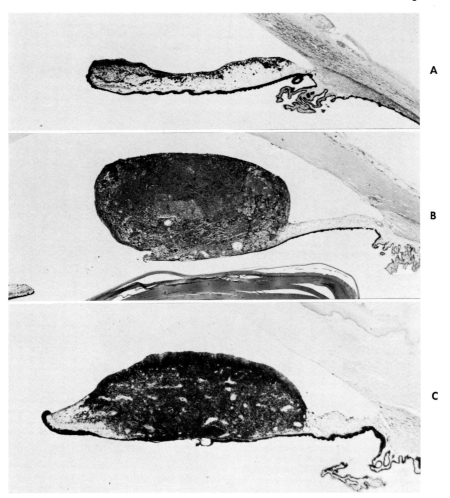

Fig. 4-1. Examples of melanomas of the iris that could have been removed by iridectomy. In none of these cases is the chamber angle or ciliary body involved by the tumor. (**A,** H & E ×16, Neg. No. 62-4718. **B,** H & E ×13, Neg. No. 58-5126; from Zimmerman, L. E.: Clinical pathology of iris tumors, Amer. J. Clin. Path. **39:**214, 1963. **C,** H & E ×21, Neg. No. 66-9130; from Zimmerman, L. E.: Changing concepts concerning the malignancy of ocular tumors, Arch. Ophthal. **78:**166, 1967.)

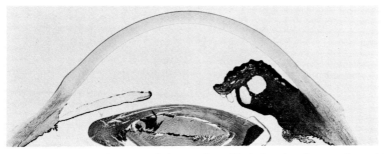

Fig. 4-2. This malignant melanoma of the iris has filled the chamber angle and invaded the pars plicata of the ciliary body. (H & E ×6, Neg. No. 98199)

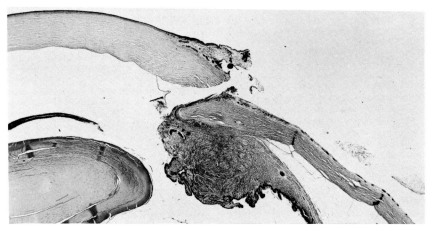

Fig. 4-3. The tumor-containing iris has been excised, but residual melanoma is present in the pars plicata of the ciliary body. (H & E ×12, Neg. No. 64-2883)

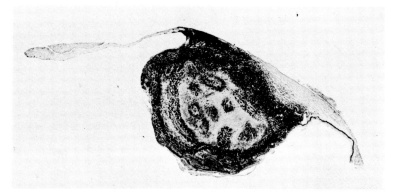

Fig. 4-4. This malignant melanoma of the iris and pars plicata ciliaris has been removed by iridocyclectomy. The specimen was contributed by Dr. O. E. Lund, of Bonn, Germany, from one of the cases reported by Müller and associates. (H & E ×14, Neg. No. 60-6374) (From Zimmerman, L. E.: Changing concepts concerning the malignancy of ocular tumors, Arch. Ophthal. **78:**166, 1967.)

in the treatment of enlarging ciliary body tumors that are believed to be benign.[10] Certainly I cannot disagree with this point of view, but it has been my experience that clinicians are very often incorrect in their preoperative impressions. We have seen many benign lesions that clinically were thought to be malignant melanomas of the iris and/or ciliary body. In his excellent statistical study of this problem, Ferry found that 35% of eyes enucleated for presumed malignant melanomas of the iris and ciliary body proved after histopathologic study to be lesions other than a malignant melanoma.[11] A few examples of such cases are shown in Figs. 4-5 to 4-10. Fig. 4-5 reveals a localized staphyloma that was thought to be a malignant melanoma. The rest of the eye is perfectly normal. Fig. 4-6 shows a cyst of the epithelium of the iris bulging forward through the pupil, simulating a malignant melanoma. Again, the remainder of the eye looks quite normal.

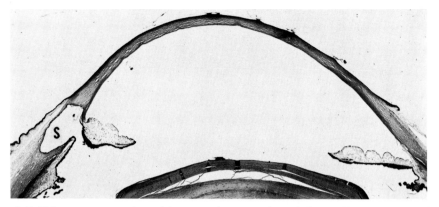

Fig. 4-5. This eye was enucleated because the corneal staphyloma *(S)* was mistaken for a malignant melanoma. (H & E ×8, Neg. No. 64-290) (From Ferry, A. P.: Lesions mistaken for malignant melanoma of the iris, Arch. Ophthal. **74:**9, 1965.)

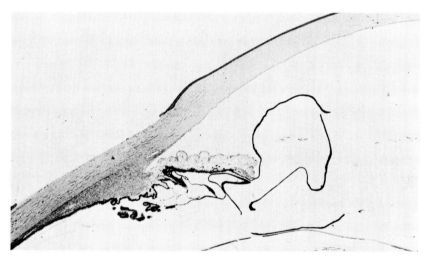

Fig. 4-6. Protruding through the pupil is a cystic proliferation of pigmented epithelium, derived from the iris and ciliary body, that was mistaken for a malignant melanoma. (H & E ×14, Neg. No. 60-6783)

Another example of a cystic lesion is shown in Fig. 4-7, but it is one in which the cyst has been carried forward by aqueous flow into the chamber angle. This little lesion was picked up in the course of routine gonioscopic examination of a perfectly normal eye, and was thought to be an early malignant melanoma.[12] The treatment that was instituted was enucleation of the eye! Fig. 4-8 reveals another example: a segmental mela-nosis of the iris. Fig. 4-9 illustrates a benign nevus, the type often referred to as a melano-cytoma.[13] Many people do not realize that these benign nevoid lesions can also fill the chamber angle and involve adjacent tissues, simulating a malignant melanoma. Still another example, a mass of ectopic lacrimal gland tissue growing in the chamber angle and in the iris, is shown in Fig. 4-10. Dr. Reese has recorded a case that serves as a

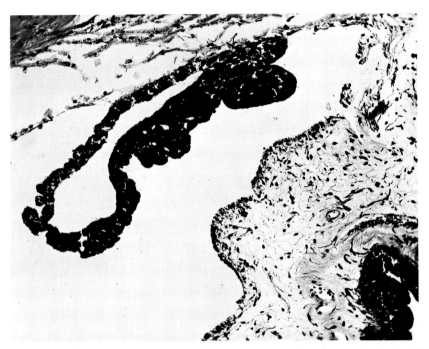

Fig. 4-7. This pigmented cyst attached to the trabecular meshwork was discovered during a routine gonioscopic examination of an otherwise normal eye. The eye was enucleated because the lesion was thought to be a malignant melanoma and resection of the involved tissues was thought to be "impractical." (H & E ×145, Neg. No. 64-6615; from Yanoff, M., and Zimmerman, L. E.: Pseudomelanoma of anterior chamber caused by implantation of iris pigment epithelium, Arch. Ophthal. **74**:302, 1965.)

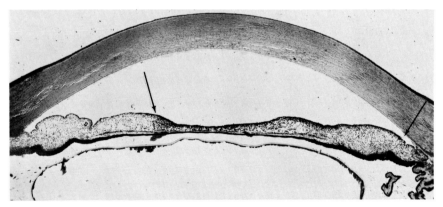

Fig. 4-8. Segmental melanosis of iris (area between arrows) simulating malignant melanoma. (H & E ×14, Neg. No. 64-555; from Ferry, A. P.: Lesions mistaken for malignant melanoma of the iris, Arch. Ophthal. **74**:9, 1965.)

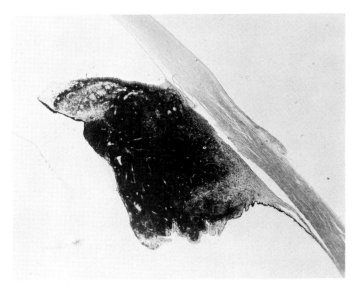

Fig. 4-9. Melanocytoma of iris and ciliary body. (H & E ×18, Neg. No. 64-6355; from Zimmerman, L. E.: Melanocytes, melanocytic nevi, and melanocytomas, Invest. Ophthal. 4:11, 1965.)

magnificent example of the point I am trying to make.[14] A 2½-year-old child had a rapidly growing mass in the ciliary body near the root of the iris. It was believed to be a diktyoma, but instead of enucleating the eye as is usually done in such cases, Dr. Reese removed the entire lesion by iridocyclectomy with corneal transplantation. Histopathologic examination revealed the lesion to be a perfectly benign congenital epidermoid cyst (Fig. 4-11).

One very valid reason for championing excisional operations whenever they are technically feasible is the fact that there are so many lesions that *simulate* malignant neoplasms. These lesions can be treated by excisional methods, rather than by enucleation of the eye.

Treatment of melanomas

I believe there are some very good reasons to suggest that melanomas of the iris are not of the same type as melanomas of the skin that are studied in medical school. The latter generally have a very poor prognosis. Melanomas of the iris are different, since they tend to grow in a very distinctive fashion and to have a very distinctive cytologic make up.

First of all, it should be remembered that there are two main categories of melanoma of the posterior uveal tract.[9] One large group, in which the tumors are made up solely of spindle shaped cells, have a very favorable prognosis. The other type is more akin to malignant melanoma of the skin. The second group of tumors are composed entirely or in part of epithelioid cells and have an unfavorable prognosis. The spindle cell melanomas may be further subdivided into two types, spindle A and spindle B. The former are the most benign but, unfortunately, in the choroid and ciliary body pure spindle A melanomas are rather rare. In the iris, however, the situation is just the reverse. The great majority of tumors of the iris and adjacent ciliary body are made up of the most benign type—the spindle A melanomas. These are tumors that grow in a very compact, cohesive fashion, and even though they may erupt through the anterior border layer into the anterior chamber, or posteriorly through the pigment epithelium and dilator

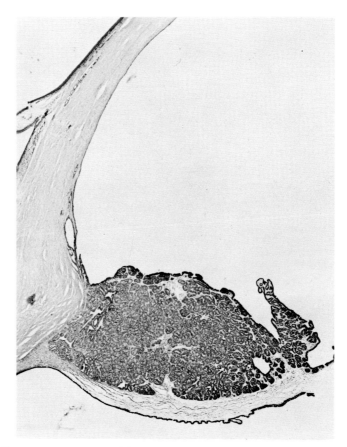

Fig. 4-10. Choristomatous mass of lacrimal gland tissue in iris and ciliary body. (H & E ×21, Neg. No. 62-78)

muscle to bulge into the posterior chamber, they tend to grow in a very compact cohesive fashion (Fig. 4-12). These are cells that tend to cling together, and are not readily disseminated upon gentle manipulation. This is a different type of cancer from the type that general surgeons usually encounter in mastectomies or exploration of the abdomen.

It has become a widely appreciated concept in general surgery to handle cancerous tissue much in the same way that an infectious lesion is handled. Contaminating the wound with tumor cells is to be avoided because the tumor is friable, the neoplastic cells are typically not cohesive, and they tend to break off and seed adjacent tissues. One

might wonder, therefore, why this is not also the case with tumors of the iris. Why is it that the ophthalmologist removing a tumor of the iris does not, in the course of doing an iridectomy, shake loose tumor cells into the aqueous, and why do not these cells then become seeded onto the other parts of the iris and into the chamber angle? One would expect, if he knew nothing about the cytology and general histopathologic features of iris melanomas, that every iridectomy would be followed by dissemination of tumor cells throughout the anterior chamber. And yet this is not the case! The prognosis for iris tumors treated by simple iridectomy is excellent.

However, there are rare melanomas of the

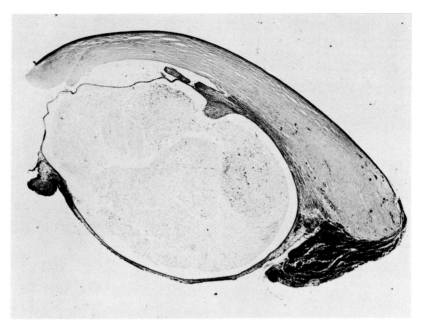

Fig. 4-11. Epidermoid cyst of iris and ciliary body removed by corneoscleroiridocyclectomy. (H & E ×21, Neg. No. 68-8069) (Courtesy Dr. A. B. Reese.)

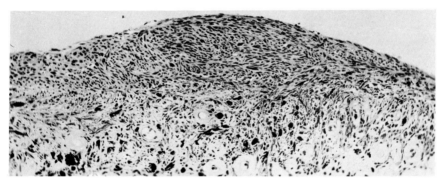

Fig. 4-12. Typical spindle A melanoma of iris. Observe that the tumor cells exhibit a compact cohesive manner of growth. (H & E ×115, Neg. No. 63-6515; from Zimmerman, L. E.: Melanocytes, melanocytic nevi, and melanocytomas, Invest. Ophthal. **4:**11, 1965.)

iris that are made up of epithelioid cells (Fig. 4-13). These cells are not cohesive and they tend to become dispersed even without the added trauma of iridectomy or iridocyclectomy. When one tries to do an iridectomy on a tumor of this type he will shake cells loose. These cells will become implanted on the iris and will be dispersed throughout the anterior chamber. With such tumors an early recurrence can be expected. But the odds are all in favor of the ophthalmologist, because this is a rare type of tumor in the iris; the great majority are spindle cell melanomas that grow in the compact cohesive fashion previously mentioned. Following iridectomy the results are excellent. In a study

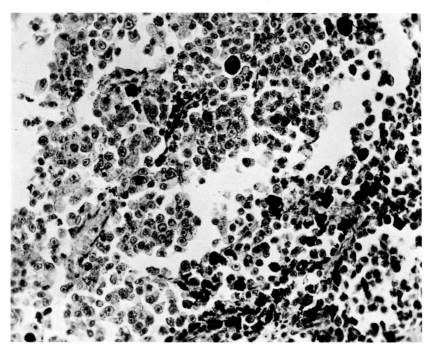

Fig. 4-13. Rare epithelioid cell melanoma of iris. The tumor cells typically exhibit a loss of cohesiveness with spontaneous desquamation into the aqueous humor, with dissemination throughout the anterior chamber. (H & E ×285, Neg. No. 55-23351)

that Rones and I made a few years ago, we found that following iridectomy, recurrence is unusual and tumor deaths are very few: less than 5% 16 years after iridectomy.[15] Other investigators have also been impressed by the relative benignity of melanotic tumors of the iris.[4, 16-18] Of course, some problems can be anticipated if the tumor is not completely removed. I am asked now and then whether there is evidence of a change in cell type and what the prognosis is following recurrence. Based on my experience, I must say that although the eye may ultimately be destroyed, the prognosis for life is not worsened by incomplete excision.

The case reported a few years ago by Cleasby[19] is a good one to illustrate the point: A 45-year-old woman had had a hemorrhage into the anterior chamber from a tumor of the iris that dated back to early childhood. The tumor was removed by iridectomy and the initial histopathologic study led to a diagnosis of leiomyoma. Six years later a dark spot was noted at the limbus adjacent to the surgical coloboma, but over a long period of observation this did not change significantly. Seventeen years after iridectomy a new lesion appeared inside the eye within the colobomatous area. The patient was observed by a number of ophthalmologists during the following year. Some recommended enucleation, and 18 years after the original tumor was removed the patient decided to have the eye enucleated. Microscopic examination revealed the intraocular tumor to be a recurrent amelanotic melanoma that closely resembled the original tumor. The tumor had also invaded along the surgical scar of the cornea, and the epibulbar lesion that had been observed for 12 years was found to be an extraocular extension of the tumor. This epibulbar portion, while just as benign in its cytologic appearance as the original tumor, did show considerable melanotic pigmentation of the tumor cells, clearly establishing the diagnosis of spindle A melanoma.

Summary

In summary, histopathologic studies have shown that many eyes suspected of containing a malignant melanoma of the iris or ciliary body actually have a benign lesion, and in many instances the lesion could have been excised by iridocyclectomy. Histopathologic and follow-up studies have repeatedly demonstrated that the vast majority of melanotic tumors of the iris are either benign nevi or very low grade spindle cell melanomas that rarely, if ever, metastasize.

In view of these facts, I believe that ophthalmic surgeons should be encouraged to broaden the scope of excisional methods used in the treatment of tumors of the iris and ciliary body.

REFERENCES

1. Henry, R. S.: The Armed Forces Institute of Pathology; its first century, 1964, Washington, D. C., U.S. Government Printing Office.
2. Müller, H. K., Söllner, F., and Lund, O. E.: Erfahrungen bei der operatinen Entfernung von Tumoren der Iriswurzel und des Ciliarkörpers, Berichte ü 63 Zusam Deutsch Ophth Bes, Heidelberg, 1960, pp. 194-199.
3. Stallard, H. B.: Partial cyclectomy, Brit. J. Ophthal. 45:797, 1961.
4. Reese, A. B., Jones, I. S., and Cooper, W. C.: Surgery for tumors of the iris and ciliary body, Amer. J. Ophthal. 66:173, 1968.
5. Cleasby, G. W.: Malignant melanoma of the iris and ciliary body; surgical excisions, Trans. Amer. Acad. Ophthal. Otolaryng. 67:710, 1963.
6. Winter, F. C.: Iridocyclectomy for malignant melanoma of the iris and ciliary body. In Boniuk, M., editor: Ocular and adnexal tumors, St. Louis, 1964, The C. V. Mosby Co.
7. Diamond, S., Borley, W. E., and Miller, W. W.: Partial iridocyclectomy for chamber angle tumors, Amer. J. Ophthal. 57:88, 1964.
8. Zimmerman, L. E.: Clinical pathology of iris tumors, Amer. J. Ophthal. 56:183, 1963.
9. Zimmerman, L. E.: Changing concepts concerning the malignancy of ocular tumors, Arch. Ophthal. 78:166, 1967.
10. Burch, P. G., and Maumenee, A. E.: Iridocyclectomy for benign tumors of the ciliary body, Amer. J. Ophthal. 63:447, 1967.
11. Ferry, A. P.: Lesions mistaken for malignant melanoma of the iris, Arch. Ophthal. 74:9, 1965.
12. Yanoff, M., and Zimmerman, L. E.: Pseudomelanoma of anterior chamber caused by implantation of iris pigment epithelium, Arch. Ophthal. 74:302, 1965.
13. Zimmerman, L. E.: Melanocytes, melanocytic nevi, and melanocytomas, Invest. Ophthal. 4:11, 1965.
14. Reese, A. B.: Epidermal cyst of the iris and ciliary body, Amer. J. Ophthal. 65:450, 1968.
15. Rones, B., and Zimmerman, L. E.: The prognosis of primary tumors of the iris treated by iridectomy, Arch. Ophthal. 60:193, 1958.
16. Duke, J. R., and Dunn, S. N.: Primary tumors of the iris, Arch. Ophthal. 59:204, 1958.
17. Reese, A. B., and Cleasby, G. W.: The treatment of iris melanoma, Amer. J. Ophthal. 47:118, 1959.
18. Ashton, N.: Primary tumors of the iris, Brit. J. Ophthal. 48:650, 1964.
19. Cleasby, G. W.: Recurrent malignant melanoma of the iris, Arch. Ophthal. 72:332, 1964.

Extirpation

Algernon B. Reese

The type and extent of the excision of a tumor depend on its size and on whether or not it is malignant. A tumor may be malignant in the sense that it infiltrates, metastasizes, or both. An essentially infiltrating tumor may be cytologically benign but clinically malignant, if it destroys the eye or becomes lethal by infiltrating nonexpendable or vital areas. For such tumors total excision should prove curative. Included in this group are melanomas of the iris and ciliary body, epitheliomas of the lid, glioma of the optic nerve, benign mixed tumors of the lacrimal gland, and so on.

Metastasizing tumors require early radical treatment. Into this group fall most melanomas, retinoblastoma, rhabdomyosarcoma, adnexal carcinoma of the lid, and carcinoma of the lacrimal gland.

Ophthalmologists are increasingly aware that the tenets which apply to tumors in general oncology do not necessarily apply to comparable ocular tumors. An important reason for establishing separate criteria is the fact that ocular tumors are overt and produce symptoms and, therefore, are detected at an early stage. Because of this advantage in ophthalmology, a relatively good prognosis can be anticipated in dealing with such malignant tumors as rhabdomyosarcoma and malignant lymphoma of the orbit, retinoblastoma, and some melanomas of the uvea and the conjunctiva. An exception to this is found in the case of the mixed tumors of the salivary glands as contrasted with those of the lacrimal gland. In the salivary glands the tumor is benign; however, in the lacrimal gland the tumor is malignant because it is occult, frequently arises from ectopic glands, and, most important of all, it is in close relation to bone which it invades early.

Malignant melanomas of the conjunctiva are diagnosed unusually early. However, mistakes in the treatment of these tumors can be summed up by the trite phrase, too little too late. The difficulty lies in deciding what to do and when.

Sometimes extirpation of a tumor is attempted when not indicated. This usually happens in dealing with malignant lymphomas of the orbit, neurofibromas, lymphangiomas, infantile hemangiomas, and granulomas.

Malignant melanomas and retinoblastomas are very high on the list of cancers that may show spontaneous regression and even a cure. Cancer cells in general, and malignant melanomas and retinoblastomas in particular, have antigenic properties and provoke an autoimmune reaction which acount for varying degrees of host resistance. Therefore, the cancer should be excised even though the excision may prove to be incomplete. This is advocated in order to keep the bulk of the tumor under control. Then the tumor (the antigen) will not overcome the host before its antigenic properties can help stay the process.

A great deal of evidence is accumulating in support of an autoimmune response to cancer. Cancer cells frequently get into the peripheral blood and are implanted over the body but fail to grow. Autopsies show that many people have subclinical cancer which is static. Many well-documented cases of spontaneous cures of cancer are reported, and the serum of such a cured patient may promote a cure when given to a patient with advanced cancer of the same type.

What can be accomplished in the surgical treatment of orbital tumors? There are several advantages to such treatment. The tumor may be completely excised, leaving little or no blemish (adult hemangioma, neurilemoma, angiosarcoma, dermoid cyst, some epithelial tumors of the lacrimal gland). Biopsy tissue may be obtained which directs the treatment toward radiation, radical surgery, or temporizing. Exploration of the orbit may rule out an expanding tumor.

However, there are also disadvantages to this treatment. Normal preoperative vision may be reduced even to blindness. This may occur as a result of occlusion of the central retinal artery or vein, especially from surgery in the inferior portion of the orbit in the area where vessels enter the optic nerve. It may occur as a result of macular pathology provoked by trauma of the short posterior ciliary arteries, or it may result from a pressure dressing so tight that it causes atresia of the central retinal artery. Deviation of the eye from injury to extraocular muscles may occur, ptosis from damage of the levator muscle may ensue, or keratitis sicca from removing too much of the lacrimal gland may be extremely annoying.

The most important, as well as the most difficult, feature of orbital surgery is the recognition of that moment when one has reached the point of diminishing returns. Will the possible good that accrues to the patient justify the price he will pay?

The surgical procedures for orbital tumors

range from simple local excision to extensive local excision to exenteration. There is a big jump from excision to exenteration. This gap can be narrowed by various degrees of subtotal exenteration.

There are many variations of subtotal exenteration. For example, in dealing with cancerous melanosis, one may leave the skin and cilia of both lids, the periosteum, the fat in the apex of the orbit and the extraocular muscles, placing an implant in the muscle funnel. This results in the appearance of a closed eye. For lid epithelioma which is out of control and is invading the orbit, one may leave intact the upper or lower half of the orbit as well as the eyeball and muscles, excising the entire upper or lower lid and adjacent orbital contents including the periosteum if necessary. Repair may be made by a Hughes procedure if the lower half of the orbit is excised, or by a reverse Hughes procedure if the upper half of the orbit is excised. This results in the appearance of closed lids. For some cases of neurofibroma, fibroxanthoma, hemangiopericytoma, and hemangioendothelioma, one may leave the entire upper and lower lids, all of the palpebral and bulbar conjunctiva, the extraocular muscles, and apical fat. An implant is put in the muscle funnel. This results in a conjunctival-lined socket for a prosthesis.

In total exenteration the periosteum may be left, which is used to insert an implant; nothing except the skin of the lids with or without cilia may be left and the implant may be secured with temporalis muscle. A socket for a prosthesis can be left by leaving the conjunctiva and lids and securing the implant with the temporalis muscle. By leaving only the halved lids, the implant can be secured with the temporalis muscle. The orbit can be restored later with a half-thickness graft.

Conclusion

Tumors are malignant in two senses, and treatment varies accordingly. Cancers in ophthalmology may have better prognoses than comparable tumors in general oncology. Some tumors, such as lymphomas, neurofibromas, lymphangiomas, infantile hemangiomas, and granulomas, should not be excised. Cancer cells are foreign, or antigenic, to the host and provoke an autoimmune reaction. Therefore, partial excision may be salutary. Surgery of the orbit has its advantages as well as its drawbacks. It is important for the surgeon to weigh these carefully. The long distance between local excision and total exenteration may sometimes be bridged by various forms of subtotal exenteration.

Cryosurgery in the management of intraocular tumors

Harvey Lincoff
John McLean

Cryosurgery has played only a small role in the management of intraocular tumors. There are three areas in which it has had some value. (1) Freezing has obliterated some small retinoblastomas. (Treatment of other tumors has been precluded for reasons which will be discussed.) (2) The cryosurgical lesion has been useful for localizing and de-fining the shape of malignant melanomas for treatment by the cobalt 60 plaque technique. It is to be preferred for this purpose over diathermy, particularly penetrating diathermy. (3) Cryosurgical probing has proved of value in the diagnosis of intraocular tumors. This discussion will concentrate on the latter use.

In the course of an investigation into the treatment of intraocular tumors by cryosurgery, we became aware that the penetration time and the appearance of ice on the surface of a tumor were distinct and differed from that which occurred in normal retina. We compared the appearance of ice on the surface of other lesions that might be confused with tumor and concluded that with some experience characteristic patterns could be recognized which were consistent and would aid in the differential diagnosis of intraocular lesions.

It is not our intention to review the results of the attempt to treat tumors, except to mention aspects of the investigation which are relevant to the present subject. The incentive for treating intraocular tumors came about with the realization that the cryosurgical application could penetrate sclera and selectively destroy retinal and choroidal elements without damaging the integrity of the scleral wall. Thus it might be possible to attack intraocular tumors without risking dissemination of surviving tumor cells through a necrotic wall. Reassurance against hematogenous spread was provided by the observation that capillaries were thrombosed and larger vessels remained unbroken after cryosurgical probing.

Experimental treatment of intraocular tumors

Regrettably there was no satisfactory animal model for investigating intraocular tumors as there had been for investigating retinal detachment. Therefore after some preliminary measurements on the size of the ice mass intrusion that might be expected from various probe temperatures, we proceeded to freeze a small retinoblastoma in an infant. A retinoblastoma was chosen for the initial trial because an extraordinary vulnerability of rods and cones to freezing had been observed in the normal animal retina. A small peripheral retinoblastoma was frozen transconjunctivally with probe temperatures beginning at –20° C. (Fig. 4-14). Ice appeared in the retina around the tumor in a few seconds. The wall of the infant eye is rapidly penetrated by freezing. However, a temperature of –60° C. was required to make the ice ascend to the apex of the tumor.

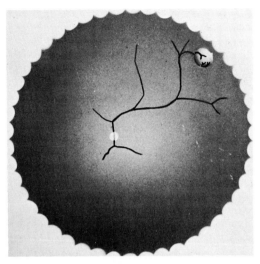

Fig. 4-14. Small peripheral blastoma.

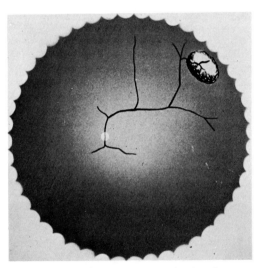

Fig. 4-15. Retinoblastoma 1 week after freezing at –60° C.

Within a week the tumor mass disappeared and left a pale atrophic scar (Fig. 4-15). Subsequently two larger retinoblastomas were frozen, one at –30° C. and the second at –90° C. These tumors also absorbed, with the exception of calcium remnants which persisted in the vitreous above the chorioretinal scar. In retrospect it is important to emphasize that a child's eye is rapidly penetrated by cryosurgical application at –20° C. Penetration of a retinoblastoma requires a lower temperature corresponding with its height. The tumor offers little resistance to the uniform spread and intrusion of the ice mass.

Encouraged by the results of treating retinoblastoma we attempted the cryosurgical destruction of intraocular metastatic carcinoma and later malignant melanoma. The adult human retina is ordinarily frozen by probe temperatures ranging from -30° C. to -50° C. depending upon the thickness of the scleral wall and the vascularity at the site of application. In our attempts to freeze carcinoma, a relatively flat tumor, ice could not be made to penetrate even the periphery of the carcinoma until temperatures below -100° C. were sustained from 30 to 60 seconds. To penetrate the center of the lesions would frequently require a sustained -180° C., the lower limit of the probe. The center of large tumors resisted -180° C. regardless of how long it was sustained. Subsequently, malignant melanoma showed the same resistance to freezing. The resistance of these tumor masses to freezing was unexpected. Retinoblastoma has accepted ice intrusion as calculated in the animal eye. Differences in the thickness of sclera and choroid could not account for the magnitude of the disparity. The explanation, we believe, lies in the warmth and, indirectly, in the vascularity of the tumor. Adenocarcinoma and malignant melanoma are warmer vascular tumors, whereas retinoblastoma is relatively avascular, even though the vessels are visible on the surface of the tumor. The tumors frequently outgrow their blood supply and become necrotic and calcified. It is to be emphasized that carcinoma and melanoma show a resistance to penetration by freezing out of proportion to their thickness.

In a report to the Gonin Society in 1966 we detailed our experience in freezing 16 intraocular tumors and concluded that freezing would be useful for the treatment of retinoblastoma, but was not satisfactory for malignant melanoma or metastatic carcinoma.[1, 2] Other factors besides their resistance

to freezing precluded further efforts in the direction of melanoma and carcinoma. Resistance to ice intrusion could have been overcome by building a larger capacity probe, but the products of acute necrosis from extensively freezing these tumors resulted in such a severe inflammatory response in the vitreous that useful vision was destroyed. This is in contrast to the products of acute necrosis from retinoblastoma, which are absorbed with relatively little inflammatory response.

Diagnostic probing

While we have ceased the cryosurgical treatment of adult intraocular tumors, we have continued cryosurgical probing of suspect lesions for diagnostic purposes, using as criteria the observations just described. The criteria have been expanded to include nevi, subretinal hemorrhage, and retinal cyst.

Metastatic carcinoma. Fig. 4-16 shows a cryosurgical application for diagnostic purposes at the edge of metastatic carcinoma to choroid. At -40° C. a semicircle of white appeared in the retina on the edge of the lesion in 3 seconds. Sustaining the probe at this temperature increased the amount of snow on the retinal surface, but never penetrated the lesion. The edge of the tumor blanched when the probe temperature was reduced to -100° C., and ice crystals appeared on the tumor surface at -120° C. When the probe was applied more to the center of the tumor a temperature of -180° C. for 18 seconds was required to penetrate. Prior to its appearance on the surface, ice tended to spread along the edge of the tumor. These developments gave the impression that one was probing a dense and vascular mass.

Malignant melanoma. Fig. 4-17 demonstrates a -40° C. application for diagnostic purposes on the edge of a malignant melanoma after 4 seconds. The tumor periphery was not penetrated until the temperature was lowered to -120° C. The center could not be penetrated at all with our instrument,

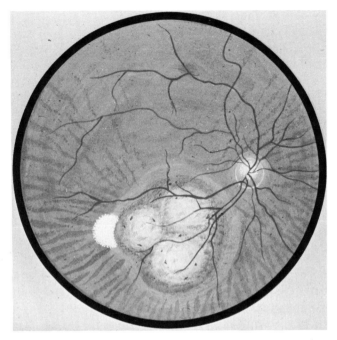

Fig. 4-16. Cryosurgical probing at −40° C. to −100° C. on the edge of metastatic carcinoma to choroid.

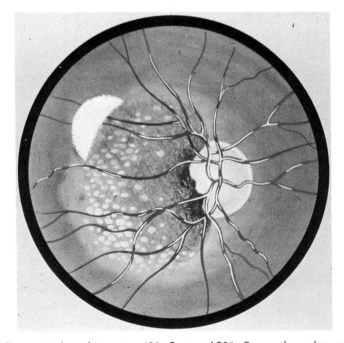

Fig. 4-17. Cryosurgical probing at −40° C. to −120° C. on the edge of malignant melanoma.

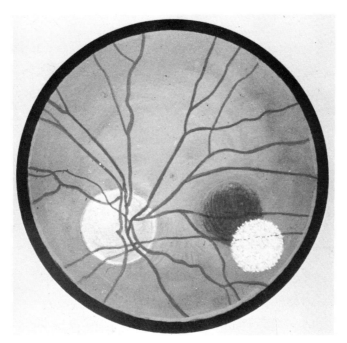

Fig. 4-18. Cryosurgical probing on the edge of benign pigment epithelial hyperplasia of the retina. The white lesion appeared uniformly at –40° C. after 4 seconds.

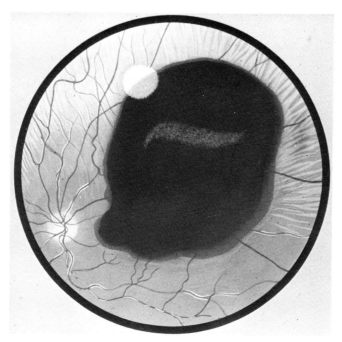

Fig. 4-19. Cryosurgical probing between –40° C. and –70° C. on the edge of a subretinal hemorrhage.

an indication that this relatively high lesion was both dense and vascular. Cryosurgical probing was not an important adjunct to the diagnosis of this particular tumor which had a solid and typical ophthalmoscopic appearance. The probing has been more useful when it revealed the density of a neoplasm in which the ophthalmoscopic appearance was confounded by overlying detached or cystic retina.

Nevus. Fig. 4-18 portrays the application of the cryosurgical probe at –40° C. to the edge of an area of benign pigment hyperplasia. Snow appeared simultaneously throughout the lesion in 4 seconds. The uniform whiteness and rapid appearance of snow on the surface indicated that the lesion was flat and avascular and confirmed its benign nature.

Subretinal hemorrhage. Fig. 4-19 shows the application of the cryosurgical probe to the edge of a subretinal hemorrhage. The probing was characterized by the gradual spread of snow into the hemorrhage as the temperature was lowered to –70° C. Initially, as the ice made its way to the surface of the lesion, it had the pink appearance which one might expect from freezing a mass of blood. Ice could be made to appear more centrally in the lesion at –80° C. in 10 seconds. The delay in appearance was proportional to the elevation (unlike in neoplasm in which the delay was disproportionately long) and indicated that the mass was homogenous and lacked an active circulation.

Retinal cyst. Fig. 4-20 portrays the exploration of a retinal cyst with the cryosurgical probe at –40° C. As one might expect, a white lesion appeared within a few seconds in the external wall of the cyst. The appearance time coincided with the appearance time in the adjacent normal retina. (It should be pointed out that the appearance time of a lesion in choroid beneath a detached retina would be longer because retina turns white before choroid.) As the ice first

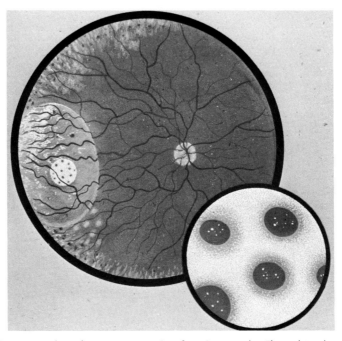

Fig. 4-20. Cryosurgical probing at –40° C. after 3 seconds. The white lesion is in the external wall of the cyst.

appeared in the wall of the cyst it revealed a mottled pattern in the external wall. The whiter areas are composed of remnants of retinal tissue; the areas in which the tissue is thin are darker and the contrasting choroid shows through. The mottled pattern which is pigskin-like is not revealed everywhere in the base of a cyst, but we have found it in some portion of the 7 cysts that have been examined, and we think it is sufficiently unique to be noteworthy. The pattern can be more perfectly defined if the freezing is done slowly at warmer temperatures, such as –30° C. Too rapid penetration freezes the choroid, eliminates the contrast of a dark background, and results in a uniform white lesion.

Technique

For the surgeons who already use cryosurgery to treat retinal detachment, the technique for cryosurgical probing will present no difficulty. It is essentially the same as that used for prophylactic cryopexy. A retrobulbar block is advisable if the lesion to be examined is posterior to the equator. Anterior lesions can be probed transconjunctivally using topical anesthesia. In the observations described here the Linde CE-3 instrument was used. Its broad range of temperatures (+37° C. to –180° C.) is advantageous; however, the –70° C. instruments so widely employed for detachment surgery will still be useful, particularly for probing the edges of a lesion where the sharpest contrasts are obtained.

Conclusion

We have presented observations from cryosurgical probing of five types of intraocular lesions. We suggest that the development and appearance of ice at the edge and on the surface of lesions is sufficiently characteristic to be of diagnostic value. The temperatures and appearance times should not be interpreted too rigidly. They are intended to serve only as guidelines in differentiating solid from cystic, elevated from flat, and vascular from avascular. It will be a mistake if the simplicity of the concept is lost. Essentially, cryosurgical probing is a method of physical diagnosis wherein the physician must artfully interpret the appearance of ice as it is applied to intraocular lesions.

REFERENCES

1. Lincoff, H.: A report on the freezing of intraocular tumors, Mod. Probl. Ophthal. **7:**348, 1968.
2. Lincoff, H., McLean, J., and Long, R.: The cryosurgical treatment of intraocular tumors, Amer. J. Ophthal. **63:**389, 1967.

Heliotherapy

Jules François

Since we at the Ophthalmological Clinic of the University of Ghent are not sufficiently experienced in the treatment of conjunctival or iridociliary tumors, I will speak only of heliotherapy in the management of malignant melanoma of the choroid and retinoblastoma.

We have only used the ruby laser coagulator in rabbits. The M-10 model of Optics Technology has several disadvantages. The illumination for ophthalmoscopy is not sufficient. During the production of the lesion, the response to coagulation is not immediately visible to the operator. He does not know the intensity of the flash, since the energy in joules is not indicated. Even with divergent rays, the coagulations are very small, so that it takes a long time to treat a large area. Lesions of the retinal vessels cannot be managed with the laser, because its beam is composed of red light.

The histologic study of laser-produced lesions of the retina shows that these are smaller and involve less destruction of the membrane than the ones produced by the xenon-arc photocoagulator. At the periphery of the lesion, only the external layers of the retina are destroyed; in the center of the lesion, both the internal and external layers are altered, but the choroid is only slightly affected and the sclera is not affected at all. Moreover, there is often a reaction within the vitreous overlying the lesion. Finally, the chorioretinal scar that results from laser coagulation is not as durable or as strong as the one obtained with conventional light coagulation.

For all these reasons, we have used only the xenon-arc light coagulator after Meyer-Schwickerath in the management of intraocular tumors.

Malignant melanoma of the choroid

The conservative treatment of malignant melanoma of the choroid has always been considered with skepticism and must be attempted only with great prudence. It must nevertheless be recognized that enucleation has not been especially successful. Reese's important statistics concerning 600 malignant melanomas of the uvea treated by removal of the eyeball show that 48% of patients died from metastases within 5 years and that, in a group of 200 enucleated patients followed for 10 years, the mortality was 66%.[1] Therefore, we have not hesitated to treat malignant melanoma of the choroid and, we think, it is now demonstrated that light coagulation can cure these tumors.

Indications for light coagulation

The melanoma which does not exceed 5 to 6 disc diameters in size, is not elevated more than 9 to 10 diopters, and is not accompanied by retinal detachment, is susceptible to destruction by light coagulation. The smaller the tumor and the less elevation, the better the prognosis.[2]

Of course not all small tumors are malignant; some are benign melanomas of the choroid, hyperplasias of the pigment epithelium, angiomata of the choroid, and so on. Nevertheless, in all the histopathologic examinations that have been made in our department (more than 250), we have been mistaken only two times in establishing the clinical diagnosis of malignant melanoma.

Contraindications

Contraindications of light coagulation include tumors that are more than 6 disc diameters and more than 10 diopters and tumors in which the anterior border cannot be reached (in these cases diathermy can nevertheless be associated). Light coagulation is also contraindicated in cases in which the secondary retinal detachment does not disappear after the first light coagulation or in which the detachment on the contrary develops after the latter. There are also tumors in which destruction will cause too important a loss of central or peripheral vision.

Technique

Maximum dilatation of the pupil is obtained by instillations of atropine and phenylephrine (10%). To obtain a complete immobilization of the eyeball, a retrobulbar injection is done of 5 ml. xylocaine with adrenalin and hyaluronidase.

The procedure is always begun with a barrage of two rows of light coagulations in healthy tissue around the tumor (diaphragm 6, intensity V/II). When this barrage is achieved, the tumor itself is coagulated, first using intensity V/II and then intensity V/III.

In case of retinal detachment the barrage is impossible, but rather often the detachment disappears after coagulation of the tumor surface, at least in the cases in which it is not too extensive. The barrage can then be realized in the second session. When this is not the case, light coagulation is contraindicated.

Sometimes light coagulation produces an exudative detachment, which heals spontaneously after 1 to 3 weeks. This kind of detachment is generally prevented by the barrage. If it persists, it would also be a contraindication to light coagulation.

The second session of light coagulation takes place after 4 weeks, when the tumor recovers a grayish hue. Often during further light coagulations, one sees not only a retraction of the tumor, but also a real tissular burst with gaseous bubbles; and the whole tumor can explode.

The number of sessions necessary to destroy the tumor depends on the extent and the thickness of the tumor, which must be destroyed layer by layer. Generally 3 to 7 sessions are needed; occasionally 8 to 10 are necessary.

Cure

A cure can be anticipated if the tumor is transformed into a brownish homogeneous area, protruding at the maximum 0.5 diopter, and surrounded by an atrophic, avascular white zone, which exposes the sclera. This girdle widens progressively toward the center, but it may take months or even years for the central pigmented area to disappear. This very slow resorption is due probably to the destruction of all the blood vessels. Occasionally, one can see the destroyed pigments migrating into the vitreous.

When light coagulation is *not successful* one sees that:

1. The elevation does not diminish, but increases

2. The tumor extends beyond the barrage
3. The vessels remain or reappear

Results

Our present study describes fifty-three patients who were followed for 2 or more years after light coagulation. In 4 cases, the diagnosis was questionable: three cases could have been nevi, since there was no perimetric defect and 1 case was perhaps a pseudotumoral macular degeneration. In this respect, one must recall that a malignant melanoma of the choroid never starts in the macula.

The 49 cases in which the diagnosis seemed sure all showed a defect in the visual field (scotoma), a negative retroillumination, and more recently a characteristic appearance after fluorescein angiography.

The tumors were divided into three groups on the basis of the size and elevation. In group I the tumor was less than 2 disc diameters in size and was elevated less than 2 diopters. In group II the tumor varied in size from 2 to 5 disc diameters and was elevated between 2 and 6 diopters, and in group III the size was more than 5 disc diameters and the elevation more than 6 diopters. No tumors have been treated in which the peripheral boundary was not visi-

Table 4-1. Results obtained in three groups of patients

	Group I	Group II	Group III	Totals
Number of cases	9	23	21	53
Number of cases cured	9 (100%)	23 (100%)	10 (47%)	
Number of years cured				
2 to 3	1	5	2	8
3 to 4	0	0	0	0
4 to 5	2	2	1	5
5 to 6	2	3	1	6
6 to 7	4	6	3	13
7 to 8	0	2	1	3
8 to 9	0	4	2	6
9 to 10	0	1	0	1
Failures	0	0	11 (53%)	

ble. We thought that it was more advisable to enucleate these eyes.

The results are shown in Table 4-1 (Fig. 4-21). In one of the cases that has been cured for 8 to 9 years, the tumor protruded 15 diopters.

One case is particularly interesting.

Case report. P. F., age 56 years, was seen in March 1966. He had a malignant melanoma of the choroid reaching the disc and extending toward the inferonasal quadrant of the fundus. The size of the tumor was 4 disc diameters and the elevation was 3 to 4 diopters. After 4 light coagulations the tumor seemed to be cured, but in December 1966 a relapse appeared just above the disc. Three further light coagulations destroyed this

A

B

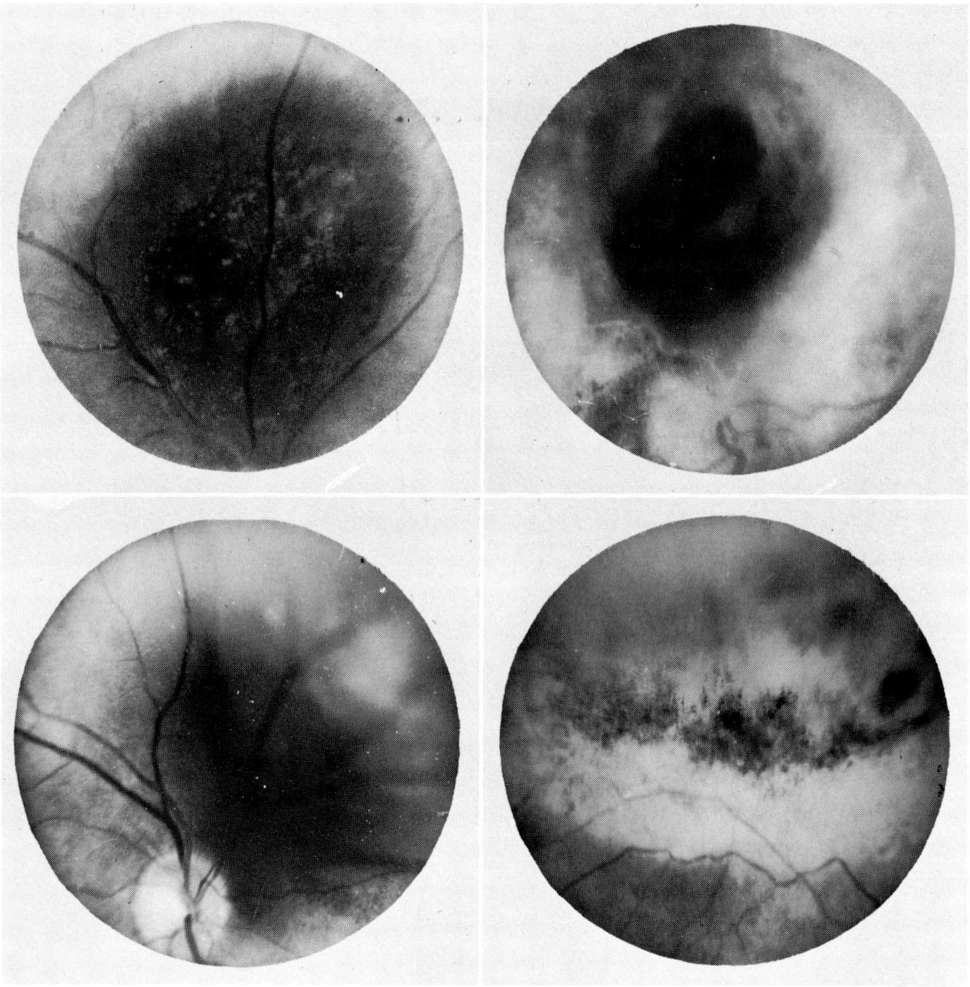

Fig. 4-21. Malignant melanoma of the choroid cured by light coagulation. **A,** At the left (12.VI.62) before, at the right (15.IX.64) after treatment. **B,** At the left (5.XI.59) before, at the right (5.IX.64) after treatment. **C,** At the left (17.X.61) before, at the right (9.IV.62) after treatment. **D,** At the left (20.XI.61) before, at the right (8.I.63) after treatment. **E,** At the left (3.IX.59) before, at the right (20.II.63) after treatment. **F,** At the left (25.VIII.59) before, at the right (5.V.64) after treatment. **G,** At the left (11.XII.61) before, at the right (2.X.63) after treatment. **H,** At the left (1.XII.59) before, at the right (12.XI.62) after treatment. **I,** At the left (18.IX.63) before, at the right (3.IX.64) after treatment. **J,** At the left (25.I.60) before, at the right (5.IX.61) after treatment.

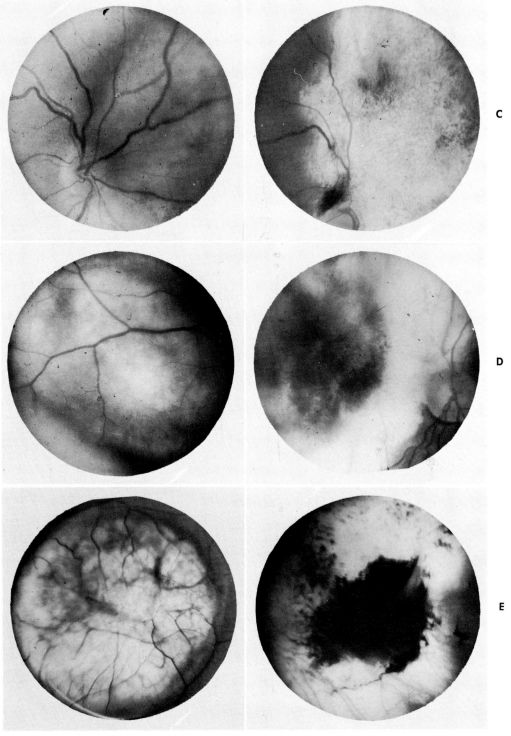

C

D

E

Continued.

Fig. 4-21, cont'd. For legend see opposite page.

F

G

H

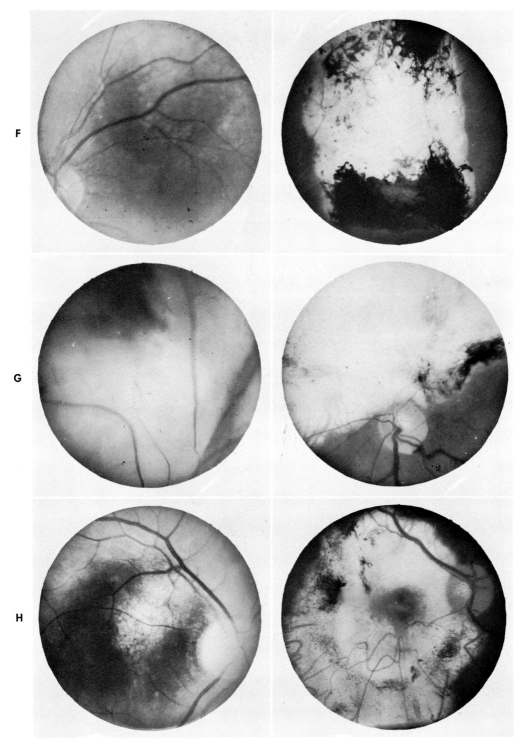

Fig. 4-21, cont'd. For legend see p. 38.

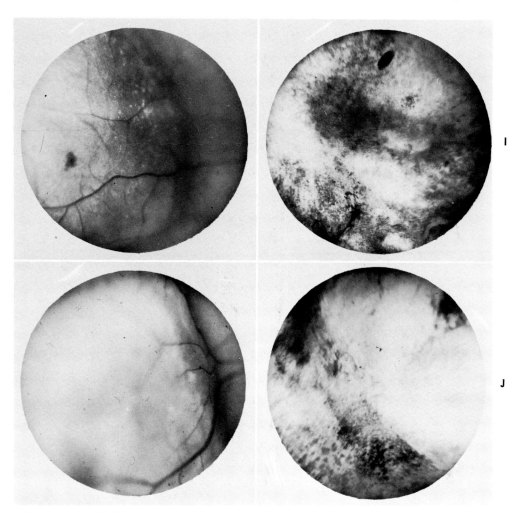

Fig. 4-21, cont'd. For legend see p. 38.

new tumor and it has seemed to be well controlled since February 1967.

All 11 failures were in group III; the size of the tumor was more than 5 disc diameters and the elevation was more than 6 diopters. This fact suggests that the smaller the tumor, the more likelihood of successful photocoagulation.

In 4 cases, despite 5 to 11 light coagulations, the tumor remained active. In 2 of these cases there was hemorrhage into the vitreous and in 2 others there was retinal detachment. Histologic examination following enucleation indicated activity of the tu-

mor. One of these patients died from hepatic metastases 18 months following the beginning of treatment. To our knowledge, this was the sole patient who died from metastases among those who were treated by light coagulation.

In 2 additional cases extensive retinal detachment followed the first light coagulation and enucleation was done. In another patient, in whom the tumor protruded more than 10 diopters, we did not believe photocoagulation was indicated following the first treatment, and therefore enucleated the eye.

Relapses occurred after 1½ to 2½ years[3]

in four patients, who initially appeared to be cured. In only 1 case was the recurrence at the level of the original tumor. In the other 3 cases it occurred in healthy tissue at the boundary of the scar, which suggests that to avoid recurrence, light coagulation barrage must go well beyond the visible limits of the tumor.

It is interesting to note that among the forty-two cured cases, there are 11 juxta-pupillary melanomas. We do not think that these tumors are prognostically so bad.

Complications

During treatment we have observed the following complications:

1. Atrophy of the iris with more or less pronounced mydriasis, probably caused by an insufficient dilation of the pupil (2 cases) (Fig. 4-22)
2. Posterior synechiae after exudative iritis (1 case)
3. Posterior subcapsular opacification of the lens of the complicated type and of late onset (1 case)
4. Intravitreous hemorrhages, occurring generally only after 4 to 6 sessions;

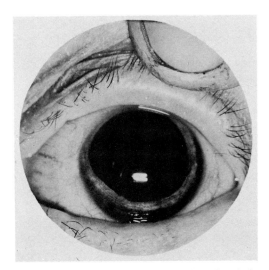

Fig. 4-22. Mydriasis and iris atrophy after light coagulation for malignant melanoma of the choroid.

they are sometimes reabsorbed slowly, sometimes not at all (5 cases)
5. Formation at the surface of the tumor of a fibrous gangue, which has been demonstrated histologically; this gangue impedes the action of the light and can be the cause of a relapse, as seen in one case
6. Traction folds in the macular region after cicatrization (1 case)
7. Transitory exudative detachment, disappearing after 1 to 3 weeks (2 cases; in 1 case there was a more important and more permanent detachment, so that we had to enucleate the eye)
8. Vitreous changes (1 case)
9. Pigment migration into the vitreous (This manifestation is frequent and without importance. It takes months and sometimes years before the pigments, which are broken away from the tumor, are reabsorbed)
10. Retinal hemorrhages around the tumor or in a retinal sector (They frequently occur, but are without any particular significance. They are probably due to the obstruction of some retinal veins)

Histopathology

We had the opportunity to examine histopathologically some cases of malignant melanoma of the choroid that were unsuccessfully treated by light coagulation.

Case 1. A man, 57 years of age, had 6 light coagulations. A few months later, however, a recurrence appeared at the border of the coagulation area. The primary tumor was completely cured and was replaced by a scar with pigment clumps, but without any living tumor cells. At the level of the transition area between this scar and the recurrence there was a zone with scattered tumor cells (Fig. 4-23).

Case 2. A man, 38 years of age, had 8 light coagulations, and seemed to be cured. Two years later at the periphery of the scar there was a recurrence which was covered by a pigmented fibrous membrane; the primary tumor was completely cured (Fig. 4-24).

Case 3. A man, 57 years of age, had 3 light coagulations. The deeper part of the tumor was not

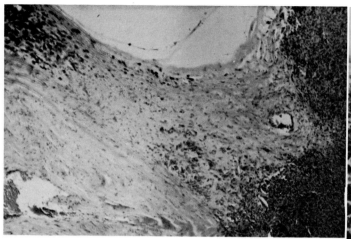

A

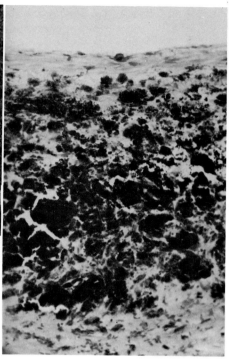

Fig. 4-23. A, Malignant melanoma of the choroid. Recurrence after light coagulation at the border of the primary tumor. This primary tumor (at the right) is completely cured. At the level of the transition area between the scar and the recurrence (at the left) there is a zone with scattered tumor cells. **B,** Malignant melanoma of the choroid treated by light coagulation. The primary tumor is cured and replaced by a scar with pigment clumps, but without any living tumor cell.

B

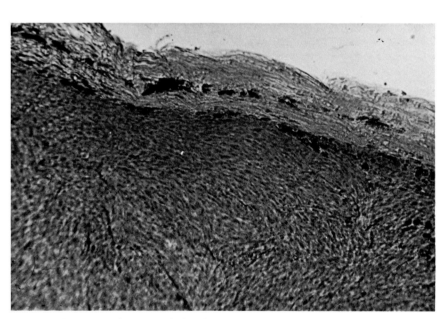

Fig. 4-24. Malignant melanoma of the choroid. After light coagulation there was a recurrence, covered by a pigmented fibrous membrane.

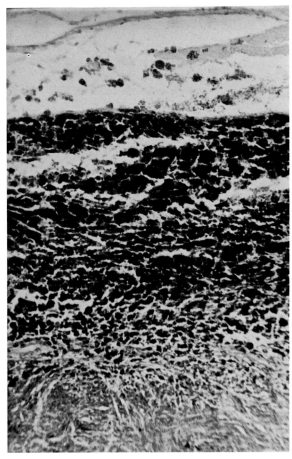

Fig. 4-25. Malignant melanoma of the choroid unsuccessfully treated by light coagulation. The deeper part of the tumor is not very pigmented, but is covered by a heavily pigmented necrotic scar. The retina is completely destroyed.

very pigmented. It was covered by a heavily pigmented necrotic scar, and the retina was completely destroyed (Fig. 4-25).

Case 4. A woman, 53 years of age, had 9 light coagulations. Two years later a recurrence appeared at the periphery of the scar. As the patient refused an enucleation, the new tumor was also coagulated. Two years later glaucoma with severe pain convinced the patient to accept an enucleation. Histologically, a dense fibrous scar covered the tumor, but it was infiltrated by tumor cells and ruptured by the proliferating cells (Fig. 4-26).

The histopathologic examination of these and 5 other tumors that have been treated by light coagulation has shown that the failure of the treatment can be ascribed to the following factors[4]:

1. Detachment of the retina

2. Absence of pigmentation of the melanoma

3. Too great size of the tumor, the thickness having more importance than the extent

4. Pigmentary crust at the level of the superficial layers of the melanoma, preventing the penetration of the radiant energy in the depth; this cicatricial necrosis may be observed even in little or nonpigmented tumors.[5]

5. Formation of a fibrous membrane at the surface of the tumor, absorbing or reflecting the rays and facilitating the scleral extension

6. Persistence of tumor cells in the chorio-

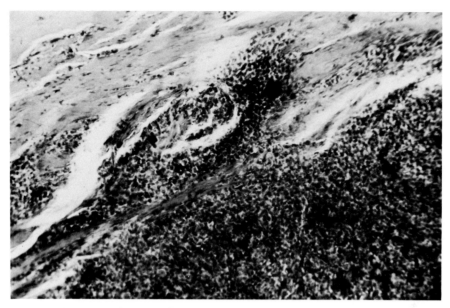

Fig. 4-26. Malignant melanoma of the choroid unsuccessfully treated by light coagulation. A dense fibrous scar covers the tumor and is already infiltrated by tumor cells.

retinal scars and even in the apparently normal choroid or sclera

7. Insufficiently broad barrage around the tumor, leaving tumor cells in the apparently normal choroid

Although our results are satisfactory, it cannot be overemphasized that one must be cautious. The treated cases have to be examined regularly and carefully. If the regression of the tumor is not obvious and progressive, or if a relapse appears, one must not hesitate to recommend an enucleation.

We have nevertheless the right to treat a malignant melanoma of the choroid by means of light coagulation if the size of the tumor does not exceed 5 to 6 disc diameters and if the elevation is not more than 9 to 10 diopters.

Indeed, all tumors, the size of which was less than 5 disc diameters and the elevation less than 6 diopters, have been cured.[6] The prognosis is worse when the volume of the tumor exceeds these values, since only 10 cases among the 21 belonging to group III have been cured (47%).

Retinoblastoma

In unilateral cases when the tumor is extensive—and this is usually the case—the only safe treatment is enucleation. The same is true for the most severely affected eye in bilateral cases.

We reserve the conservative treatment for the least affected eye in bilateral cases, when a more or less important part of the retina remains intact and when some visual function can be retained.

Indications for light coagulation

The cases are classified after Reese[1] into five groups:

Group I—Solitary tumor, less than 4 disc diameters in size, at or behind the equator *or* multiple tumors, none over 4 disc diameters in size, all at or behind the equator

Group II—Solitary tumor, 4 to 10 disc diameters in size, at or behind the equator *or* multiple tumors, 4 to 10 disc diameters in size, behind the equator

Group III—Any lesion anterior to the

equator *or* solitary tumors larger than 10 disc diameters behind the equator

Group IV—Multiple tumors, some larger than 10 disc diameters *or* any lesion extending anteriorly to the ora serrata (we have not treated cases belonging to this group)

Group V—Massive tumors involving over half the retina *or* vitreous seeding (we have not treated cases belonging to this group)

Solitary or multiple tumors which do not exceed 4 disc diameters in size and 6 diopters in elevation, and which are situated at or behind the equator (Reese's group I), as well as the relapses after radiotherapy may be treated by light coagulation alone.

Contraindications to light coagulation

Contraindications include tumors that extend anteriorly to the equator, so that a barrage in healthy tissue is impossible.

Indications for combined treatment

The combined treatment consists of light coagulations, radiotherapy (4,500 to 6,000 r, Reese's technique), and chemotherapy. It is very often necessary to start with radiotherapy and antimitotics, and to apply light coagulations only when the tumor is already sufficiently reduced.

The antimitotic we use is Endoxan (2 mg. per kilogram body weight per day orally; 2.5 to 3 mg. per kilogram have occasionally

been used). The bone marrow and the blood must of course be regularly examined, since leukopenia and thrombocytopenia can be observed. Other side effects include alopecia and exceptionally hemorrhagic cystitis.

We use the combined treatment for all the retinoblastomas that exceed 4 disc diameters in size and 6 diopters in elevation (Reese's groups II to V).

Results

We have treated 6 cases of retinoblastoma by light coagulation alone and 14 by light coagulation in combination with radiotherapy and chemotherapy (see Table 4-2).

Light coagulation alone (3 to 12 sessions). Five of the 6 cases treated by light coagulation alone have been cured for more than 6 years; 1 has been cured for more than 4 years. Four of these cases belonged to Reese's group I, 1 to group II, and 1 to group III.

This last case is interesting.

Case report. D. B. H., age 13½ months, had three tumors in the right eye. The first was a superonasal tumor of 2 discs diameters, the second was below the disc (½ disc diameter), and the third was anterior to the equator at the temporal side. Twelve light coagulations were applied within 2 years. This case has now been cured for 10 years. Visual acuity is 8/10 (Fig. 4-27).

Combined treatment. Fourteen cases have had combined treatment. One case, belonging to group II, died after 2 weeks, probably because of a cerebral metastasis.

In 2 cases, also belonging to group II, the treatment could not be continued. They are nevertheless interesting and they show how fast other independent tumors can appear.

Case report. A child, 6 months of age, had an extensive bilateral cystic formation at the posterior pole of the fundus. In the retina we could see yellowish spots, and we made the diagnosis of bilateral retinoblastoma. This child had a monozygotic twin brother who seemed to be healthy. We examined the twin also and found in the lower temporal part of the right retina a small retinoblastoma, which we photocoagulated immediately. Fourteen days later the tumor seemed to be cured but 2 others appeared in the neighboring fundus. They were also photocoagulated and were apparently cured. Nothing happened for 4 months until a fourth tumor appeared at the superior

Table 4-2. Treatment of retinoblastoma by light coagulation alone and in combination with radiotherapy and chemotherapy

Classification after Reese (1963)	Number of cases	Success	
		No.	%
Group I	4	4	100
Group II	12	6	50
Group III	4	4	100
Total	20	14	70

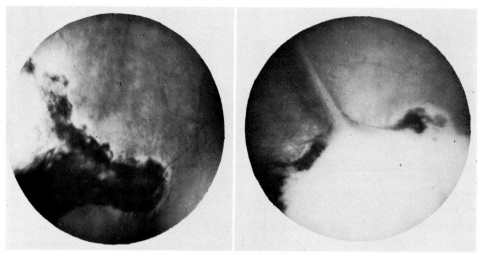

Fig. 4-27. Retinoblastoma cured by light coagulation.

periphery in the same eye. The parents refused any further treatment.

Three cases, belonging to group II, became worse in spite of combined treatment and the eyes had to be enucleated.

Eight cases (5 belonging to group II and 3 to group III) may be considered as cured for 2 or more years.

Case 1. Child, 6 months of age, with 2 important tumors, which have been photocoagulated 12 times. This case has been cured for more than 6 years.

Case 2. Girl, 10 weeks of age with a large superonasal tumor, which has been photocoagulated 6 times. This case has been cured for more than 6 years.

Case 3. Child with 3 tumors (1 near the disc, 1 in the macula, and 1 anterior to the equator). Eight light coagulations were applied. This case has also been cured for more than 6 years.

Case 4. D. W., 2½ months of age, was seen in December 1964 for bilateral retinoblastoma. The right eye was enucleated. In the left eye we found 2 tumors of 1 disc diameter in size at 7:30 o'clock; which were photocoagulated. In January 1965, we saw a new tumor of 1 disc diameter at 11 o'clock, it was also photocoagulated. In February 1965 a fourth tumor of ¼ disc diameter appeared at the temporal side of the macular region, and it was also photocoagulated. At the end of March 1965 we observed a relapse in situ at the level of the first 2 tumors at 7:30 o'clock; light coagulation was effective. In January 1966 a fifth new tumor appeared at 6 o'clock between the equator and the ora serrata; it was destroyed by diathermy, com-

bined with radiotherapy (4,500 r) and Endoxan. This case has been cured for more than 2 years.

Case 5. W. J., 17 months of age, was seen in March 1965 for bilateral retinoblastoma. The right eye was enucleated. In the left eye we found 3 tumors, a large one on the nasal side of the disc, another of 2 disc diameters in the macular region, and a third important one at the superior periphery anterior to the equator. After combined treatment with 7 light coagulations the three tumors were cured. There were no relapses, but in December 1965 a hemorrhage appeared in front of the disc and 2 weeks later one appeared in the anterior chamber. Afterward a dystrophy of the cornea developed progressively. At this time, the eye is still quiet in regard to the retinoblastoma.

Case 6. E., aged 10 months, was seen at the end of 1966 for bilateral retinoblastoma. The left eye was enucleated. The right eye showed 3 tumors: one of 2 disc diameters at the nasal side of the disc, another of 1 disc diameter above the macular region, and a third one at the superior periphery at the level of the equator. A complete cure was obtained after a combined treatment of radiotherapy (4,700 r), 10 light coagulations, and antimitotics.

Case 7. P. P., aged 2 months, was seen at the end of 1966 for bilateral retinoblastoma. The right eye was enucleated. The left eye showed, at the nasal side of the disc, a tumor of 1½ disc diameters. A complete cure was obtained after a combined treatment of radiotherapy, 7 light coagulations, and antimitotics.

Case 8. V. P., the twin brother of the previous patient, was also seen at the end of 1966 for bilateral retinoblastoma. The left eye was enucleated. The right eye showed a tumor of 2 disc diameters above the disc. A complete cure was obtained after a combined treatment of radiotherapy, 5 light coagulations, and antimitotics. At the present time, lens opacities are developing.

Complications

The principal complications we have observed are:

1. Irradiation cataract (3 cases of total cataract and 1 case of partial cataract). It must be noted that multiple light coagulations of high intensity can sometimes also produce opacities of the lens (posterior subcapsular cataract)

2. Corneal dystrophy with vascularization (1 case)
3. Intraocular hemorrhage (1 case)
4. Hyphema (1 case)
5. Atrophy of the iris with mydriasis, probably due to an insufficient dilatation of the pupil (4 cases)
6. Traction folds of the retina (several cases)

Histopathology

We had the opportunity to histopathologically examine 2 eyes that had been removed

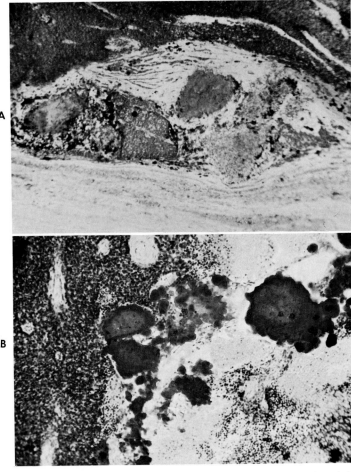

Fig. 4-28. A, Retinoblastoma treated by light coagulation. Hyalinized nodule with foci of living and necrotic tumor cells and with calcifications. **B,** Retinoblastoma treated by light coagulation. There are large areas of necrosis and calcification. A completely hyalinized vessel is seen.

for a relapse of retinoblastoma after unsuccessful light coagulation treatment. Some interesting points can be pointed out.

1. Treated tumors have the same aspect as untreated ones.
2. Hyalinized foci are found, which can still contain living tumor cells (Fig. 4-28).
3. There is no fibrous reaction in the treated tumors and this fact can probably be explained by the nervous nature of the tumor.
4. Some vessels with thickened walls are still supplying the tumor with blood.
5. At the periphery of the tumor small foci of living tumor cells can be found in apparently healthy tissue.
6. Even when the tumor seems to be completely destroyed, an infiltration of the sclera or optic nerve can be seen.

Summary

We have the right to treat the second eye in cases of bilateral retinoblastoma by light coagulation and combined treatment.[7, 8] I even think that when we have the opportunity to see a unilateral retinoblastoma at an early stage as in familial cases, we also can treat it conservatively. Indeed, we could cure 14 cases among 20 cases of bilateral retinoblastoma (70%).

The tumor in its early stage can often be cured by only one light coagulation. In further stages multiple light coagulations are necessary, combined with radiotherapy and chemotherapy.

When we find a retinoblastoma, we must always carefully and regularly examine the eye at least once a month to determine whether new tumors are developing. In apparently unilateral cases we must also carefully and regularly examine the other eye to be able to treat new tumors as soon as possible.

In bad cases, when we expect metastases from the retinoblastoma, we can sometimes predict these by examination of the bone marrow, in which we can find retinoblastoma cells. We have examined 30 bone marrows in uni- and bilateral retinoblastomata and found retinoblastoma cells in 4 cases.

Fifty-three cases of malignant melanoma of the choroid have been treated by means of light coagulation for more than 2 years. Nine cases belonged to group I, 23 to group II, and 21 to group III. All cases of groups I and II have been cured; 10 cases of group III have also been cured, but 11 cases of this group were not cured and the eyes had to be enucleated.

Twenty cases of retinoblastoma have been treated. Six were treated by light coagulation alone and these have all been cured. Fourteen cases were treated by combined photocoagulation; 8 are cured, 3 had to be enucleated, 2 have given up the treatment, and 1 died after 14 days.

REFERENCES

1. Reese, A. B. and Ellsworth, R. M.: The evaluation and current concepts of retinoblastoma therapy, Trans. Amer. Acad. Ophthal. Otolaryn. **67:**164, 1963.
2. François, J.: Treatment of retinoblastoma. In Boniuk, M., editor: Ocular and adnexal tumors; new and controversial aspects, St. Louis, 1964, The C. V. Mosby Co.
3. François, J.: Treatment of malignant melanoma of the choroid by photo-coagulation. In Boniuk, M., editor: Ocular and adnexal tumors; new and controversial aspects, St. Louis, 1964, The C. V. Mosby Co.
4. François, J.: Treatment of malignant melanoma of the choroid by light-coagulation, Trans. Ophthal. Soc. U. K. **85:**179, 1965.
5. François, J.: Disappearance of pigment after light-coagulation of malignant melanoma of the choroid, Amer. J. Ophthal. **66:**443, 1968.
6. François, J.: Traitement des mélanomes malins de la choroide par la photocoagulation. Modern problems in ophthalmology, Vol. 7. Symposium Club Gonin, Munich, 1966, Basel, Karger, 1968, pp. 8-15.
7. François, J.: Traitement du rétinoblastome par la photocoagulation. Modern problems in ophthalmology. Vol. 7, Symposium Club Gonin, Munich, 1966, Basel, Karger, 1968, pp. 204-207.
8. François, J., and Weekers, R.: La photocoagulatoin en ophthalmologie, Bull. Soc. Belge Ophthal. **139:**1, 1965.

Radiation of fundus tumors

M. A. Bedford*

In London during the last few years there has been an increasing liaison between eye surgeons, radiotherapists, and physicists. Radiation now has become increasingly important in the treatment of intraocular tumors particularly with regard to retinoblastoma and malignant melanoma.

Retinoblastoma

Three radiation techniques may be used— the cobalt plaque, the cobalt beam, and the linear accelerator.

Cobalt plaques. Cobalt plaques are discs of radioactive cobalt sealed in platinum with projecting lugs which can be sewn to the sclera after localization.[1] They were designed to prevent the very hot spots given by radon seeds when they were sewn to the outside of the eye to give an adequate dose to the tumor within. Because side effects were frequent and much scarring ensued, the use of radon seeds is not justified. The cobalt plaques with their sophisticated and localized irradiation dose are the ideal treatment for the optimum sized tumor.[2]

In 1 week a plaque will deliver a tumor-lethal dose of 4,000 r to the cells of the summit of the neoplasm with very little involvement of the tissues adjacent. The choroid and sclera underneath receive enormous doses which are relatively well tolerated. The fact that the choroid is heavily irradiated is probably of great importance, as there is little doubt that the incidence of metastasis is directly related to choroidal invasion.[3] The effect of such a localized large dose of radia-

tion is dramatic and certain. Side effects are few with the exception that the plaques, when applied near the optic nerve, may cause troublesome hemorrhages or exudates from the large retinal vessels months later. Current indications for the application of a cobalt plaque are:

1. Single tumors less than 13 mm. in diameter
2. Two separate tumors or groups of tumors that require not more than one 10 mm. plaque on each group (providing that the plaque does not have to be placed nearer than 5 mm. to the optic disc)

With larger tumors and those adjacent to the optic disc regardless of their size the cobalt beam or linear accelerator may be necessary.

Cobalt beam. A direct anterior field can be used and it can be shown that the relevant iso-dose curve occupies the greater part of the eye including the lens. The optic nerve does not receive a high dose of radiation, as can happen with a plaque. The course of treatment using this technique produces a complete regression of the tumor, and in many cases secondary detachments reattach completely.[4] However, all cases develop a radiation cataract in 2 years. Because of this complication other techniques have been developed, particularly the use of the linear accelerator.[5]

Linear accelerator. Using the linear accelerator technique the source of radiation is tilted horizontally. With the sharp "cut-off" inherent with this source of radiation, the lens and, to a greater or lesser extent, the retrolental portion of the vitreous may be spared. There are certain problems to be considered when using this method of treatment, such as the build-up of an adequate tumorcidal dose to the retina on the temporal side, and the dose that the other eye receives if it is present. Some workers have reported the use of a tilted field to miss the other eye,[6] but this could involve the parotid and teeth of this same side. Nevertheless it

*My thanks are due Mr. H. B. Stallard for his constant help and encouragement, to Professor Barrie Jones for allowing me access to beds at Moorfields and to Dr. Lederman and Mr. Williams, the radiotherapists at Moorfields Eye Hospital and St. Bartholomew's Hospital, London.

does seem that the linear accelerator can be of great use in certain cases.

Summary. The cobalt beam with the direct anterior field is indicated when (1) a tumor greater than 13 mm. in diameter is present, (2) when the tumor is adjacent to the optic nerve regardless of size, and (3) where there are free floating neoplastic cells in the vitreous. The indications for the linear accelerator with a temporal field are much the same except that no tumor cells must lie adjacent to the lens as it and its adjacent structures are not irradiated.

It can be argued that the whole retina should be irradiated during the primary treatment. It can be seen, however, from Table 4-3 that the number of recurrences following cobalt beam treatment is exactly the same as those following localized radiation techniques with a cobalt plaque. Some cases may require both forms of radiation, together with perhaps light coagulation or cryosurgery. Each eye should be considered on its own merit and the appropriate therapeutic agent administered. In the vast majority of cases the eye will be saved (Table 4-4).

Malignant melanoma

Malignant melanomas may respond remarkably to treatment with a cobalt plaque.[2] The plaque is left in twice as long as is normal for retinoblastoma so that the summit of the tumor receives at least 8,000 r; the base receives 40,000 r which the eye will certainly tolerate. Effects may take months to manifest themselves and one may have to wait from 9 months to a year before the outcome is certain. At present the indications for cobalt plaque therapy for these tumors seem to be:

1. Tumors that do not directly involve the macula
2. Tumors with an overlying serous retinal detachment that involves the macula
3. Tumors that do not involve the ciliary body

In all cases the ideal tumor for treatment

Table 4-3. Analysis of cases of retinoblastoma (125 cases)

Treatment	Number of eyes
Cobalt plaque	39
Further treatment needed	15 (38%)
Radiation of whole retina	61
Further treatment needed	26 (42%)

Table 4-4. Results of treatment for retinoblastoma (100 eyes)

Results	Number of eyes
Enucleations after treatment	19
Deaths	5
Eye saved	76

is from 10 to 12 mm. in diameter. Contraindications to treatment are:

1. Tumors adjacent to the optic disc
2. Gross involvement of the ciliary body
3. Evidence of dissemination

Follow-up must be prolonged; 1 case had a recurrence 7 years after an apparent cure. The cobalt beam with a direct anterior field is of no use in treating larger tumors. The eye will not tolerate the tumor-lethal dose necessary for malignant melanoma administered with this source of external irradiation. Such an attempt will lead to complete xerosis, glaucoma, and cataract. However, external beam therapy can be used in combating malignant melanoma in the treatment of extrascleral extension noted clinically or histologically after enucleation. Such cases should be immediately treated by a course of radiation, and if this is carried out with a plastic shell in the socket there will be no shrinkage of the conjunctival sac and a prosthesis may be easily worn.

Summary. In summary, approximately 60% of malignant melanomata will respond to local radiation. Unfortunately only 1 in every 4 cases referred to us has proved a suitable case for local radiation techniques. It can be seen in Table 4-5 that if one's criteria are sufficiently stringent, the cure rate

Table 4-5. Analysis of cases of malignant melanoma (29 cases)

Suitable for treatment	25%
Overall cure rate (Stallard)	60%
Cure rate for tumors under 10 mm. in diameter	90% (10 of the 29 cases; 9 reacted)

will rise to approximately 90%. However, this is not a plea for all malignant melanomata to be irradiated with local techniques. Certainly, in most of them enucleation is the correct form of treatment; two-thirds of those selected for treatment may respond to local radiation, and one-third almost certainly will respond.

Discussion

Moderator:

Frank H. Constantine

Dr. Constantine: In the very interesting presentations that we have just heard I recall hearing the term fluorescein angiography used only once, and I wonder what the members of the panel think of it. Prof. François, do you find it useful in differential diagnosis of tumors?

Prof. François: Yes, because in tumors, when you do fluorescein angiography, very often you see beautiful fluorescence and you can make the differentiation between a malignant tumor which is rather vascularized and a benign tumor which is not vascularized.

Dr. Constantine: Dr. Lincoff, would you like to comment on that? Do you find the differential diagnosis that sharp?

Dr. Lincoff: Yes, I do. We are fluorescing all of our tumors and trying to prove that this is so. Our experience is the same as that of Prof. François.

Mr. Bedford: Actually we use it as a routine, and we are also investigating the postoperative appearance with fluorescein.

REFERENCES

1. Innes, G. S.: The application of physics in the treatment of ocular neoplasms. In Boniuk, M., editor: Ocular and adnexal tumors. New and controversial aspects, St. Louis, 1964, The C. V. Mosby Co.
2. Stallard, H. B.: The treatment of retinoblastoma, Ophthalmologica (Basel) **151:**214, 1966.
3. Brown, D. H.: The clinicopathology of retinoblastoma, Amer. J.. Ophthal. **61:**508, 1966.
4. Skeggs, D. B., and Williams, I. G.: The treatment of advanced retinoblastoma by means of external irradiation combined with chemotherapy, Clin. Radiol. **17:**169, 1966.
5. Reese, A., and Ellsworth, R.: Trans. Amer. Acad. Ophthal. Otolaryng. **70:**949, 1966.
6. Bagshaw, M. A., and Kaplan, H. S.: Retinoblastoma, megavoltage, therapy, and unilateral disease, Trans. Amer. Acad. Ophthal. Otolaryng. **70:**944, 1966.

Dr. Constantine: Mr. Bedford, have you had any experience with the use of ultrasound in the differential diagnosis of ocular tumors?

Mr. Bedford: None at all.

Prof. François: Yes, we use ultrasound routinely now. We find it really helpful as you can easily make the differentiation between a detachment of the retina, for example, and a dense tumor.

Dr. Constantine: I would like to ask Prof. François if he has found radioactive phosphorus useful in the diagnosis of ocular tumors?

Prof. François: I have had no experience with this diagnostic procedure.

Mr. Bedford: We have actually given up using it. We find that it is hopelessly inaccurate.

Dr. Constantine: I see you agree, Dr. Lincoff, you are nodding your head. Dr. Reese, do you find any use for the phosphorus test?

Dr. Reese: No.

Dr. Constantine: Does the immediate enucleation of a choroidal malignant melanoma increase the percentage of 5 year survivals?

Dr. Reese: There have been some figures

published which suggest that possibility; however, I have not come to any conclusion.

Dr. Zimmerman: I am just not aware of any controlled study where people have matched up comparable tumors for size and every other characteristic and treated one group by enucleation and followed the others. Without such a controlled study I don't know how one could answer that question.

Dr. Constantine: Dr. Reese, would you list your indications for exenteration of an orbit containing a malignant melanoma of the uveal tract?

Dr. Reese: There are two modes of extension of a melanoma from the uveal tract to the orbit. One accompanies necrosis of the sclera; this involves the orbit diffusely and certainly requires exenteration. The second method of invasion of the orbit is through the scleral channels which transmit the emissary vessels. If one leaves some tumor in the orbit due to an extension through an emissary, I think a subtotal exenteration could be done.

Mr. Bedford: May I add something to that? Recently we have been giving a course of beam therapy to the orbit if there has been either clinical or histologic evidence of extrascleral spread. We have no figures on it yet, and conclusions will be derived only after many years of follow-up.

Dr. Zimmerman: I would like to know if you have been able to correlate the cell type with radiosensitivity. In other words, will a pure spindle melanoma be as responsive to cobalt as other highly malignant types?

Mr. Bedford: We have attempted to make such a correlation, but without success. Tumor size appears to be of prime importance. The smaller the tumor the better the prognosis. Therefore, we are confining our treatment to smaller tumors. We no longer radiate the big ones which we might have treated 3 or 4 years ago in London.

Dr. Constantine: Dr. Reese, if you have a patient who has had 1 eye enucleated for a retinoblastoma, and later develops a similar tumor in the remaining eye, how would you handle it?

Dr. Reese: Eighty-five percent of the patients we have seen with retinoblastoma show multiple origins. These are best handled by blanket betatron therapy to the retina. I think that type of case is not suitable for the cobalt applicator.

Prof. François: If the second eye displays a tumor behind the equator, less than 4 disc diameter in size and not elevated more than 6 diopters, light coagulation is sufficient. But when the blastoma is larger we have to employ a combination of therapy, consisting of photocoagulation, cryotherapy, and chemotherapy.

Dr. Zimmerman: I would like to question this because if this is the second eye, you know you are dealing with a multicentric tumor; and just because you can see only one that is smaller than 4 mm. it doesn't preclude there being the seeds of others that you cannot yet see. So doesn't Dr. Reese's suggestion of blanketing the whole retina with radiation make more sense, prophylactically?

Prof. François: First, you have to carefully examine your patient under general anesthesia. In the beginning, you must repeat this every 14 days; afterward every month, and later, every 3 months, then 6 months, and so on. If you see another tumor appearing you can immediately coagulate it with light. By following this system I have cured several cases.

Dr. Constantine: I would like to ask Mr. Bedford if he has tried the method of Drs. McLean and Lincoff for diagnosing and defining neoplasms by freezing before commencing treatment.

Mr. Bedford: No, not at all. But I would like to endorse what Dr. Lincoff said about the way retinoblastomas respond to cryosurgery. After discussing this with him in New York last year, I have used it on a half dozen cases. The response has been remarkably satisfactory.

Dr. Constantine: It is generally believed that the black race is practically immune to the development of not only malignant melanoma but also sympathetic ophthalmia. In closing this session, I would like to ask our panelists if any relationship exists between these facts. Dr. Zimmerman?

Dr. Zimmerman: I definitely think there is a possible relationship. Both of these conditions are thought to be related to melanocytic cells: sympathetic ophthalmia is assumed to be an acquired antosensitivity to some antigenic material, associated with melanocytic cells; the other being neoplasm of melanocytic cells. In this sense there is a possible relationship.

On the other hand, from my own experience I have not been nearly as impressed as many others have been, with the relative immunity of non-Caucasians to sympathetic ophthalmia. We have seen many instances of sympathetic ophthalmia in non-Caucasians.

I am very much impressed with the relative immunity of non-Caucasians to the development of malignant melanoma; we find this to be an exceedingly rare tumor in all non-Caucasian races in all parts of the world—Asiatic groups, Negro groups, and so on. Still, the tumor does occur in these populations and you have to always be alert for it. We have even seen a Negro child 7 years of age with a large malignant melanoma of the choroid.

Dr. Constantine: I am glad to hear you mention that it is possible to have malignant melanoma or sympathetic ophthalmia in non-Caucasians. This has been a common misconception that can lead to a false sense of security regarding the need for enucleation after trauma in the Negro.

Dr. Reese, would you like to comment about the fact that they seem to be relatively immune from sympathetic ophthalmia and from the melanomas?

Dr. Reese: I wouldn't like to take on the sympathetic aspect of the question, but I would like to comment on the incidence of melanoma in the Negro race. I think one can say roughly that melanomas are more or less in inverse proportion to the amount of pigment, that is, the Scandinavian countries have the highest incidence, and then it is more or less graded down to the amount of pigment of the Negro race which is almost immune to it.

It is interesting that in cases of melanosis oculi in a Caucasian, the incidence of melanoma in that type of eye, which would be perfectly normal for a Negro, is definitely higher than in the fellow eye which has less pigment. Now how can you explain that? It seems to me a possible explanation is that the Negro develops an immunity by the continuous fabrication of melanin, and it must act as an antigen and give them a resistance to it.

On the other hand, if a Caucasian gets a dark eye he doesn't have this inherent immunity, and then a melanoma is liable to appear.

Dr. Constantine: Professor François, do you have any thoughts along this line?

Prof. François: I have no special thoughts on this because I do not see many people who are non-Caucasian. I might mention that in the Congo carcinomas are very frequent in black people.

Dr. Zimmerman: You are referring now to the sole of the feet, not to the uveal tract.

Dr. Constantine: On behalf of Manhattan Eye, Ear and Throat Hospital I wish to express my profound appreciation to Dr. Lorenz Zimmerman, Dr. Algernon Reese, Dr. Harvey Lincoff, Professor Jules François, and to Mr. Michael Bedford for their valued participation in this Centennial Symposium.

CONTROVERSIAL AREAS IN OCULAR SURGERY

Presiding Chairman: **Walter S. Schachat**

Chapter 5

Refractive keratoplasty

Herbert M. Katzin

Refractive keratoplasty is a new experimental method with which we have been working for some time. Surgical intervention in the correction of myopia and ametropia in general has been treated extensively in the literature. Among the many methods described are altering the shape of the globe by shortening the sclera, removing the crystalline lens in high myopia, introducing plastic lenses into the globe, and changing the refractive power of the cornea. I shall confine myself to the latter method.

One surgical procedure, called double slicing, removes corneal substance from the stroma to render the cornea flatter to reduce myopia. Conversely, addition of corneal substance to make the surface more convex will correct hyperopia. This is done with a modified pocket type of graft. Astigmatic errors are also subject to correction by removing, rotating, and replacing a cylindrical layer of the cornea.

The optics for correcting ametropia have been worked out in our laboratory* by Dr. Milton Kaplan. We have favored the technique of double slicing. I believe that Dr. Barraquer favors layer carving. However, the theoretical basis is the same. Myopic astigmatism requires removal of corneal tissue for correction. Hyperopic astigmatism requires stromal addition. In the measure of astigmatism, the spherical equivalent is the pertinent value.

The limits for correcting myopia depend upon the amount of cornea that can be removed. The normal central corneal thickness is said to be 0.56 mm. to 0.60 mm.

*Laboratory of The Eye Bank for Sight Restoration

We have determined that the safe minimum residual thickness of the cornea should be 0.15 mm. The minimum edge thickness of a corneal slice is 0.12 mm. Allowing for a 10% error in the thickness of the slice, as much as 0.40 mm. may be removed from the center of the cornea, and 0.12 mm. of it replaced.

The residual central thickness of the corneal bed would be 0.15 mm., plus 0.12 mm. of the original slice, for a total of 0.27 mm. Our calculations reveal that a correction of 15 diopters of myopia is possible, with a 6 mm. maximum disc diameter.

As far as hyperopia is concerned, the use of the donor material to implant a pocket type disc makes the method quite flexible. As much as 20 diopters of correction may be easily obtained. In the correction of corneal astigmatism, a plano-convex or plano-concave corneal lens can be removed by employing a toric semiapplanation plate.

Since the only way that a cylindrical slice can be taken from the cornea is along the 180th meridian, there are certain axes of astigmatism which cannot be corrected. It may be seen from the graph in Fig. 5-1 that as the axis approaches 45 or 135 degrees a greater power of cylinder must be removed to correct 1 diopter of astigmatism. This cylinder, after rotation, can effect the cylindrical correction.

Thus far, in humans, we have performed only lamellar transplants *without* change of power. Refractive changes have been made only in rabbits. There have been 25 human lamellar grafts done to date, using the autokeratome on the patient's eye as well as on the donor eye.

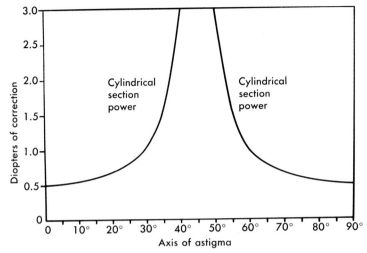

Fig. 5-1. As the axis approaches 45 or 135 degrees, a greater power of cylinder must be removed to correct one diopter of astigmatism.

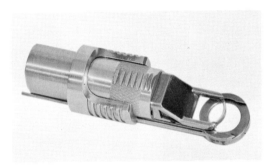

Fig. 5-2. Suction ring and microkeratome.

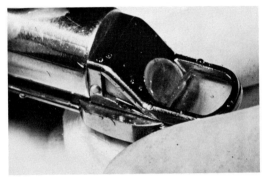

Fig. 5-3. Corneal disc lying on take-off surface of the microkeratome.

The preparation of the autokeratome begins with sterilization. A new blade is cleaned with alcohol and a plastic applanation plate is selected for the desired corneal thickness. Both are inserted into the Elkat autokeratome and sterilized with rings of several sizes and the vacuum hose in an ethylene oxide sterilizer. In the operating room the appropriate ring is fitted and centered on the cornea of the donor eye. The suction is applied and the motorhead assembly is inserted into the guides and moved forward, so that the transparent plate shows the applanated disc of the cornea. If the disc diameter is not the desired size, the ring is exchanged until the proper size applanation is achieved. The motor is then switched on and the dissection is made by steadily advancing the head across the cornea. This requires only 3 or 4 seconds. When the cut is complete, the motor is stopped, the vacuum is released, and the whole instrument is removed from the eye. In experimental work, or in the first few cases, one may wish to instill a drop of fluorescein on the bed from which the graft has been removed, so that the regularity of the cut can be observed. The disc is picked up by sliding a spatula under it and lifting it into a Petri dish. The same method is used on the recipient eye.

Fig. 5-2 shows the suction ring and the microkeratome. In Fig. 5-3 an eye has been cut and the corneal disc is lying on the take-off surface.

Most of the patients who have had this type of operation required a lamellar graft for therapeutic reasons, but 4 have been done for optical improvement—patients with Buecklers' dystrophy or superficial scars of various kinds. The visual results are far better than those we used to obtain with manual dissection of the patient's cornea.

Refractive keratoplasty as a practical clinical reality is still in the future, as far as our work is concerned. In the meantime, I regard the autokeratome as a vastly superior way to perform routine lamellar transplants.

Chapter 6

Keratomileusis and keratophakia: indications, complications, and results

José I. Barraquer

Keratomileusis and keratophakia are two surgical techniques of refractive keratoplasty for correcting refractive errors by modifying the corneal shape.[1]

Cryosurgery of the cornea was applied for the first time in the development of these techniques, as was the extracorporeal modification of a function (refraction).[2]

The word "keratomileusis" comes from two Greek roots that mean cornea and chiseling. Consequently, it means carved, chiseled, or modeled cornea. The word "keratophakia" comes from the Greek roots meaning cornea and lens.

It is easy to understand that interventions with these characteristics require special knowledge and techniques, many of which are unfamiliar to the ophthalmic surgeon. Knowledge of optics, mathematics, physics, manufacture of lenses, cryobiology, and mechanics, in addition to the already specialized corneal surgery and microsurgery, are necessary to perform an operation of this kind successfully.

In keratomileusis a parallel-faced corneal disc is separated from the ocular globe.[3] A tissue lens of the exact value and opposite sign of the ametropia to be corrected is carved on the exposed parenchyma, and the cornea is then reconstructed (Fig. 6-1). Great care and precision are required during all the operative procedures to obtain good results.

The resection of the parenchymatous lens can be done in the excised tissue disc (extracorporeal carving) or in the layers or the exposed parenchyma of the ocular globe (optical carving over the eyeball).[4]

The first process is the one I usually work with, as it allows more precision, and this discussion will refer only to this technique.

For resection of the parenchymatous lens in the excised tissue disc the eye is fixed with a pneumatic ring, through which a microelectrokeratome passes, which operates on the principle of the carpenter's plane. A round parallel-faced corneal disc is shaved from the anterior layers of the patient's own cornea.[5] From this corneal tissue disc, a lens of the necessary optical power is carved on a lathe similar to those used in the manufacture of corneal contact lenses. The conditions of the carving are mathematically calculated for each specific case, either preoperatively or at the time of the operation.

In order to obtain the corneal tissue lens, the corneal tissue disc is placed on its epithelial side, over a concave or convex, spheric or toric lap as required, and carved on its parenchymatous side. For this step to be possible, the tissue must be firmly fixed to the lap and hardened, which is done by freezing the tissue. This principle, used for many years in the freezing microtome, has been applied for the first time in human surgery in keratomileusis (Fig. 6-2). Once

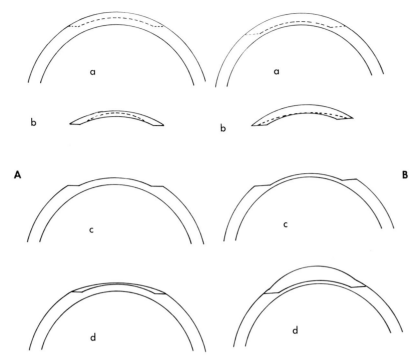

Fig. 6-1. A, Myopia correction. **B,** Hyperopia correction. **a,** Resection of a circular corneal tissue disc, thin in myopic cases, thick in hyperopic cases. **b,** The corneal tissue disc is carved on its parenchymatous side, in the center or in the border, according to the case. **c,** Aspect of the receiving bed. **d,** The corneal tissue lens is replaced, modifying the curvature of the anterior surface of the cornea.

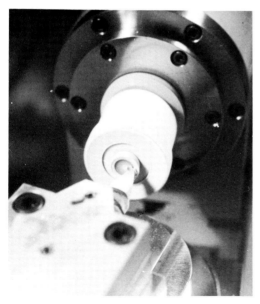

Fig. 6-2. Optical carving of a frozen tissue disc.

carved, the corneal tissue lens is replaced into its bed, and is stitched and covered with a reversed conjunctival flap to compress and protect the corneal tissue.

In keratophakia a parallel-faced corneal disc is separated from the ocular globe (Fig. 6-3, *A*). On the exposed interface, a homoplastic corneal tissue lens of the exact value and of the same sign of the ametropia to be corrected is placed (Fig. 6-3, *B*), centered, and finally covered by the previously resected corneal disc, which is then carefully stitched to the cornea (Fig. 6-3, *C*).[2, 3, 6, 7]

The corneal tissue lens is ground out of the parenchyma of a donor's cornea with the same technique as in keratomileusis (Fig. 6-2). It may also be obtained without freezing or lathe forming, by using only the microkeratome technique on the donor's eye (Fig. 6-3, *D-F*).[5]

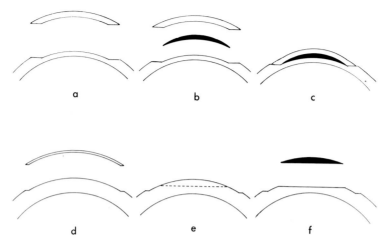

Fig. 6-3. Keratophakia for the correction of hyperopia and aphakia. **a,** Resection of a corneal tissue disc, about one-half of the corneal thickness. **b,** A corneal tissue lens is placed in the interface. **c,** Reconstruction. Notice the sliding of the coaptation edge. **d,** Obtaining a corneal tissue lens with the microkeratome. Superficial resection of the anterior layers of the cornea (epithelium and Bowman). **e,** Flat section with the microkeratome. **f,** The corneal tissue lens thus obtained.

This corneal tissue lens, a living lens, is placed in the center of the operated cornea, the interface of which has been exposed by means of a microkeratome section. It is then covered by the anteriorly resected corneal layers, which are fixed to the cornea by a continuous Perlon suture.

Keratomileusis is an operation by subtraction of tissue, while keratophakia is performed by tissue addition.[8] For this reason keratomileusis is an autoplastic operation; keratophakia is a homoplastic one.

The techniques of these interventions have been described elsewhere.[3, 9] I shall refer only to the results obtained after more than 15 years of animal research and 4½ years of clinical work.

Indications
Keratomileusis

The general indication for keratomileusis is aniseikonia with or without strabismus, and intolerance to contact lenses. Myopia correction is up to 10 diopters vertex power, and hyperopia correction is up to 6 diopters vertex power.

The specific indications for keratomileusis are the following:

1. Anisometropia by nonprogressive myopia
2. Myopic anisometropia with strabismus in children
3. Anisometropia, postkeratoplasty
4. Hyperopic anisometropia (up to 6 diopters)
5. Horror fusionis with diplopia, after squint surgery, by extraocular aniseikonia

The astigmatic correction, with toric base, is indicated when the astigmatic degree is of some significance in relation to the spheric ametropia.

Contraindications. Contraindications to keratomileusis are:

1. Anterior segment and corneal surgery
2. Ametropia by keratoconus—even incipient—and keratectasia
3. Thinner cornea
4. Flat cornea in myopia correction; steep cornea in hyperopic correction
5. Leukomatous cornea in pupillary area
6. Cornea of irregular thickness

Table 6-1. Keratomileusis—operative accidents and postoperative complications in the first 100 cases after observation of 3 years minimum

Complications	Number of cases
Operative accidents	
Irregular resection	1
Thin resection	3
Deep resection	6
Irregular thickness	3
Postoperative complications	
Infection	1
Tissue lens displacement	3
Tissue lens loss	1
Vascularization	0
Central opacities	1
Peripheral opacities	15
Foreign bodies in the interface	25
Ectasia (correction loss)	12
Filamentary keratitis	2

Table 6-2. Keratomileusis—operative accidents and postoperative complications in the following 200 cases after observation of 1 year minimum

Complications	Number of cases	Percent
Operating accidents		
Irregular resection	3	1.5
Thin resection	2	1
Deep resection	9	4.5
Small resection	2	1
Irregular thickness disc	3	1.5
Decentered resection	4	2
Two freezings of the tissue	3	1.5
Three freezings of the tissue	2	1
Lenticle perforation	2	1
Postoperative complications		
Infection	0	0
Vascularization	0	0
Central opacities	2	1
Peripheral opacities	4	2
Foreign bodies in the interface	5	2.5
Tissue lens opacification	1	0.5
Ectasia (correction loss)	24	12
Epithelial grow at the interface	1	0.5
Pterygium	1	0.5
Filamentary keratitis	1	0.5

Keratophakia

The general indication for keratophakia is aniseikonia with great anisometropia, in cases of poor tolerance to contact lenses. Hyperopia correction is over 6 diopters vertex power. Myopia correction is over 10 diopters vertex power. The upper limit has not been determined.

Specific indications are:

1. Anisometropia with amblyopia, with or without excentric fixation and strabismus
2. Monocular aphakia
3. Monocular aphakia, posttraumatic cataract in children
4. Aniseikonia

The astigmatic correction, when necessary, may take place in the inclusion tissue lens or in the corneal tissue disc with the keratomileusis technique.

Contraindications. Contraindications to keratophakia are:

1. Anterior segment and corneal surgery
2. Leukomatous corneas in the central area
3. Very thin corneas
4. Corneas with irregular thickness

Complications
Keratomileusis

Complications of keratomileusis are listed in Tables 6-1 and 6-2. The former makes reference to the first 100 cases after an observation period between 3 and 4½ years; the second table refers to the following 200 cases after a minimal observation period of 1 year.

Operative complications. In the case of an irregular resection (Fig. 6-4), the corneal disc is replaced and the operation is postponed. Some months later the procedure may be performed again.

The conditions for an irregular section are:

1. Intraocular low pressure
2. Intraocular pressure variations during keratectomy
3. Absence of uniformity during the microkeratome's translation motion
4. Withdrawal of the microkeratome be-

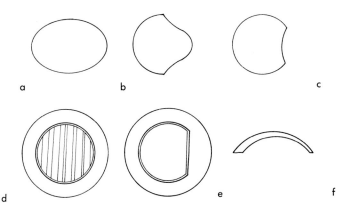

Fig. 6-4. Irregular resection. **a,** Oval; **b,** piriform; **c,** kidney-shaped; **d,** fluted bed; **e,** section in the final third; **f,** irregular thickness.

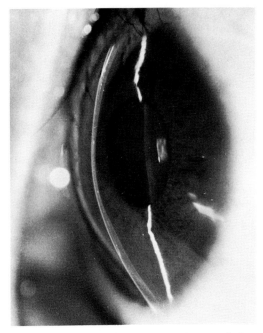

Fig. 6-5. Ectasia of the posterior layers of the cornea, following a too deep resection in myopia correction.

fore completing the section of the disc while the motor is still running

Thin resection is caused by a low intraocular pressure. The available tissue thickness may not be sufficient to obtain the necessary correction. Very anterior sections heal with opacity.

Deep resection is caused by an excess of pressure in the globe at the moment of the keratectomy. Deep resections heal without opacity but allow ectasia of the posterior layers of the cornea (Fig. 6-5).

The cause of irregular thickness in the resection (Fig. 6-4) is an uneven speed in the motion of the microkeratome. This determines postoperative astigmatisms.

A small resection is either caused by taking the dimension of the applanation over a wet cornea or by a defective adaptation of the applanation lens over the ring surface.

Decentered resection is due to a defective placement of the pneumatic fixation ring. If the ring cannot be centered adequately with the cornea, the conjunctiva must be recessed near the limbus on the opposite side of the ring displacement, in order to allow a correct placement of the ring. A small decentration of less than 1 mm. does not seem to have consequences optically. Multiple freezings of the corneal tissue have not proved to have any side effect on the final result.

Perforation of the lenticle may result from a faulty regulation of the lathe. In our experience it happened in two instances in which the tissue was preserved by desiccation instead of glycerine solution and dimethyl sulfoxide. These 2 cases coincide with

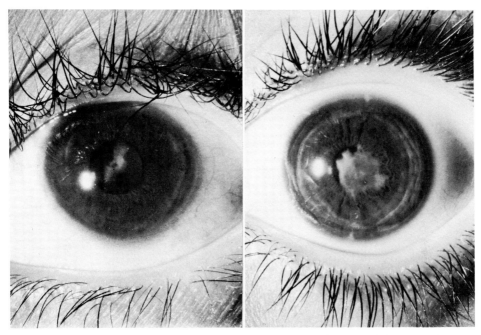

Fig. 6-6. Two cases of superficial central scar, following perforation of the corneal tissue lens at the time of carving.

those in which there were central opacities (Fig. 6-6). They will need a lamellar refractive keratoplasty.

Postoperative complications. In the case in which infection occurred the corneal tissue lens and the fixation contact lens were removed; treatment was with antibiotics. Healing occurred with superficial leukoma. Three months later, a lamellar refractive keratoplasty was performed.[9]

Preoperative vision: –16.00 sphere = 0.05
Postoperative vision: – 2.00 sphere = 0.30.

With the use of an edge-to-edge suture and/or the reversed conjunctival flap, there have been no other cases of infection.

Corneal tissue lens displacement was treated with border-to-border suture and there were no further complications. However, the loss of the tissue lens required the immediate application of a homoplastic lens with the same characteristics, and a border-to-border suture.

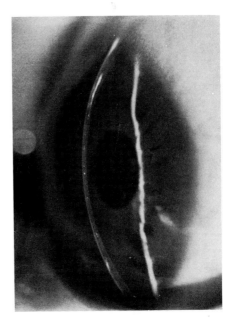

Fig. 6-7. Foreign bodies (dust?) in the interface in myopia correction.

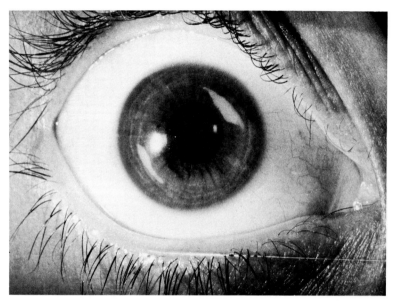

Fig. 6-8. Liquid deposit in the interface.

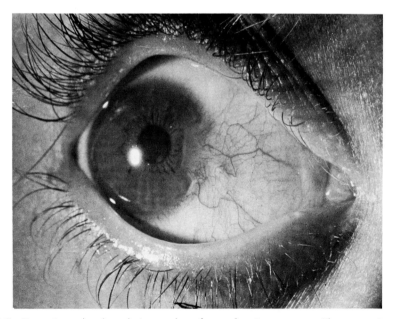

Fig. 6-9. Pterygium developed 6 months after refractive surgery. The pterygium head arrives just at the slightly elevated edge of the corneal tissue lens.

Foreign bodies in the interface have been the most frequent complication in this first series (Fig. 6-7). Twenty-five of the cases required that the interface be washed with a balanced salt solution before the stitches were removed.[10] A high percentage of foreign bodies in the interface are avoided at present by taking maximum care and practicing biomicroscopic control under a slit lamp at the time of surgery.

Peripheral interlamellar opacities outside the area of the pupil, formed by liquid deposits, have been avoided with the use of the reversed conjunctival flap or the use of a pressure bandage placed 2 or 3 days after surgery (Fig. 6-8). The deposits may be evacuated by puncture and expression.

The case of tissue lens opacification was caused by a superficial resection.

Central opacity (Fig. 6-6) followed in both cases a central perforation of the corneal tissue lens at the carving time.

Epithelial growth at the interface was caused by bad coaptation at the border. The tissue lens was withdrawn, the interface carefully cleaned of epithelial remains, and the tissue lens was replaced by a homoplastic one. Border-to-border sutures were inserted and there have been no further complications.

One patient with a small nasal pinguecula developed a nasal pterygium 6 months after surgery (Fig. 6-9), caused by a slight elevation in the border of the corneal tissue lens. This increased the discontinuity of the prelacrimal film in the area between the pinguecula and the border of the lenticle.[11]

Ectasia is the specific complication of the keratomileusis for correction of myopia. In general, it is caused by too high a correction or too deep a resection. The ectasia may begin during the first postoperative weeks, or even 1 or 2 years later. Until the present, only in 1 case has the cornea reached a steeper curvature than before surgery.

Table 6-3. Keratophakia—operative accidents and postoperative complications in the first 50 cases after observation of 3 months minimum

Complications	Number of cases	Percent
Operative accidents		
Irregular resection	1	2
Small resection	1	2
Decentered resection	3	6
Anterior chamber perforation	0	0
Postoperative complications		
Infection	0	0
Vascularization	0	0
Opacification (immune reaction)	0	0
Foreign bodies in the interface	4	8
Epithelial remains (dead) in the interface	1	2
Corneal herpes over the disc	1	2
Wound rupture after suture removal	2	4
Ectasia	0	0

Table 6-4. Keratomileusis: results in myopia correction

Record number	Months of control	Preoperative		Postoperative	
		Refraction at 12 mm.	Acuity	Refraction at 12 mm.	Acuity
31.131	54	− 4.50 to 2.00 × 95°	0.33	Neut. to 1.50 × 45°	0.80
22.316	42	−13.50 to 1.00 × 189°	0.45	Neut. to 0.50 × 115°	0.90
13.192	42	−10.25 to 2.25 × 189°	0.10	−2.00	0.67
18.214	33	−10.00 to 2.50 × 95°	0.67	+0.50 to 1.75 × 90°	0.80
52.696	32	−11.50 to 2.00 × 5°	0.45	+0.50 to 3.50 × 7°	0.90
52.421	31	− 4.00 to 2.75 × 135°	0.40	+0.75 to 1.00 × 155°	0.67
52.778	31	− 8.00 to 3.00 × 180°	0.10	+2.00 to 1.00 × 0°	0.30
61.082	24	− 7.00 to 1.50 × 180°	0.29	Neut. to 1.25 × 90°	0.90
54.090	23	− 6.25 to 2.00 × 160°	0.80	+1.00 to 2.00 × 150°	0.80
21.783	18	− 4.75 to 2.75 × 40°	1.00	+1.75 to 2.50 × 15°	1.00

Table 6-5. Keratomileusis: results in hyperopia correction

Record number	Months of control	Preoperative		Postoperative	
		Refraction at 12 mm.	Acuity	Refraction at 12 mm.	Acuity
60.952	28	+5.00 to 1.75 × 180°	0.45	+2.00 to 0.75 × 165°	0.70
61.684	22	+6.50 to 1.00 × 180°	0.10	+1.75 to 0.50 × 15°	0.80
61.923	21	+4.25 to 3.00 × 20°	0.25	+1.50 to 2.50 × 30°	0.30
20.459	17	+8.00 to 2.25	Fingers	+2.00 to 3.00 × 55°	0.10
62.510	16	+5.25 to 4.50 × 15°	0.40	+1.00 to 4.00 × 15°	0.80
34.342*	13	+5.00 to 0.50 × 5°	0.10	−0.50 to 2.00 × 135°*	0.10
34.605	12	+8.50 to 1.00 × 90°	0.10	+2.50 to 1.25 × 105°	0.67
34.673†	5	+8.00	Fingers	+4.50 to 2.00 × 110°†	0.10

*Other eye myopic −0.75.
†Patient is 48 years old, other eye hyperopic +3.50 to 0.50 × 180 degrees. Exotropia healing.

Table 6-6. Keratophakia: results in aphakia correction*

Record number	Months of control	Preoperative		Postoperative	
		Refraction at 12 mm.	Acuity	Refraction at 12 mm.	Acuity
60.999	29	+18.00	P.L.	+6.00	P.L.
12.590	26	+11.75 to 2.00 × 150°	0.30	+6.00 to 1.00 × 135°	0.30
20.240	23	+15.00	P.L.	+2.00	P.L.
56.561	11	A.L. = 23.00 mm.	P.L.	+2.00	0.80
100.215	11	12.75 to 1.50 × 180°	0.80	+2.00 to 1.50 × 135°	0.80
54.286	9	A.L. = 20.00 mm.	P.L.	+4.00 to 1.00 × 180°	0.90
57.154	9	+ 9.75 to 2.00 × 60°	0.06	+1.00 to 1.50 × 180°	0.33
63.540	8	+15.00 (estimated)	P.L.	+9.00 to 6.00 × 90°	0.80
63.804	6	+12.75 to 1.50 × 175°	0.80	Neut. to 2.00 × 15°	0.80
61.020	6	+ 7.50 to 2.50 × 20°	0.70	Neut. to 1.58 × 85°	0.90

*A.L. = Axial length in millimeters in cases of complete cataract

Table 6-7. Keratophakia: results in aphakia correction*

Record number	Preoperative		Postoperative	
	Refraction at 12 mm.	Ri	Refraction at 12 mm.	Rf
60.999	+18.00	8.0	+6.00	6.6
56.626	+ 7.25	7.9	−0.75	6.2
20.240	+15.00	8.2	+2.00	6.2
100.260	A.L. = 24.50	7.5	−3.25	5.6
22.691	+ 9.00	8.3	−1.00	6.3
62.845	+10.25	7.8	+2.25	6.3
62.885	+10.25	7.2	−2.00	5.5
34.600	+ 9.50	7.6	+0.50	5.8
56.561	A.L. = 23.00	8.0	+2.00	6.1
54.286 R.	A.L. = 20.00	7.9	+6.00	6.5
54.286 L.	A.L. = 20.00	7.8	+4.50	6.3
57.336 R.	A.L. = 21.30	8.0	+3.00	6.4
57.336 L.	A.L. = 21.30	8.0	+2.50	6.3

*Key to table:
   A.L. = Axial length in millimeters in cases of complete cataract
   Ri = Initial corneal radius
   Rf = Final corneal radius (postoperative)
   Refraction at 12 mm. of the corneal vertex, expressed in spherical equivalent

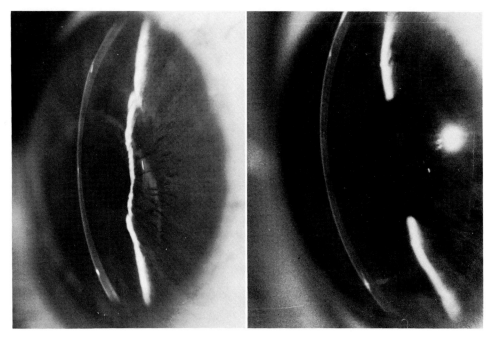

Fig. 6-10. Keratomileusis for myopia correction. Result 1 year after surgery. Left: strong correction. Right: small correction.

Keratophakia

The complications of the first 50 cases of keratophakia, employing the actual technique, are listed in Table 6-3.

Operative complications. In case of irregular or small resection, the disc must be placed in its bed and sutured and the operation postponed.

When the resection is decentered, the same procedures described for keratomileusis must be done. Since we employ resections of 8.25 mm., the decentration is never too large.

Postoperative complications. Case No. 100.215 developed a corneal herpes 50 days after the operation, which was healed with idoxuridine treatment.

We consider that the wound rupture after removing the stitches was caused by excessive use of corticosteroids during the postoperative period. A new lenticle was applied and the tissue disc was sutured once again to the wound. There were no further complications.

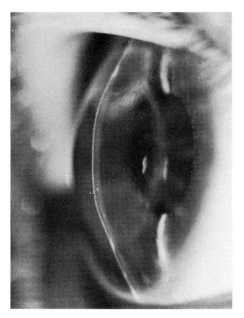

Fig. 6-11. Keratophakia for myopia correction. Result 6 months after surgery.

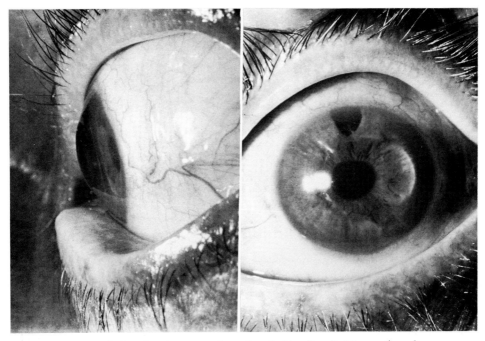

Fig. 6-12. Keratophakia for the correction of aphakia. Result 15 months after surgery. Right: Notice the diffraction of the light, as with a keratoconus.

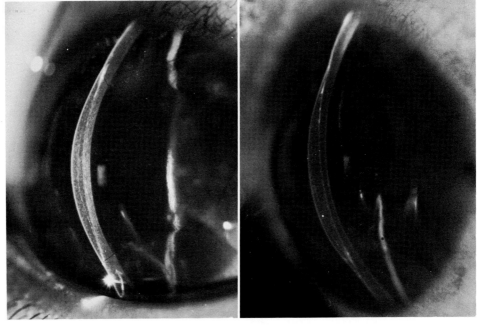

Fig. 6-13. Keratophakia for the correction of aphakia. Left: 15 days after surgery. Right: 1 year after surgery.

Results

Examples of the results obtained with the keratomileusis technique in the correction of myopic and hyperopic ametropias are shown in Tables 6-4, 6-5, and Fig. 6-10. The results of keratophakia for myopia are shown in Fig. 6-11 and results that may be obtained with keratophakia for aphakia correction are shown in Tables 6-6 and 6-7, and Figs. 6-12 and 6-13. The postoperative astigmatisms are similar to those after cataract intervention. In cases in which the lenticle was carved on the lathe, the astigmatism was less severe than when it was obtained by microkeratome. The operated patient is able to walk around easily without glasses, and in some cases the vision reaches 20/40 or better without correction.

In cases of monocular aphakia, the binocular vision is restored. If the aphakia is associated with exotropia, the orthotropia is obtained after refractive surgery only, or after some muscle procedure.

The recovery of vision is more rapid when a fresh donor cornea is used, than if a precarved lenticle that has been preserved by Payrau's or Urretz Zavalía's method is used. Fig. 6-13 shows the change of thickness and curve of the operated cornea induced by the surgery.

Summary

Refractive keratoplasty is a difficult and highly specialized technique, nevertheless not 1 eye has been lost. The complications have been less severe and less frequent than in other routine surgery. This surgery allows the correction of some problems that up to now have had no satisfactory solution by other methods.

REFERENCES

1. Barraquer, J. I.: Refractive keratoplasty. Estudios e informaciones, Oftalmológicas 2:8, 1949.
2. Barraquer, J. I.: Method for cutting lamellar grafts in frozen cornea. New orientation for refractive surgery (Previous note), Arch. Soc. Amer. Oftal. Optom. 1:271, 1958.
3. Barraquer, J. I.: Queratomileusis para la Corrección de la Miopía, Ann. Inst. Barr. 5: 206.
4. Barraquer, J. I.: Basis of refractive keratoplasty, Arch. Soc. Amer. Oftal. Optom. 6:21, 1967.
5. Barraquer, J. I.: El microqueratomo en cirugía corneal, Arch. Soc. Amer. Oftal. Optom. 6:69, 1966.
6. Barraquer, J. I.: Keratomileusis and keratophakia. II. Corneoplastic Conference, London, 1967 (In press).
7. Barraquer, J. I.: Modification of refraction by means of intracorneal inclusions, Int. Ophthal. Clin. 6:58, 1966.
8. Barraquer, J. I.: Conducta de la cornea frente a los cambios de espesor (contribución a la cirugía refractiva), Arch. Soc. Amer. Oftal. Optom. 5:81, 1964.
9. Barraquer, J. I.: Keratoplasty—special methods. In Proceedings of the World Congress on Cornea, Washington, D. C., 1965, Butterworth, Inc.
10. Barraquer, J. I.: Evaluation of balanced salt solution in keratomileusis, Arch. Soc. Amer. Oftal. Optom. 5:219, 1965.
11. Barraquer, J. I.: La discontinuité localisée du film lacrymal précornéen, Ophthalmologica 150:111, 1964.

Chapter 7

Posttraumatic pseudophakia in children

Cornelius D. Binkhorst, Marc H. Gobin, and Paul A. M. Leonard

Unilateral eye injuries in children are not uncommon. Stintzy, in a review of 450 cases, reported the development of cataract in 26%.[1] Traumatic cataract, if not complicated by severe damage to other structures of the eye, and if successfully treated by surgery, presents the surgeon and the child with the problems of unilateral aphakia. The optical correction of the latter is the crux of successful functional recovery.

In the adult aphakic patient visual acuity can be, and usually is, preserved for long periods, even without optical correction. Binocularity has also been demonstrated in adults who were fitted with a contact lens or a lens implant several decades after lens injury. This, however, does not hold true in case of lens injury in infancy and childhood. The younger the child and the longer the interval between injury and clearing of the pupil, the more the chance of irreparable loss of visual acuity and binocularity. Loss of visual acuity and binocularity is the rule when no correction at all is prescribed or when the eye is equipped only with a spectacle glass.[2, 3]

The development of contact lenses seemed to offer more hope to the unilateral aphakic child. Experiences have been reported by a number of authors.[4-12] The type of contact lens generally used for this purpose today is the corneal lens. However, it is recognized that high plus corneal lenses tend to become displaced downward, thus causing vertical diplopia.[13] Several authors, therefore, prefer the corneoscleral lens.[4-6, 11, 14, 15] Because of their increased weight, however, the latter

also can give rise to vertical phoria and diplopia.

Although we fitted young children and even infants with contact lenses, as did others,[6, 8, 14-17] it is generally agreed that fitting children under a certain age has little practical value (F. Ridley, under 10 years; Spaeth and O'Neill, under 10 years; Magnard and colleagues, under 7 years; Saraux, under 6 years; Bonnet and colleagues, under 7 years; Bronner, under 8 years; Offret and colleagues, under 5 years).* Several authors also mention major difficulties in children above these age limits. Wearing possibilities remain largely dependent on the cooperation not only of the child but also of the parents. Many unilateral aphakic patients give up wearing their contact lens sooner or later. Bonnet and colleagues found that out of 308 adult unilateral aphakics, nearly 80% had given up wearing the contact lens after 10 years.[11] It is difficult to understand why the results in children should be better than in adults, and in a child, even temporary discontinuation of the contact lens can be disastrous.[19]

There are good reasons for future functional failure even in the child who has been successfully fitted and who has good visual acuity and parallel eyes. The main reason for failure is the strong tendency in children toward suppression. This tendency results from the generally underdeveloped binocular capacity in infancy and childhood. Any time the child finds it difficult to fuse the images

---

*See references 4, 5, 7, 10-12, 18.

of both eyes, he escapes from the problem by way of suppression. This may already be the case at relatively low levels of aniseikonia, which is more likely to occur in contact lens correction than in pseudophakia. In a comparative study of Girard and colleagues and ourselves an average of 1.9% image size difference was found in pseudophakia, and an average of 6.9% image size difference in contact lens correction. Suppression may also occur in case of contact lens–induced image disparity, especially in vertical direction. Thus the child will stay monocular and become amblyopic in the long run, and squint may result. It is recognized by experienced authors that orthoptic training in these cases is seldom successful.[5, 20]

If contact lens wearing in many children cannot prevent suppression and squint, it is readily understood that the curative effect of the contact lens in these cases is negligible. Traumatic cataract in children very frequently gives rise to suppression and development of squint at an early stage.[21] There are a few isolated reports of a straightening effect of contact lenses,[22] but generally contact lens treatment was unsuccessful even when accompanied by the prescription of prisms, by muscle surgery, or by orthoptic training. On the contrary, a contact lens has been reported as the origin of squint or as the cause of an unfavorable change in preexisting squint in quite a few instances.* Our own experiences with ten children are most significant. In every case either suppression or persistent diplopia occurred. Deviation of the eyeball was never cured, either spontaneously or after muscle surgery. In a 10-year-old child esotropia was initiated by the contact lens. In a 3-year-old child esotropia was present as long as the contact lens was worn, and disappeared after its removal. In another 10-year-old child esotropia was aggravated significantly on the application of the contact lens, and in two 3-year-old children initial exotropia turned into esotropia

*See references 5-7, 9, 11, 14, 20, 21, 23.

with the contact lens. In the beginning it was thought that in every case of unilateral aphakia the patient should be given a chance with a contact lens; however, today it is felt that in children such a trial should be abandoned, since it reduces the chance of binocular reeducation.[21, 23]

Pseudophakoi

In the last 20 years intraocular lenses (pseudophakoi) have been used for the correction of aphakia. Pseudophakoi, of course, have many practical advantages over contact lenses, and there is no doubt that the optics of pseudophakoi are superior to the optics of contact lenses. A well-fixated and well-centered pseudophakos produces a stable retinal image with stable space localization. Pseudophakoi can be made to give the unilateral pseudophakic patient a fair chance for iseikonia or at least for a minimal and tolerable aniseikonia.[23, 24] Pseudophakoi offer maximal chances for reestablishment of binocularity in case of loss of a crystalline lens. In children in which binocularity is readily lost and difficult to restore, there is even a strong indication for the use of pseudophakoi. The younger the child, the stronger the indication.

Many techniques of pseudophakos implantation failed to give reliable long-term results, which was, of course, responsible for a generally negative attitude toward this kind of therapy. Reports about unilateral pseudo-

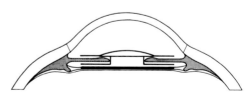

Fig. 7-1. Iris clip lens in pseudophakia after extracapsular cataract operation. The optical part is in the anterior chamber. The haptic part consists of two pairs of wire loops with the iris between them. The posterior wire loops are located in the iridocapsular cleft. The posterior capsule is intact.

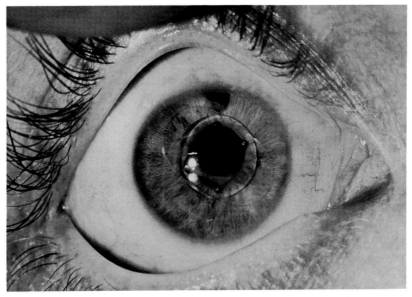

Fig. 7-2. Patient H. N. was injured at the age of 11 years. Implantation of iris clip lens 3 years later. Clear posterior capsule. No posterior synechiae were formed. Miotics are being used for extra stability.

phakia in children, moreover, are particularly scarce.[19, 21, 23] In the 14 earliest cases of the series presented here, the anterior chamber lens with angle fixation according to Dannheim was used. In the other cases anterior chamber lenses with diaphragm fixation were used. We feel that diaphragm fixation of pseudophakoi is a safe procedure and gives good stability and centering.[25-27]

The iris clip lens has proved its value in over 200 implantations in adult patients.[28] Although the iris clip lens is mainly used after intracapsular cataract extraction, it can be used after extracapsular cataract extraction as well. After intracapsular cataract extraction it is nearly completely held in place by the iris diaphragm; after extracapsular cataract extraction it is supported by the iris diaphragm and as well by the secondary membrane diaphragm (Fig. 7-1). In children this type of pseudophakos is indicated when posterior synechiae fail to form after extracapsular cataract extraction. The anterior chamber should be deep enough to prevent

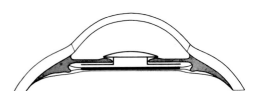

Fig. 7-3. Iridocapsular lens in pseudophakia after extracapsular cataract operation. The optical part is in the anterior chamber. The haptic part is a pair of wire loops located in the iridocapsular cleft and embedded by posterior iris synechiae. The posterior capsule is intact.

endothelial touch by the anterior wire loops, since the secondary membrane may be responsible for a slightly more forward position than after intracapsular cataract extraction. The iris clip lens has been used in only one child of the series presented here (Fig. 7-2).

During the past 3 years the iridocapsular lens has been used satisfactorily in nearly 50 implantations at all ages and in all types of cataract. It is exclusively used for combined iris diaphragm and secondary membrane

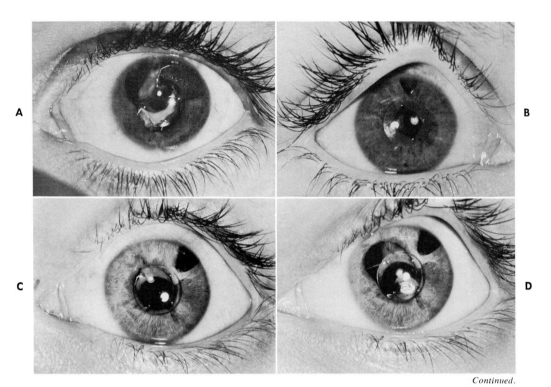

Continued.

Fig. 7-4. A, Case 3 (J. D.). Severe injury at the age of 3 years. Sector coloboma after excision of iris prolapse. Implantation of iridocapsular lens 1½ years later. Secondary membrane with clear center. Posterior synechiae keep the pseudophakos in place. **B,** Case 9 (N. P.). Injury at the age of 5 years. Implantation of iridocapsular lens 3 years later. Clear posterior capsule. The pseudophakos has to be kept in place with miotics, as no posterior synechiae developed. **C** and **D,** Case 11 (J. J.). Injury at the age of 6 years. Implantation of iridocapsular lens 1 year later. Secondary membrane with clear center. The pseudophakos is kept in place by posterior synechiae. **C,** Without mydriatic. **D,** With mydriatic to show the extent of posterior synechiae. **E** and **F,** Case 12 (M. G.). Injury at the age of 7 years. Implantation of iridocapsular lens 1½ years later. Clear posterior capsule. The pseudophakos is held in place by posterior synechiae. **E,** Without mydriatic. **F,** With mydriatic to show the extent of posterior synechiae. **G,** Case 15 (J. E.). Injury at the age of 8 years. Implantation of iridocapsular lens 12 years later. Secondary membrane with clear center. The pseudophakos is held in place by posterior synechiae. **H** and **I,** Case 16 (W. R.). Injury at the age of 10 years. Implantation of iridocapsular pseudophakos 9 years later. The pseudophakos is held in place by posterior synechiae. The thick secondary membrane has partly been excised after implantation. **H,** Without mydriatic. **I,** With mydriatic to show more of the secondary membrane and the presence of posterior synechiae. **J,** Case 22 (S. H.). Injury at the age of 12 years. Implantation of iridocapsular lens 2 months later. Clear posterior capsule. The pseudophakos is held in place by posterior synechiae. **K,** Case 25 (L. K.). Injury at the age of 14 years. Implantation of iridocapsular lens 3 years later. Secondary membrane with clear center. The pseudophakos is held in place by posterior synechiae. **L** and **M,** Case 26 (P. G.). Injury at the age of 14 years. Implantation of iridocapsular lens 6 months later. Secondary membrane with clear center. The pseudophakos is held in place by posterior synechiae. **L,** Without mydriatic. **M,** With mydriatic to show the extent of posterior synechiae.

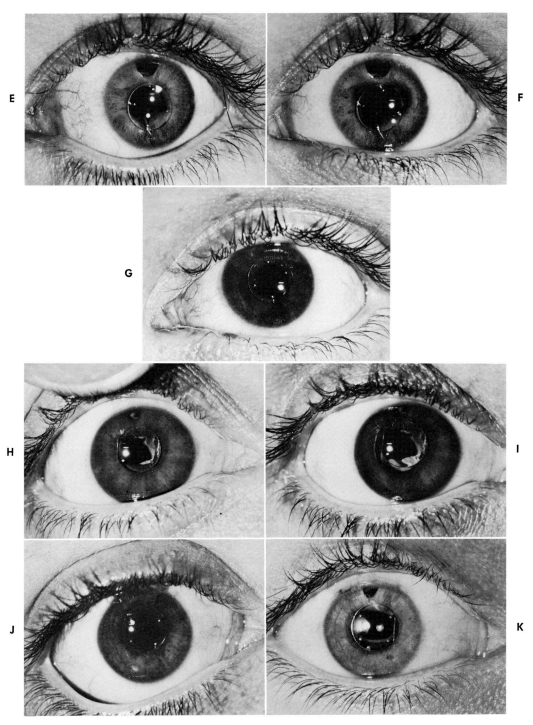

Fig. 7-4, cont'd. For legend see p. 75.

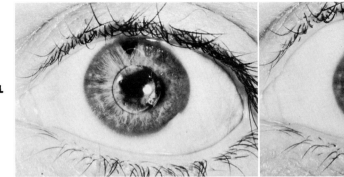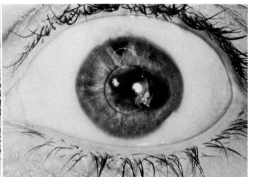

L   M

Fig. 7-4, cont'd. For legend see p. 75.

fixation. It is supported by one pair of wire loops, buried in the partially obliterated iridocapsular cleft (Fig. 7-3). The iridocapsular lens was used in eleven children of the series presented here (Fig. 7-4). We feel that this type of pseudophakos is most satisfactory for the vast majority of children with traumatic cataract.

Surgical techniques in children

Iris clip lens. Although the iris clip lens can be manufactured to individual specifications, we have generally used a standard type. Its optical part is designed as a simple plano-convex acrylic lens with a diameter of 4 to 5 mm., a center thickness of 0.5 mm., and a radius of curvature of the anterior surface of 7.6 mm. Its equivalent power in aqueous is 20.26 diopters. It is entirely located in the anterior chamber, immediately in front of the pupil, and does not touch the iris. It carries one pair of 0.1 mm. Supramid wire loops level with the lens that lie in front of the iris diaphragm, and one pair of 0.2 mm. loops at a slightly posterior level lying behind the iris diaphragm. The clearance between the loops on each side is from 0.5 to 0.75 mm., allowing just enough room for the iris to lie between them (Fig. 7-1). The distance between the tips of the loops is 9 mm. The wire loops act as safeguards against forward or backward displacement, but the actual fixation and cen-

tering are performed by the iris sphincter muscle at the four posterior loop attachments. For this purpose 2% pilocarpine eye drops are prescribed continuously twice daily. Only in rare cases, in which adhesions develop between the iris and the posterior loop attachments, is this not necessary.

The operation is performed under general anesthesia. The iris clip lens in children is used in two-stage surgery and only in the special case in which extracapsular cataract extraction has failed to form adhesions between iris and secondary membrane. The usual measures for intraocular surgery are taken. The only special precautions in implantation surgery are the preoperative administration of a broad-spectrum antibiotic and instillation every 3 hours of a 0.1% solution of dexamethasone 21-phosphate (Decadron). Preoperative mydriasis is produced by instillation of homatropine. An ab externo incision, made with a knife and scissors, must be wide enough to make the insertion maneuver comfortable. If not already present, a peripheral iris coloboma is cut. As a rule the pseudophakos is held with the loops in a horizontal direction and maneuvered into position by zig-zag movements; the forceps is then removed and the anterior chamber is irrigated with a 1:100 acetylcholine solution or with 1% pilocarpine. The anterior chamber is irrigated with acetylcholine before removing the forceps only in the case of a very wide pupil. If the pupil is small the pseudophakos is held with the loops vertically and the upper iris sector is carefully placed between the two pairs of loops with a blunt iris hook, while the corneal flap is lifted. Fedorov proposed a modification of the iris clip lens having the anterior and posterior loops placed crossed. This design may be slightly easier to insert in case of absolute absence of the anterior chamber.[29] Before the wound is closed, the anterior chamber is completely filled with air to prevent the implant from rubbing the corneal endothelium during suturing. There is no risk of migration of air behind the iris. The wound is closed with at least 5 virgin silk end-to-end sutures and is covered by the limbal-based conjunctival flap. The eye is not padded, but is protected by an eye-shield, and if lid closure is insufficient, the cornea is protected by pilocarpine 2% ointment. The eye can be observed and treated through the 1.5 to 2 cm. central hole in the shield. Postoperative treatment consists of instillation of a 0.1% solution of dexamethasone 21-phosphate (Decadron) every 3 hours for the first week, gradually diminishing to 4 times daily for 6 to 8 weeks, and the continuous use of 2% pilocarpine eyedrops twice daily.

Iridocapsular lens. A standard implant is usually used in this procedure also. The optical part is the same as in the iris clip lens, and it is also located entirely in the anterior chamber immediately in front of pupil without touching the iris. The fixation mechanism requires a strong secondary membrane and adhesions between this membrane and the iris. The iridocapsular lens has only one pair of wire loops, which lie posterior to the lens and are buried in the iridocapsular cleft (Fig. 7-3). Iridocapsular adhesions embedding the loops guarantee excellent stability and even prevent inadequate mydriasis. The usual distance between the tips of the loops is 9 mm., but this can be slightly modified by the surgeon if necessary. Again, contact between the implant and the eye is minimal.

In cases of soft cataract, one-stage surgery is time-saving and hence sometimes advisable. Preparatory needling is recommended a few days to a week before the removal of the cataract. Immediately after insertion, the pupil should be made to fit firmly around the four loop attachments, producing ideal centering and giving extra support to the pseudophakos. This pupillary action should be maintained until iridocapsular adhesions have formed. Careful administration of mydriatics is then started to give the aqueous as much access to the lens remnants as possible in order to clear the pupil without affecting the stability of the lens. The effectiveness of the iridocapsular adhesions can be tested under maximal mydriasis.

In two-stage surgery, to ensure that efficient iridocapsular adhesions embed the wire loops, the latter should be placed exactly where adhesions had to be cut. If no adhesions are present, one may decide to use the iris clip lens instead.

The iridocapsular lens has the advantage of reducing the risk of touching the cornea if the secondary membrane tends to push the lens a little more forward. This is important in eyes of young children or infants as well as in eyes with a shallow anterior chamber or with eccentric pupil. Because of the firm fixation in the iridocapsular cleft, it can even be used in case of colobomatous iris.

An inert metal wire (platina-iridium) has been chosen for the loops. As compared with Supramid, it slightly increases the total weight of the pseudophakos, but this is easily tolerated if the pseudophakos is fixated to a rigid secondary membrane.

Summary. The insertion of an iris clip lens or an iridocapsular lens into the aphakic eye is to be considered as an easy and a safe procedure as long as the posterior capsule of the crystalline lens is intact, and there is no possibility for the vitreous to enter the anterior chamber. Though not impossible,

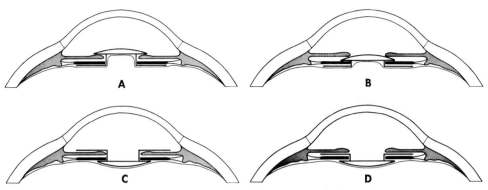

Fig. 7-5. A, Iridocapsular lens in pseudophakia after extracapsular cataract operation. The optical part is in the anterior chamber. The wire loops are inserted through a hole in the posterior capsule. **B,** Iridocapsular lens in pseudophakia after extracapsular cataract operation. The optical part is in the iridocapsular cleft. The wire loops are inserted through a hole in the posterior capsule. **C,** Iridocapsular lens in pseudophakia after extracapsular cataract operation. The optical part is inserted through a hole in the posterior capsule. The wire loops are situated in front of the iris. **D,** Iridocapsular lens in pseudophakia after extracapsular cataract operation. The optical part is inserted through a hole in the posterior capsule. The wire loops are situated in the iridocapsular cleft.

insertion becomes at least hazardous if the posterior capsule has been perforated either at the time of the injury, during cataract extraction, or as a result of needling the secondary membrane. In this case severe complications, such as corneal dystrophy, uveitis, and secondary glaucoma, may be caused by the presence of vitreous in the anterior chamber. The vitreous may also interfere with the position of the pseudophakos.

If needling or excision of the secondary membrane is necessary, therefore, it should always be done at a later stage, after the insertion of the pseudophakos. With this pseudophakos in place it is a simple and a safe procedure, since the vitreous is kept out of the anterior chamber by the pseudophakos.

For the same reason the use of techniques of iridocapsular and capsular fixation other than those described here should be considered with hesitation. It is possible to insert the posterior wire loops or the lens body through a central hole in the secondary membrane. In the first case the lens body and in the second case the wire loops come to lie on the anterior surface of the iris or on the anterior surface of the secondary membrane (Fig. 7-5). The pigment epithelium layer of the iris is therefore protected against pseudophakos touch by the secondary membrane, but the insertion of the pseudophakos is more difficult and more liable to give rise to early or late complications caused by a free access of vitreous into the anterior chamber. Yet in case of vast destruction of the iris diaphragm (coloboma, irreparable anterior synechia) and in presence of a solid secondary membrane, mere capsular fixation of the pseudophakos, as advised by Fedorov, can work out well.

Results and comment

From July 1959 to May 1967 a total of twenty-six children were treated with a lens implant because of unilateral traumatic cataract. The results of all cases are given; no preselection was made. Age at the time of injury varied from 2 years to 14 years. The follow-up period ranges from almost 9 years to at least 1 year (Table 7-1).

Only one child with severe perforating in-

Table 7-1. Results in twenty-six children with unilateral posttraumatic pseudophakia

Case and age at injury	Time interval between injury and implantation	Corrected visual acuity fixation	Residual deviation (degrees)	First degree fusion	Second degree fusion (degrees)	Binocular performances Third degree fusion		
						Synoptophore	Fly test	Wirt test (dec. score)
1. E. K. 2 yrs.	3 yrs.	0.01 excentric fixation	+5	−	—	−	−	—
2. C. R. 2 yrs.	4 mos.	0.8	+13	−	—	−	−	—
3. J. D. 3 yrs.	1½ yrs.	0.1 perifoveal fixation	+2 L/R 3	−	—	−	−	—
4. W. H. 3 yrs.	1 yr.	1.0	0	+	−6 to +6	+	+	0.1
5. R. S. 3 yrs.	4 mos.	1.0	0	+	−3 to +2	+	+	0.6
6. C. W. 3 yrs.	5 mos.	1.25	0	+	0 to −2	−	−	—
7. L. E. 3 yrs.	4 mos.	0.6	0	+	—	−	−	—
8. J. V. 4 yrs.	3 mos.	0.6	0	+	−6 to +3	+	+	0.5
9. N. P. 5 yrs.	3 yrs.	0.3	−5	+	—	−	−	—
10. W. H. 6 yrs.	3 mos.	0.8	0	+	−4 to +6	+	+	0.8
11. J. J. 6 yrs.	1 yr.	0.5	0	+	+3 to +17	−	−	—
12. M. G. 7 yrs.	1½ yrs.	1.0	0	+	−7 to 0	−	+	0.7
13. J. S. 8 yrs.	1½ yrs.	0.8	0	+	0 to +30	+	+	0.5
14. J. I. 8 yrs.	5 mos.	1.25	0	+	−2 to +8	+	+	1.4
15. J. E. 8 yrs.	12 yrs.	1.0	0	+	+3 to +7	+	−	—
16. L. F. 9 yrs.	1 yr.	0.3	0	+	−3 to +8	−	−	—
17. A. C. 10 yrs.	2 yrs.	0.6	0	+	−2 to +7	+	+	—
18. T. W. 10 yrs.	1 yr.	0.8	0	+	0 to +15	+	+	0.6
19. W. R. 10 yrs.	9 yrs.	1.0	0	+	−4 to +8	−	+	0.6
20. A. J. 10 yrs.	1 yr.	1.25	0	+	−4 to +9	−	+	0.3
21. H. N. 11 yrs.	3 yrs.	1.6	0	+	−2 to +10	+	+	0.7
22. S. H. 12 yrs.	2 mos.	2.0	0	+	−8 to +15	+	+	0.8
23. V. S. 13 yrs.	6 yrs.	1.6	0	+	−6 to +20	−	+	0.7
24. M. H. 13 yrs.	6 yrs.	0.6	0	+	−3 to +10	+	+	—
25. L. K. 14 yrs.	3 yrs.	1.25	0	+	−4 to +14	−	−	—
26. P. G. 14 yrs.	6 mos.	1.6	0	+	−7 to +16	+	−	0.5

jury was treated by us from the beginning; all other children were referred to us after they had been variously treated elsewhere for shorter or longer periods of time. Some children came with partially resorbed traumatic cataracts; others as aphakics with a dense secondary membrane or with a clear pupil. Sometimes vitreous was present in the anterior chamber as a result of the injury or as a result of surgery (needling or extraction of the secondary membrane). In many children the neglect of any functional training had led to deep amblyopia and squint. In a few instances the child had been equipped with a contact lens without any

orthoptic control. The inevitable result was that in many children the interval between injury and implantation was unnecessarily long, which was more disadvantageous to the younger children. It is beyond doubt that the ultimate results would have been still better if the directions for the treatment of lens injury and traumatic cataract in children outlined in previous publications had been followed.[21, 23]

Implantation took place at the earliest 2 months and at the longest 12 years after the injury.

Visual acuity was measured with Snellen's E-test at 5 meters distance (Fig. 7-6). In two

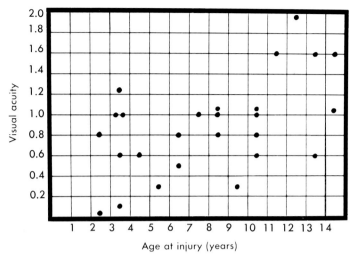

Fig. 7-6. Visual acuity, measured with Snellen's E test, in twenty-six unilateral pseudo-phakic children, injured at ages varying from 2 to 14 years.

children final visual acuity and fixation were bad. The first child came under treatment 3 years after injury, and in both children the occlusion which had been prescribed was neglected. In all other children visual acuity was reasonable to good. There is a slight tendency to better visual acuity in older children. In most cases weak additional spectacle correction is worn and in one case with central scarring of the cornea, visual acuity improved with a plano-contact lens.

Recovery of visual acuity partly depends on factors beyond our control, such as the nature of the injury and the success of surgical intervention. Especially in children, however, it largely depends on quick and efficient functional reeducation. We feel that this is best effected with pseudophakos implantation, which requires minimal cooperation and produces no discomfort. In many young children amblyopia is already very deep after a few weeks. It is evident that suppression starts at the time of injury.[21] Even in seemingly hopeless cases, however, we have witnessed cure of amblyopia after pseudophakos implantation and with prolonged occlusion of the other eye. Six out of eight children under the age of 5 years

regained reasonable to good visual acuity. Reports on unilateral aphakic children equipped with a contact lens mention good visual acuity only in older children. Bonnet and colleagues frankly admit that visual acuity under the age of 7 years usually was bad.[11]

The better visual acuity is, or at least the more it equals that of the other eye, the better the chance is of reestablishment and maintenance of binocular vision. Visual acuity of at least 0.5 is generally estimated as giving a chance of fusion. Visual acuity of at least 0.5 was present in twenty-one out of our twenty-six children. Yet there is good evidence that for third degree fusion a still better visual acuity is necessary. Offret and colleagues found stereopsis only in case of 0.7 to 0.8 visual acuity.[12] Bronner and Gerhard found "useful stereopsis" only in patients with 0.8 to 1.0 visual acuity.[30] These patients were adults and it is likely that in children such high levels of visual acuity are even more stringent than in adults. Visual acuity of at least 1.0 was present in eleven out of our twenty-six children.

We learned that during reeducation it is very important to check visual acuity carefully and at regular intervals for early discovery and treatment in case of lowering due to anatomic (secondary membrane formation) or sensorial factors (suppression).

The position of the eye was tested with Maddox's cross at a distance of 1 meter. In only four of the younger children a residual deviation is reported, in three children convergent squint, and in one child divergent squint. In one child convergent squint was accompanied by vertical deviation. Although the resistant cases evidently have to be reported among the youngest children, it is worth mentioning that five out of eight children under the age of 5 years had no residual deviation.

Squint appeared to be a frequent complication. There were deviation problems in all but five children. Twenty children already had deviation of the eye before cataract surgery. This fact may support our opinion that suppression starts with cataract development and that the injured eye should be occluded.[21] The high incidence and early occurrence of squint in unilateral traumatic cataract is also mentioned by Magnard and colleagues, Rougier, Maurer, and Ruben.[7, 17, 31, 32] Magnard and colleagues mention divergent squint in all but one case, and convergent squint in only one case. We, however, found divergent and convergent squint equally divided among our patients who were significantly younger. In one of our children convergent squint was initiated by contact lens correction of the aphakic eye. We could not confirm the opinion of Keith Lyle, Magnard and colleagues, and Maurer, that vertical squint is common in these patients.[7, 20, 32] It is not at all impossible that the occurrence of vertical deviation must be explained by the very application of contact lenses. Our only patient with a residual vertical deviation had been fitted with a contact lens prior to implantation.

There was a spontaneous cure of squint in nine out of twenty-one squinting children

after pseudophakos implantation without any orthoptic training. We have never seen this with contact lens application, even with intensive orthoptic training. Some authors report the same negative experience,[18, 33] whereas others, in older patients, had positive experience.[4, 7, 20, 34, 35] Eight children had the deviation corrected with muscle surgery, most of them some time after pseudophakos implantation. In one child a recession of the external muscle was performed at the same time as the implantation.

All children were tested for first, second, and third degree fusion.

First degree fusion (simultaneous perception) could be demonstrated at the synoptophore in twenty-three out of the twenty-six children. The three youngest children, all having residual convergent squint, were suppressing.

Second degree fusion was present at the synoptophore in twenty-one out of twenty-six children. The fusional amplitude, as registered at the very first examination and without insisting, varied from 2 to 30 degrees, with an average of 13.5 degrees. Fusion in unilateral pseudophakic patients is stable and vision is comfortable. If unilateral pseudophakics complain about diplopia, it is only for very short periods after the implantation, whereas contact lens patients may suffer from persistent diplopia,[7] from periodic break of fusion,[9] or from "visual discomfort."[36] Fusion in unilateral pseudophakic patients is unconditional, because of the absence of obstacles that are inherent to contact lens correction. It is less affected by such factors as the absence of accommodation or loss of interest, and is not so easily broken by provocative measures as occlusion or weak prisms. This characteristic of pseudophakoi is especially valuable in children in whom fusion capacity is still underdeveloped and suppression tendency is strong.

To what degree the absence of accommodation in one eye unfavorably influences the stability of fusion, is a matter of discussion.

Most authors dealing with unilateral aphakic patients wearing a contact lens think it is an important obstacle in binocular reeducation,[7, 13, 37, 38, 39] whereas others do not.[22, 40] It is evident that suppression is most likely to occur in children in which a static aphakic or pseudophakic eye has to compete with a highly dynamic phakic eye. The absence of accommodation in one eye produces not only retinal images of different acuity, but also of considerable size difference. Both factors are liable to provoke diplopia or suppression. Visual acuity difference can be eliminated with a bifocal spectacle glass, preferably with a large lower segment, or, as we did in a few children, by prescribing one single glass that is slightly overpowered for distance and slightly underpowered for near, thus giving tolerable performance at all distances. The prescription of gradient glasses (Varilux) has been suggested by Apers.[41] The prescription of near addition for both eyes is strongly advised to counteract accommodation–induced aniseikonia.

Third degree fusion (stereopic capacity) was tested at the synoptophore, with the Polaroid fly stereo-test and with the Wirt stereo-test. We found a positive performance at the synoptophore in 13 children, with the Polaroid fly stereo-test in fifteen children, and with the Wirt stereo-test in fourteen children. Decimal scores varied from 0.1 to 1.4. In seventeen children one or more stereo-tests were positive. According to Bronner and Gerhard the tests used, even for adults, are not the easiest to appreciate. We must also keep in mind that stereoscopic capacity is probably only fully developed at the age of 8 years, and that it was completely unknown how the children had performed before the accident.[30] These facts may partly account for negative test results. There were positive tests in the youngest children as well as negative tests in the older children. In quite a few children we observed how initial negative test performances became positive in the course of years without any orthoptic training. The results mentioned should be evaluated against the opinion that contact lens correction in young children definitively fails as to binocular reeducation, even with intensive orthoptic training.[10, 18, 20, 38] Pseudophakic children thus have not only psychologic and social advantages over children with contact lenses, but may also benefit throughout their life as far as profession is concerned. Finally we feel, as do others, that the achievement of binocular vision is the best guarantee against suppression, and therefore against amblyopia and squint.[11]

Conclusions

The general attitude toward unilateral traumatic cataract in children is changing. This condition is no longer considered identical with the practical loss of visual acuity and binocularity. It is recognized, however, that treatment should start as soon as possible, and not only consist of clearing of the pupil in the shortest possible time, but also of giving the most adequate correction and functional guiding to the aphakic eye. The case should not be dismissed unless maximal visual acuity and full binocularity have been regained.

Although contact lens fitting of adult unilateral aphakic patients may give better results, it gives definitely insufficient results in children. Even with maximal cooperation of everyone concerned, contact lenses too often produce invincible obstacles for fusion in children, who, as a result, respond with suppression, amblyopia, and squint. Not one good result has been reported in children under 5 years of age.

The development of safe diaphragm-fixated pseudophakoi offers better chances on complete functional recovery of children with unilateral traumatic cataract. This is due to their optical advantages and to the fact that they do not require a great amount of cooperation.

In twenty-six children with unilateral traumatic cataract, injured at ages varying from

Table 7-2. Amblyopia and deviation prevention and treatment scheme for children with unilateral lens injury

Phase	Preventive and therapeutic measures		
	Correction	*Occlusion*	*Muscle surgery*
Opaque pupil		Injured eye 24 hrs.	
Clear pupil			
Improving vision	Pseudophakos	Other eye 24 hrs.*	
	Spectacle glass	Other eye 24 hrs.*	
	Contact lens	Other eye 24 hrs.*	
Stationary vision			
Subnormal	Pseudophakos	Other eye 3 × 1 hr.	Long-standing deviation: without delay.
	Spectacle glass	Alternative	Recently developed deviation: within
	Contact lens	Alternative	6 weeks
Normal	Pseudophakos	Other eye 1 hr.	Long-standing deviation: without delay.
	Spectacle glass	Alternative	Recently developed deviation: within
	Contact lens	Alternative	6 weeks

*Thorough control of fixation and visual acuity of this eye is necessary and eventually short alternative occlusion of the injured eye is indicated.

2 to 14 years, reasonable to good results were obtained in the vast majority of cases with pseudophakic implantation. This notwithstanding the fact that in most children the onset of treatment was considerably delayed and many children had developed amblyopia and squint that could possibly have been prevented with earlier treatment. In the vast majority of the children we succeeded in restoring and maintaining visual acuity and demonstrating varying degree of binocularity. In several children it took some time before third degree fusion could be demonstrated. In a few, demonstrable stereopic capacity developed only after several years.

It is highly important to compensate for the absence of accommodation with the best means available, as this also helps to stabilize fusion.

The functional reeducation was effected mainly with occlusion and sustained by muscle surgery, but there was no orthoptic training. Table 7-2 gives the measures taken in different phases of functional reeducation.

Although we agree with Ogle and colleagues that favorable test performances do not necessarily mean a complete cure, we feel that binocular vision can reach a higher level more easily in the pseudophakic child than can be done in the unilaterally aphakic child with contact lenses. In order to prove this statement further, we intend to subject all children to finer stereopic tests in the future.

Summary

Unilateral traumatic cataract in children brings its own specific functional problems: amblyopia, monocularity, and deviation. Contact lens fitting fails in too many instances to solve these problems, because of physical, social, educational, and optical reasons. The implantation of an artificial lenticulus (pseudophakos) seems to give better results and safe techniques for producing pseudophakia have been described.

In case of lens injury in children, the following line of treatment is advised:

1. First aid surgery, if necessary
2. Occlusion of the injured eye
3. Immediate reference to a center in which pseudophakic implantation can be performed and orthoptic control is available
4. Clearing of the pupil and implantation of a pseudophakos as soon as possible
5. Occlusion of the fellow eye until visual acuity is maximal
6. Careful binocular reeducation by gradual reduction of occlusion

7. Muscle surgery if deviation is present and not likely to be cured spontaneously
8. Periodic control of visual acuity for early detection of secondary cataract or suppression

REFERENCES

1. Stintzy: Quoted by Bonnet, R., Gerhard, J. P., and Massin, M.: Les verres de contact, Bull. Soc. Ophtal. Franc. Suppl.: 1-265, 1966.
2. Juler, F. A.: Amblyopia from disuse; visual acuity after traumatic cataract in children, Trans. Ophthal. Soc. U. K. **41:**129, 1921.
3. McKinna, A. J.: Results of treatment of traumatic cataract in children, Amer. J. Ophthal. **52:**43, 1961.
4. Ridley, F.: Contact lenses in unilateral aphakia, Trans. Ophthal. Soc. U. K. **73:**373, 1953.
5. Spaeth, P. G., and O'Neill, P.: Functional results with contact lenses in unilateral congenital cataracts, high myopia and traumatic cataracts, Amer. J. Ophthal. **49:**548, 1960.
6. Blaxter, P. L.: The use of contact lenses in infants, Trans. Ophthal. Soc. U. K. **83:**41, 1963.
7. Magnard, P., Hugonnier-Clayette, J. R., Hugonnier, R., Bourelly, M.: Cataracte traumatique et vision binoculaire, Bull. Soc. Ophtal. Franc., pp. 203-208, 1963.
8. Ruben, C. M.: Discussion of Blaxter, Trans. Ophthal. Soc. U. K. **83:**49-50, 1963.
9. Riehm, E., and Thiel, H. J.: Funktionelle Ergebnisse bei einseitig aphaken Kontaktlinsenträgern, Klin. Mbl. Augenhk. **146:**589, 1965.
10. Bronner, A.: Problèmes posés par l'adaptation des lentilles de contact, Bull. Soc. Ophtal. de Franc., pp. 607-632, 1966.
11. Bonnet, R., Gerhard, J. P., and Massin, M.: Les verres de contact, Bull. Soc. Ophtal. Franc. Suppl.:1-265, 1966.
12. Offret, G., Coscas, G., and Huet, M.: Essais de correction optique des enfants aphaques par des verres de contact (31 cas), Bull. Soc. Belge ophtal. **145:**221, 1967.
13. Bronner, A., and Gerhard, J. P.: Verres de contact et lentilles précornéennes, Bull. Soc. Ophtal. Franc. **1:**77, 1958.
14. Lake, L. H., and Manson, N.: The treatment of infantile aphakia with contact lenses, Trans. Ophthal. Soc. U. K. **84:**687, 1964.
15. Girard, L. H.: Quoted by Lake, L. H., and Manson, N.: The treatment of infantile aphakia with contact lenses, Trans. Ophthal. Soc. U. K. **84:**687, 1964.
16. Cassady, J. R.: Quoted by Lake, L. H., and Manson, N.: The treatment of infantile aphakia with contact lenses, Trans. Ophthal. Soc. U. K. **84:**687, 1964.
17. Ruben, C. M.: Quoted by Magnard, P., and others: Cataracte traumatique et vision binoculaire, Bull. Soc. Ophtal. Franc. pp. 203-208, 1963.
18. Saraux, H.: Les verres de contact dans les cataractes unilatérales de l'enfant, Bull. Soc. Ophtal. Franc. **66:**1069, 1966.
19. Choyce, P.: Intraocular lenses and implants, London, 1964, H. K. Lewis and Co., Ltd.
20. Keith Lyle, T.: The importance of orthoptic investigation before contact lens fitting in unilateral aphakia; a preliminary report, Trans. Ophthal. Soc. U. K. **73:**387, 1953.
21. Binkhorst, C. D., and Gobin, M. H.: Pseudophakia after lens injury in children, Ophthalmologica **154:**81-87, 1967.
22. Ogle, K. N., Burian, H. M., and Bannon, R. E.: On the correction of unilateral aphakia with contact lenses, Arch. Ophthal. **59:**639, 1958.
23. Binkhorst, C. D., and Gobin, M. H.: Injuries to the eye with lens opacity in young children, Ophthalmologica **148:**169, 1964.
24. Girard, L. J., Friedman, B., Moore, C. D., Blau, R. J., Binkhorst, C. D., and Gobin, M. H.: Intraocular implants and contact lenses, Arch. Ophthal. **68:**762, 1962.
25. Binkhorst, C. D.: Eigene Verfahren der Pseudophakie; iris clip Pseudophakos und irido-kapsulärer Pseudophakos, Klin. Mbl. Augenhk. **151:**21, 1967.
26. Binkhorst, C. D.: Iris-clip and irido-capsular lens implants (pseudophakoi), Brit. J. Ophthal. **51:**767, 1967.
27. Binkhorst, C. D.: Iris-supported artificial pseudophakia; a new development in intraocular artificial lens surgery (iris-clip lens), Trans. Ophthal. Soc. U. K. **79:**569, 1959.
28. Binkhorst, C. D., and Leonard, P. A. M.: Results in 208 iris clip pseudophakos implantations, Amer. J. Ophthal. **64:**947, 1967.
29. Fedorov, S.: Quoted by Binkhorst, C. D.: Lens implants (pseudophakoi) classified according to method of fixation, Brit. J. Ophthal. **51:** 772, 1967.
30. Bronner, A., and Gerhard, J. P.: La vision binoculaire chez l'aphake unilatéral porteur de verres de contact. Incidences médico-légales et médico-sociales, Bull. Soc. Ophtal. France, pp. 703-706, 1959.
31. Rougier, J.: Quoted by Magnard, P., and others: Cataracte traumatique et vision binoculaire, Bull. Soc. Ophtal. Franc., pp. 203-208, 1963.
32. Maurer: Quoted by Magnard?, and others: Cataracte traumatique et vision binoculaire, Bull. Soc. Ophtal. Franc., pp. 203-208, 1963.
33. François, J.: Quoted by Bronner, A., and Gerhard, J. P.: Verres de contact et lentilles précornéennes, Bull. Soc. Ophtal. Franc. **1:** 77, 1958.
34. Constantine, E. F., and McLean, J. M.: Contact lenses in aphakia, Arch. Ophthal. **51:**212, 1954.
35. Gettes, B. C., and Ravdin, E. M.: Monocular

aphakia and exotropia corrected by contact lens, Amer. J. Ophthal. **32:**850, 1949.

36. Fontan, P., Thalabard, J., and Robert, C.: Appareillage par prothèse de contact dan l'aphakie posttraumatique unilatérale, Ann. Oculist. (Paris) **195:**248, 1962.

37. Cowan, A.: Aphakia, Amer. J. Ophthal. **32:** 419, 1949.

38. Cowan, A.: Monocular aphakia, Arch. Ophthal. **50:**16, 1953.

39. Cross, A. G.: Quoted by Hirtenstein, A.: Contact lens in unilateral aphakia, Brit. J. Ophthal. **34:**668, 1950.

40. Hirtenstein, A.: Contact lens in unilateral aphakia, Brit. J. Ophthal. **34:**668, 1950.

41. Apers, R.: Personal communication.

Chapter 8

Intraocular manipulation in retinal detachment surgery*

Edward Okun

Intravitreal procedures should not be undertaken in retinal detachment surgery unless it becomes apparent that a cure cannot be obtained by more routine ab externo procedures. The conditions that most frequently require intravitreal surgery are retinal detachments complicated by massive preretinal retraction (Fig. 8-1) or by giant tears with rolled-over retina (Fig. 8-2).

Massive preretinal retraction

Massive preretinal retraction had been considered a hopeless condition prior to the accomplishment of vitreoretinal membrane separation by Paul Cibis in 1961.[1, 2] At that time, he utilized the water immiscible property of liquid silicone to separate a semitransparent membrane from the surface of the retina, thus allowing it to settle back into its normal position. At the present time, after trying unsuccessfully to accomplish the same feat by other techniques, we are left with essentially the same procedure. Long-term follow-up of patients who have received liquid silicone has revealed many complications. However, when the silicone has remained properly positioned, it has been extremely well tolerated. For this reason we have continued to refine the techniques of intravitreal membrane separation utilizing liquid silicone.

*This investigation was supported in part by a research grant, NB-01789, from the National Institute of Neurological Diseases and Blindness, National Institutes of Health, Bethesda, Maryland.

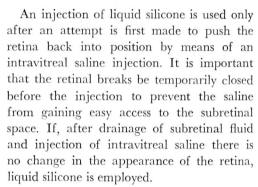

An injection of liquid silicone is used only after an attempt is first made to push the retina back into position by means of an intravitreal saline injection. It is important that the retinal breaks be temporarily closed before the injection to prevent the saline from gaining easy access to the subretinal space. If, after drainage of subretinal fluid and injection of intravitreal saline there is no change in the appearance of the retina, liquid silicone is employed.

The drainage sclerotomy is shelved in such a way that slight pressure on the inner flap results in drainage, while pressure on the outer flap stops the flow of subretinal fluid (Fig. 8-3). The eye should not be allowed to become too soft since this would impair proper visualization of the intravitreal maneuvers. Enough subretinal fluid is released to allow for the injection of approximately 0.05 ml. of liquid silicone without excessive elevation of the intraocular tension. The anterior sclerotomy is made with a Graefe knife in the pars plana just anterior to the ora serrata (5 to 6 mm. posterior to the limbus). The knife is directed radially and carried into the center of the vitreous where the tip of the blade must be seen free of tissue. It is then removed, and a 20 gauge blunt needle is inserted through this sclerotomy to the same point in the center of the vitreous cavity (Fig. 8-4). The tip of this needle is then directed into the center of the funnel toward the optic disc. After the gummy, transparent membrane that covers the funnel has been penetrated, one drop of

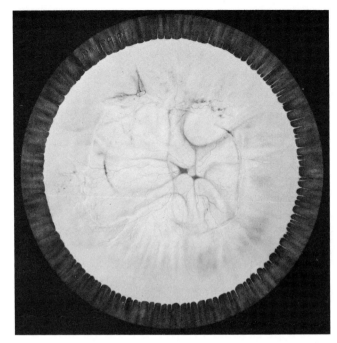

Fig. 8-1. Drawing of retinal detachment complicated by massive preretinal retraction. (From Cibis, P. A.: Vitreous cavity and retinal detachment, Mod. Prob. Ophthal. **5:**89, 1967.)

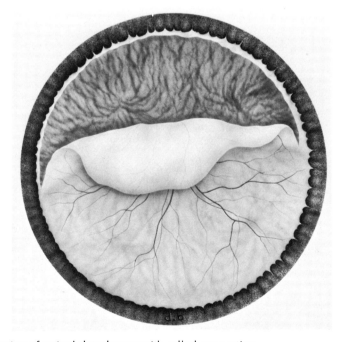

Fig. 8-2. Drawing of retinal detachment with rolled-over retina.

liquid silicone is expressed. If properly placed, the drop will remain trapped deep to the membrane. If the drop escapes, the needle tip must penetrate more deeply toward the disc. The patient's head is turned to one side during the injection so that an escaping globule of liquid silicone will not interfere with visualization during the injection. Since the specific gravity of medical fluid No. 360 (liquid silicone) is 0.972, escaping bubbles will float up and away from the needle tip. When the needle is properly placed, further injection of liquid silicone will push the funnel apart and allow the optic disc to be visualized for the first time through the silicone globule. After the injection of approximately 0.05 ml., the intraocular tension becomes normalized (Fig. 8-5, *A-D*).

The assistant carefully tests the intraocular tension during the injection by means of palpation with a muscle hook. At this point in the procedure complete drainage of subretinal fluid can be accomplished. The injection is then completed by replacing the injection needle back inside the silicone bubble which is deep to the partially separated membrane. The injection is completed when the retina appears flattened and the intraocular tension is between 10 and 17. This usually requires 1 to 2 ml. of liquid silicone.

Occasionally it is necessary to sever a

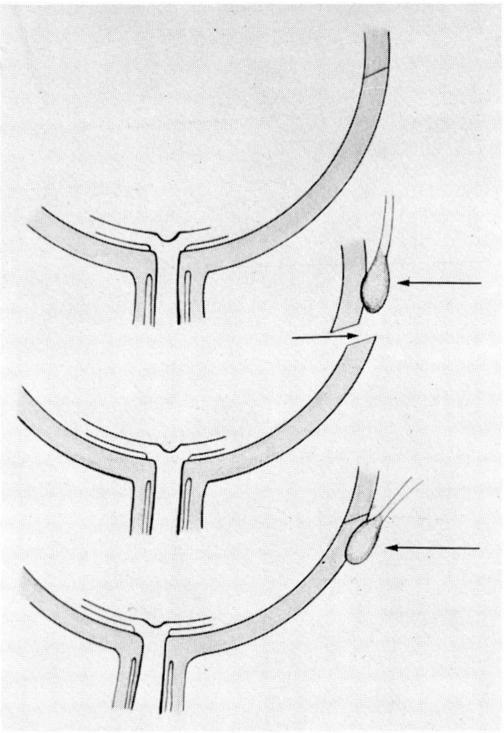

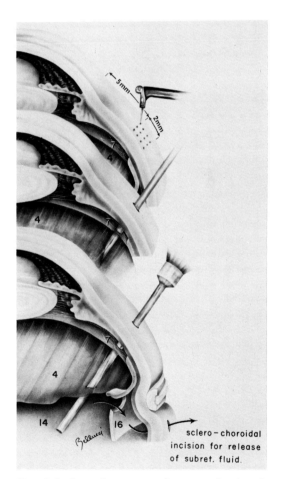

Fig. 8-3. Sketch showing shelved sclerotomy and effect of depressing inner and outer shelves. Note the subretinal fluid drainage with depression of inner shelf.

Fig. 8-4. Site of anterior sclerotomy for liquid silicone injection. (From Cibis, P. A.: Vitreous cavity and retinal detachment, Mod. Prob. Ophthal. **5:**70, 1967.)

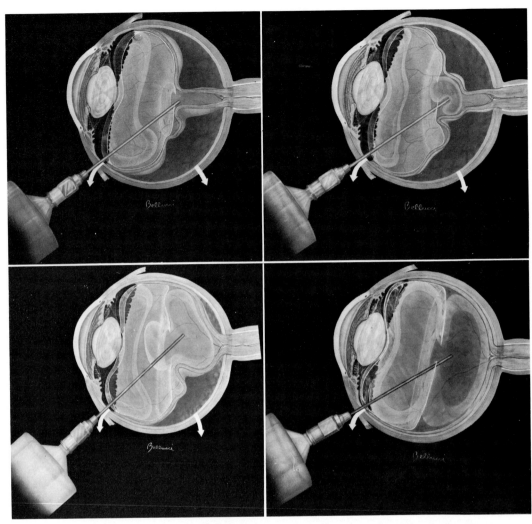

Fig. 8-5. Progressive steps in intravitreal liquid silicone surgery. (From Cibis, P. A.: Vitreous transfer and silicone injections, Trans. Amer. Acad. Ophthal. Otolaryng. **68:**983, 1964.)

vitreous band that holds two bullae together. This is done after the liquid silicone injection has separated the bullae as much as is possible. Either the Cibis vitreous cutter (Fig. 8-6) or a needle knife is used to cut these bands. Although it is difficult to completely sever these bands, the combination of a liquid silicone injection plus the initiation of the dissection with sharp instruments has resulted in reattachment of the retina in instances in which either technique alone had not been able to accomplish the task.

The injection of liquid silicone has been greatly facilitated by the development of a foot-operated pump. This pump allows the rate of injeciton to be determined by the force applied to the foot pedal, which frees the hand to perform the delicate tasks of teasing and dissecting the vitreous membranes (Fig. 8-7). It is essential for every step of this procedure to be under constant stereoscopic ophthalmoscopic control. For this purpose, we have used the indirect ophthalmoscope worn on the head.

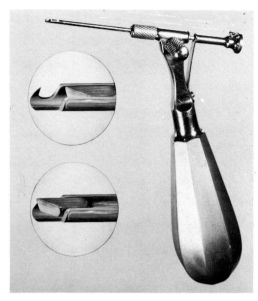

Fig. 8-6. Cibis vitreous cutter. (From Cibis, P. A.: Vitreous transfer and silicone injections, Trans. Amer. Acad. Ophthal. Otolaryng. **68:**997, 1964.)

Results

To date, intravitreal surgery utilizing liquid silicone has been used in 311 patients. Immediate anatomic improvement has been accomplished in 186 (60%). Fifty-one (16%) of the patients showed no visual improvement despite the reapposition of the retina. Fifty-four (17%) showed early improvement in visual function, which subsequently deteriorated secondary to either recurrent retinal detachment or other complications. Seventy-nine of 267 patients (34%) followed 6 months to 6 years have maintained visual acuity of counting fingers or better (walking vision). Fifty patients of 219 patients with continuous follow-up have maintained usable vision, some for 6 and 7 years. Eight patients have maintained visual acuity of 20/200 or better for more than 4 years. Forty-four patients have been lost to follow-up, and of the eleven who have been followed less than 6 months, 31% were visually improved when last seen. Nine patients have died during the follow-up period, and in all cases in which the cause of death is known, the disease

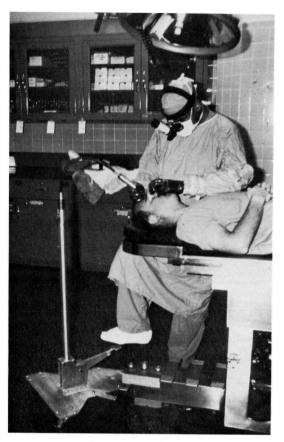

Fig. 8-7. Demonstration of foot-operated liquid silicone pump.

process which led to death anteceded the liquid silicone injection (Fig. 8-8).

Complications

Complications of intravitreal surgery can be divided into those occurring during the surgical procedure and those occurring postoperatively. At the time of surgery the injection can be poorly placed so that most of the silicone goes anterior to the membrane. This usually results in persistent retinal detachment (Fig. 8-9). Too vigorous an injection or excessive tug against the vitreous membranes can result in iatrogenic retinal breaks. Other retinal breaks can be produced either by too posterior an entry incision or by direct trauma from the delivery needle. Liquid silicone may gain access to the sub-

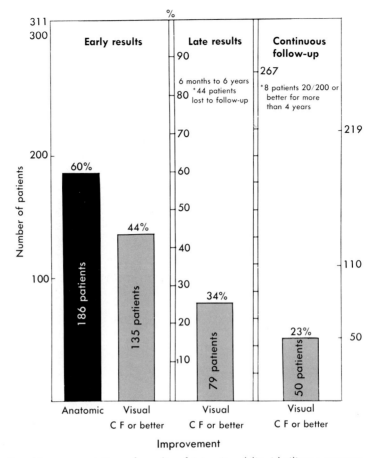

Fig. 8-8. Graphic representation of results of intravitreal liquid silicone surgery.

retinal space either through one of these iatrogenic breaks or through one which had not been closed, which leads to failure. Vitreous hemorrhages can occur at the injection site if a large ciliary vessel is inadvertantly injured. A poorly directed injection needle can cause lens injury either at the time of injection or during its removal. Overfilling with liquid silicone can push the membrane too far anteriorly and lead to an extrusion of the vitreous base and subsequent disinsertion of the retina.

Late complications have included recurrent retinal detachment, usually inferior (Fig. 8-10). This type of recurrence was observed frequently in patients treated with liquid silicone (Dow-Corning No. 360 fluid) viscosity 2,000 cs. with specific gravity .972. An-

other complication was cataract formation which occurred in 51% of the patients. The usual cataract seen is a combination of nuclear sclerosis and posterior subcapsular opacification. It took from 6 months to 3 years to develop enough opacity to alter the patient's visual acuity. A third complication, corneal dystrophy, occurred in 17% of the aphakic patients. It started as a horizontal band-shaped area of edema just above the midline, and it gradually spread to involve the entire cornea (Fig. 8-11). Many of these patients also developed secondary glaucoma. The fourth complication was secondary glaucoma, which occurred in thirty-one of the 304 patients. All but three of the patients were aphakic. The superior angle in these eyes always showed peripheral anterior sy-

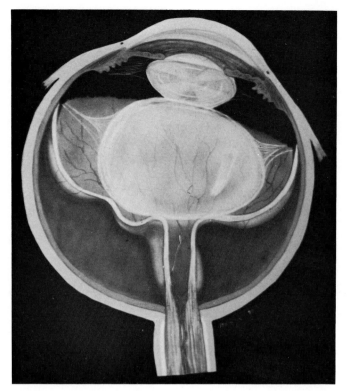

Fig. 8-9. Drawing of incorrectly placed liquid silicone, anterior to preretinal membrane.

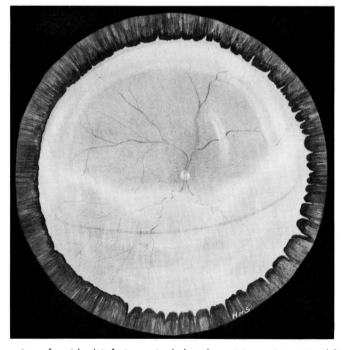

Fig. 8-10. Drawing of residual inferior retinal detachment in an intravitreal liquid silicone case.

nechiae and, in addition, many contained fine, foamy-appearing globules of liquid silicone (Table 8-1).

Comments

The most significant finding that comes from this critical review of surgery with liquid silicone is that some patients continued to do quite well and were still walking about on their own 4 or 5 years after surgery. A critical study of these patients reveals:

1. The silicone has remained posterior to the transvitreal membrane

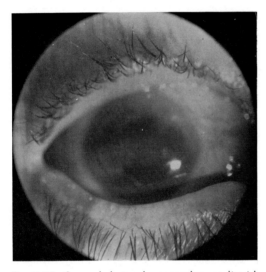

Fig. 8-11. Corneal dystrophy secondary to liquid silicone in anterior chamber. (From Cibis, P. A.: Vitreoretinal pathology and surgery in retinal detachment, St. Louis, 1965, The C. V. Mosby Co.)

2. The retina flattened without residual fixed folds
3. The silicone remains in one large globule

In general, the earlier one intervened in the process of preretinal fibroplasia, the better and more durable the functional results. In the present series no eyes were treated with liquid silicone if it was felt there was a chance of cure by any other procedure. Poor functional results are built into such a series. There was a high incidence of complications, and the visual results were frequently less than we had been accustomed to seeing after perfect anatomic reattachment of the retina. However, these were eyes that were considered hopeless from the start, and the return of any vision makes the procedure worthwhile in a one-eyed individual. The two-eyed patients in the present study have found it very annoying and exasperating when late complications requiring active therapy have occurred in the eye they were not using. For this reason, we have limited our intravitreal surgery to essentially one-eyed patients.

We are hopeful that new materials and techniques will be forthcoming that will produce results less plagued by complications than liquid silicone; but until this comes about, liquid silicone will continue to be used in the treatment of those hopeless cases of retinal detachment complicated by massive preretinal retraction.

Table 8-1. Late complications—intravitreal liquid silicone

Cataracts	Corneal dystrophy	Glaucoma	Enucleations	Recurrent retinal detachments

78/152 phakic (51%)
 	
10/78 cataract extraction
5 extracapsular
  1 glaucoma
5 intracapsular
  2 corneal dystrophy
  1 glaucoma
	(Only in aphakia) 27/162 (17%)-2, in otherwise successful cases	31 (all but 3 aphakic)	10	45 (recurrence requiring revision and refill)

Giant tears with rolled-over retina

Giant tears with inverted posterior flaps are very difficult to close by routine techniques and, not infrequently, require intravitreal maneuvers. Giant disinsertions (greater than 90 degrees) without rolled-over posterior margins carry a good prognosis with routine ab externo surgery and will not, therefore, be included in this report. Factors of importance in the preoperative evaluation of these complicated retinal detachments are:

(1) the circumferential extent of the giant break; (2) the extent of posterior inversion; (3) the posterior extent of an associated radial tear; (4) the mobility of the flap as determined by postural change and movement of the eye; and (5) the degree of preretinal fibroplasia and vitreous band and strand formation associated with the giant tear.

Giant breaks which usually require intravitreal manipulations are: (1) those that

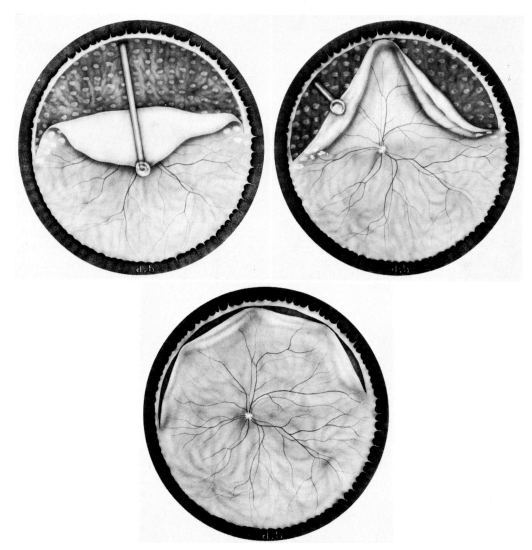

Fig. 8-12. Drawing of intravitreal cryoprobe used to reposition rolled-over retinal flap.

extend circumferentially for greater than 200 degrees and are hinged posterior to the equator; (2) those that contain extremely posterior radial tears and are hinged at the posterior edge of the tear; and (3) those that are complicated by preretinal fibroplasia.

In general, any large flap that can be influenced dramatically by position change should be treated by an ab externo technique, including a wide, shallow buckle. If drainage of subretinal fluid is required, most of the volume of fluid is best made up with an air injection followed by postoperative positioning of the patient so that the air bubble lies against the repositioned flap. If the inverted flap is mobile but the edge appears to be pulled firmly inward, minimal incarceration at the drainage site is advisable.

The intravitreal maneuvers resorted to in these extremely difficult cases include: (1) well-positioned air bubbles; (2) posterior flap manipulation and incarceration by means of suction or intravitreal cryoadhesions; and (3) liquid silicone injections.

When a rolled-over flap appears immobile and the edge has moved to the opposite side of the globe, intravitreal maneuvers must be used to elevate the edge of the flap. Once this is accomplished, a large air bubble can be placed under the flap. If the air bubble begins to escape and the flap remains stationary, direct incarcerating procedures are tried. Sclerotomies are prepared at an equatorial level within a wide lamellar bed, approximately 45 degrees apart, and a 22 gauge needle is introduced through the central sclerotomy into the vitreous with the aid of diathermy. Under ophthalmoscopic control, this needle is brought close to the central edge of the inverted flap and suction is created. While a minimal amount of vitreous is being withdrawn, the flap is gradually pulled into the incarceration site. The sclerotomy is then temporarily closed. The same procedure is repeated at the other sclerotomy sites. Air is then injected into the vitreous and the remainder of the ab externo procedure is completed.

If the suction technique does not budge

the inverted flap, the Cibis intravitreal cryoprobe is introduced through the sclerotomy site and passed across the globe to the edge of the inverted flap, which then becomes adherent to the probe by the formation of a small ice ball (Fig. 8-12). Incarceration followed by air injection is then completed as with the suction technique.

Some cases of giant tears are complicated by preretinal fibroplasia. These eyes have usually been preoperated unsuccessfully. In these cases, intravitreal liquid silicone has been used in the same way as outlined above. The membranes in these cases have confined the liquid silicone to the posterior vitreous compartment and pushed the flap back up into a more normal position.

Results

During the past 3 years, 67 cases of giant tears with inverted posterior edges (rolledover retina) were treated by various means. Intravitreal manipulations were required in 27 of these cases, successful reattachment was accomplished in 9 (33%). Of 67 cases treated and followed for a minimum of 6 months, 44 have remained reattached. In reviewing the techniques used in those cases that were cured without intravitreal manipulations, only 2 required incarcerating procedures. Fifteen required intravitreal air injections. Twenty-one required only 1 procedure; the remainder required 2 to 4 procedures.

Summary

Intravitreal surgery should be utilized only when a cure cannot be obtained by ab externo procedures. However, when indicated, intravitreal maneuvers have made it possible to cure some otherwise hopeless cases of retinal detachment.

REFERENCES

1. Cibis, P. A., Becker, B., Okun, E., and Canaan, S.: The use of liquid silicone in retinal detachment surgery, Arch. Ophthal. 68:590, 1962.
2. Cibis, P. A.: Vitreoretinal pathology and surgery in retinal detachment, St. Louis, 1965, The C. V. Mosby Co.

Chapter 9

Indications for surgery in glaucoma

Moderator:
Raymond Harrison

Panelists:
H. Saul Sugar
Maurice H. Luntz
Adolph Posner
Rudolf Witmer

Open-angle glaucoma

H. Saul Sugar

In the field of glaucoma treatment no greater diversity of opinion exists than in the indications for surgical intervention in open-angle glaucoma. As the years have passed, a trend toward conservatism has become apparent.[1] On the negative side this is largely caused by the incidence of operative failure and the relative frequency of late postoperative complications following succesful surgery. On the positive side, the long period of 10 to 20 years between onset of open-angle glaucoma and the appearance of field and disc damage and the somewhat greater drug armamentarium available today have contributed to the trend toward conservatism.

Factors that influence decision

Among the factors that influence the decision about surgery for open-angle glaucoma are: (1) the age and general health of the patient, (2) the control of the glaucoma by medical means, (3) the presence of reduced vision or symptoms from medical treatment, (4) the dependability of the patient in using his medications, (5) the degree of disc and functional damage, (6) a family history of

damaging glaucoma, and (7) previous malignant glaucoma in the fellow eye.

Age and general health. Since it takes from 10 to 20 years to produce significant disc and field changes in open-angle glaucoma, one must be less strict about medical treatment in a patient in the seventies or older and, certainly, less strict about the indications for surgery. Goldmann's statistical study of Leydhecker's survey of 19,880 normal eyes indicates that glaucoma suspects increases linearly with age over a period of 18 years.[2, 3] This suggests that an average of 18 years is required from the initial tonometric onset to the functional evidence of glaucoma. Hollows and Graham, in a study of over 4,000 individuals in Wales, from 40 to 75 years of age, found only 13 cases of field loss among 397 patients with tonometric pressures of 21 or over in three separate observations.

In my own experience, a study of the progression of disc changes in patients with open-angle glaucoma was initiated in 1952. The thirty patients who have remained under observation and control during this time showed not a single case of progressive disc changes. It has been obvious that cases of chronic open-angle glaucoma that were diagnosed relatively early (before significant disc damage) have done well for at least up to 20 years if controlled medically. Those patients with marked functional and disc changes when first seen have usually required surgery, which, if successful in lowering tension, most often succeeded in maintaining the postoperative functional status. A few had significant functional loss associated with the surgery itself, and some had gradual post-

97

operative functional reduction in spite of good pressure control.

Control of glaucoma by medical means. Open-angle glaucoma should be treated medically as long as the visual fields show no deterioration, the nerve head changes are not progressive, and the tension does not indicate continued high elevation which might potentially damage the visual functions. Some surgeons feel that an operation should not be performed, whatever the height of the ocular pressure, unless impaired visual fields are evident; however, if the field is impaired, the operation should be done early. I feel that functional testing (visual fields) is often relatively gross and unstandardized in the hands of many examiners and may not demonstrate the actual extent of functional loss. Evaluation of field loss should include careful assessment of pupil size, cataract development, and vascular complications.

I consider drug therapy to be most effective if the ocular pressure is less than 20 mm. by applanation or Schiøtz tonometry. The tonographic coefficient of outflow should be over 0.13 and the Po/C value under 100. However, these values are not considered absolute and are considered only part of the entire picture. Personally, I consider repeated tonometry, particularly applanation tonometry, more informative than all the other observations. However, it must be fully evaluated in relation to disc and field findings. If the tension on maximal drug therapy (including topical long-acting miotics, epinephrine, and systemic carbonic anhydrase inhibitors) is constantly elevated to 30 to 35 mm. or above, surgery is to be considered.

One of the reasons for the insecurity felt by the ophthalmologist in the use of medical therapy for chronic open-angle glaucoma is his inability to always know the diurnal curve of intraocular pressure. This has been pointed out by Drance, who found that one-third of medically treated glaucomatous eyes with an intraocular pressure of 19 mm. Hg or less by applanation during office visits had peaks of intraocular pressure of 24 mm. Hg or more, some up to 37 mm. Hg. Half of these peaks occurred at 10:00 p.m. and 6:00 a.m.

Presence of reduced vision or symptoms from medical treatment. Intolerance to drugs because of side effects not infrequently leads to earlier surgery than would normally be the case. The abandonment rate for drugs such as echothiophate (Phospholine), epinephrine, and acetazolamide (Diamox) is about 25% or more.

The short-acting miotic drugs, such as pilocarpine, rarely lead to sensitivity, and even when it does occur there are other drugs that can be substituted. However, with the long-acting anticholinesterase drugs, the reason for abandonment of one is often a reason for abandoning the entire group. It is sometimes necessary to avoid using these drugs in patients who have chronic open-angle glaucoma in which the anterior chambers have become narrowed. Narrowing of the angles may become a problem after long use of these strong miotics because looseness of the zonule may lead to forward displacement of the lens.

In the presence of central lens opacities even weak miotics may not be tolerated since they reduce vision. In such cases epinephrine and carbonic anhydrase inhibitors alone may be effective. When miotics are used in the presence of central lens opacity, one must be careful to establish new base lines for visual field evaluation when the miotic and, consequently, the pupil size are changed. It is my practice to stop all miotics the night before and the morning on which visual fields are measured. Sometimes it is even necessary to use a mydriatic.

The epinephrine drugs may have to be stopped if palpitation, hypertensive crises, or allergies are produced. Even the severe headaches experienced following their initial use and the redness of the conjunctiva may lead to their abandonment. They should not be used in cases of mixed primary glaucoma.

The carbonic anhydrase inhibitors must often be given up because of gastrointestinal symptoms, weight loss, taste disturbances, psychic disturbances, and renal colic. Alopecia and potassium depletion may occasionally occur especially if digitalis or other diuretic drugs are used simultaneously.

Dependability of the patient. Sometimes, in spite of adequate explanation and discussion about the nature of the disease and its control, patients wander from one ophthalmologist to another, psychologically unable to accept either the illness or the necessary treatment. Therefore, it must be recognized that despite a relatively good array of therapeutic drugs, they are not always properly and effectively used by individual patients.

Degree of disc and functional damage. In cases with evidence of early optic atrophy with large cups and poor rim capillarity, surgery is advised much earlier and with lower pressures than in early cases. This is true even if pressure is fairly well controlled, but the field has a complete arcuate scotoma or greater defect. On the other hand, if the nerves are normal and their function is undisturbed, it is wise to be conservative and to continue medical therapy. Whether a patient without functional damage is treated medically depends on other factors, such as his psychologic attitude toward treatment and his dependability with medication. Personally, I use medical therapy (if it is unassociated with side effects) in all cases in which pressures are repeatedly in the upper 20's. Some authors are more conservative, others less.

When surgery has been done on one eye, I often postpone surgery on the second eye to reevaluate its status after the operated eye has healed. In this way a potential complication which has been encountered in the operated eye can sometimes be avoided in the fellow eye. This is particularly true in eyes with bilateral field reduction to approximately 5 degrees. If one eye is blind and the field in the second is reduced to 5 degrees I

do not advise surgical treatment but prefer to continue the most effective medical regimen feasible.

Family history. A family history of damaging glaucoma or a history of rapid damage in one eye will certainly influence one toward earlier surgery.

Previous malignant glaucoma. Previous malignant glaucoma in one eye in patients with open-angle glaucoma and shallow chambers should lead the surgeon to expect the possibility of the same condition in the fellow eye. Peripheral iridectomy, in my experience, does not prevent it. Prophylactic removal of the lens would be considered here, even if the lens opacity is less than that usually indicative of surgical treatment.

Summary

The indications for surgical treatment of open-angle glaucoma are dependent on inability to adequately control the intraocular pressure medically and the associated interference with ocular function, plus a number of other factors, such as the age and health of the patient, the degree of disc damage, a family history of damaging glaucoma, and previous malignant glaucoma in the fellow eye. A conservative approach is the current attitude, especially in early cases.

REFERENCES

1. Shaffer, R. N., and Hetherington, J., Jr.: The case for conservatism in open-angle glaucoma management. Canad. J. Ophthal. **3:**11, 1968.
2. Goldmann, H.: Some basic problems of simple glaucoma, Part 2, Amer. J. Ophthal. **48:**213, 1959.
3. Leydhecker, W., Akiyama, K., and Neumann, H. G.: Der intraokulare Druck gesunde Menschlicher, Augen. Klin. Mbl. Augenheilk. **133:**662, 1958.
4. Hollows, F. C., and Graham, P. A.: The Ferndale glaucoma survey. Proceedings of Symposium Royal College of Surgeons of England, London, 1965, E. & S. Livingstone, Ltd.

Angle-closure glaucoma*

Maurice H. Luntz

This discussion will cover the indications for surgery in primary angle-closure glaucoma, with particular emphasis on the controversial aspects. The presentation is divided into the broad indications for surgery in this disease and the specific indications influencing the choice of operation.

Perhaps the least controversial statement on this subject is that all patients who have suffered attacks of primary angle-closure glaucoma should have early surgery because of the high risk of subsequent attacks, even if the patient is on medical therapy.[1, 2] Possible exceptions are:

1. The rare case that has severe iris atrophy after an acute attack and the angle has widened considerably[1]
2. Elderly persons (80 years and over) who have been on miotic therapy for many years without symptoms of a subacute attack[1]
3. Malignant glaucoma in the other eye[2]
4. Patients who refuse surgery

Indications

There is a single broad indication for surgery in all cases of angle-closure glaucoma—evidence of acute, subacute, or chronic angle-closure glaucoma. Indications can be divided into absolute indications, relative indications, and indications for prophylactic surgery.

Absolute indications

The diagnosis of angle-closure glaucoma is indisputable and early surgery is strongly indicated if an acute attack of angle-closure glaucoma has been witnessed by the surgeon, or if primary angle closure is visualized gonioscopically in the presence of raised intraocular pressure. Congestion of the eye

*This work was supported by a University Council Research Grant and a Grant from the South African Council for Scientific and Industrial Research. I am indebted to members of my staff and to Miss Lucille Kay for assistance.

may be either present or entirely absent. Another indication is a history of acute or subacute angle-closure glaucoma or combined angle-closure and open-angle glaucoma with narrow angles and a positive dark room test. Generally, intraocular pressure is normal between attacks, but it may be raised. Medically uncontrollable chronic angle-closure glaucoma with progressive field loss is also an absolute indication for surgery.

Relative indications

The diagnosis of angle-closure glaucoma is presumed and the decision to operate may be controversial if:

1. The patient has a history of acute or subacute angle-closure glaucoma or combined angle-closure and open-angle glaucoma, but provocative tests (dark room test, mydriatic test) are negative (angle closure cannot be confirmed)
2. The patient has chronic angle-closure glaucoma with raised intraocular pressure, cupping, and field loss, but the glaucoma is controlled by medical therapy

Peripheral iridectomy will eliminate the danger of a superimposed acute attack and also permit treatment with epinephrine bitartrate (Epitrate) and the long-acting cholinesterase inhibitors (echothiophate phosphate).

Although angle closure cannot be confirmed, the history of angle-closure attacks is important, and these patients are probably as much at risk as those in the group with absolute indications for operation.[3] Hence the indication for early surgery is the high risk of subsequent acute angle closure attacks in these patients even if they have been treated with miotics. The danger of visual impairment after an acute attack outweighs the risks from a peripheral iridectomy ab externo.[1]

Prophylactic surgery

Prophylactic surgery is indicated on the second eye in a patient who has had an acute or subacute attack in one eye. It is indicated in an eye with a very narrow angle and normal intraocular pressure, in which the outflow facility is diminished by more than 25% after a mydriatic test.[4, 5] Prophylactic surgery is also indicated on the fellow eye in a patient with malignant glaucoma following a filtration operation in the first eye.

Surgeons are by no means as clear on the indications for surgery in this group as in the previous two groups. They are faced with the decision to operate on what, from the patient's viewpoint, is a normal and trouble-free eye. However, these eyes have a 39% chance of developing an acute episode of angle-closure glaucoma while on miotics, and a 78% chance if untreated.[6] Similar observations were reported by Adams, Kronfeld, and Phillips and Snow.[7-9] Therefore, the risk of surgery must be weighed against the risk of visual impairment or loss following an acute angle-closure attack.[10]

In my view the answer to this question is straightforward: peripheral iridectomy should be advised for all fellow eyes unless the angle is wide and the eye myopic. The risk of complications following a peripheral iridectomy ab externo is negligible, whereas a 39% risk of an acute attack of angle-closure glaucoma is significant.[9, 11-13] A positive dark room test is helpful as it favors a successful outcome for the operation, but surgery should still be undertaken even if this test is negative.[11] The "triple test" described by Kirsch may be useful in these cases.[14] Peripheral iridectomy offers a complete safeguard against future attacks.[12] Before operating one should always transilluminate the eye for the unseen neoplasm.

Choice of operation

The choice of operation includes operations on the ciliary body, broad iridectomy, iridotomy, lens extraction, peripheral iridectomy, and filtration operation. Aspiration of the posterior vitreous followed by mydriasis is ineffective.

Operations on ciliary body. Operations on the ciliary body are generally out of favor at present. Occasionally cyclodialysis is used in combination with peripheral iridectomy, especially in late cases, if the angle is almost totally closed.

Broad iridectomy. Von Graefe was the first ophthalmologist to cure acute glaucoma by broad iridectomy.[15] Curran, Bänziger, and Haas and Scheie pointed out that many cases of closed-angle glaucoma are caused by pupillary block, which can be cured by a peripheral iridotomy or iridectomy[16-18]; a broad iridectomy as recommended by Von Graefe would therefore be unnecessary. Since the publication of Curran's paper, broad iridectomy for the treatment of primary acute glaucoma has gradually fallen into disuse in favor of peripheral iridectomy.

Iridotomy. Iridotomy may be done in place of peripheral iridectomy. However, it is technically difficult to perform adequately, and the lens is easily damaged.

Lens extraction. Angle-closure glaucoma caused or aggravated by a large intumescent lens predisposing to pupil block and pushing the iris diaphragm forward is best treated by lens extraction with a peripheral iridectomy. The glaucoma is much easier to control after the lens has been removed.

Peripheral iridectomy and filtration operation. The peripheral iridectomy and the filtration operation are at present the two most favored operations. There are cases in which peripheral iridectomy will fail to control the disease and a drainage procedure is necessary. The choice between a drainage procedure and peripheral iridectomy in general or in the individual case is a major area of controversy, because the present indications are not selective enough to recognize when peripheral iridectomy will inevitably fail. I disagree entirely with those surgeons who use a filtration operation as a primary procedure in angle-closure glaucoma. The drainage operations are considerably more traumatic than peripheral iridectomy, they

Table 9-1. Number of eyes treated and incidence of complications in patients having acute or subacute attack of angle-closure glaucoma

Operation	Number of eyes		
Peripheral iridectomy	34		
Complications		0	
Filtration operation	20		
Complications		5	
Malignant glaucoma			2 (2 patients)
Sympathetic ophthalmia			2 (1 patient)
Bullous keratopathy			1
Eyes lost from angle-closure glaucoma	6		
	60		

require more instrumentation of the anterior chamber, and they have a higher incidence of postoperative complications that may even lead to the loss of the operated eye (Table 9-1). Peripheral iridectomy ab externo, on the other hand, is a safe procedure. The anterior chamber is usually not lost, the incidence of postoperative complications is minimal, and refractive changes do not occur postoperatively.[19]

One alternative is to do a peripheral iridectomy as a primary procedure in all cases, and to accept the fact that there will be cases in which a drainage operation will be required as a secondary procedure.

Another alternative is to attempt to define the indications for a successful peripheral iridectomy, to limit the operation to these eyes, and to subject the remainder to a drainage operation. There are, however, no such clear-cut indications, and there are many borderline cases in which this decision is difficult. There is, therefore, reason to do a peripheral iridectomy as a primary procedure.

Comparative studies of indications for peripheral iridectomy

Various clinical criteria are used to facilitate the decision to perform a peripheral iridectomy or a filtration operation. The interpretation and value of these criteria are controversial. In 1960 Redmond Smith and I analyzed the criteria then in use in a group of thirty-two patients (50 eyes) with angle-closure glaucoma from the Glaucoma Clinic of St. Mary's Hospital, London.[11]

1960 series

The overall results of peripheral iridectomy in the 50 eyes studied showed that 70% were cured, 12% were controlled (with miotics), and 18% failed. The following points emerged from this study:

1. A positive dark room test was regarded as a strong indication for peripheral iridectomy.
2. The presence of peripheral anterior synechiae appeared to be a contraindication. (This was not a statistically significant finding and no attempt was made to correlate the results with the degree of angle closure.)
3. Failure to achieve control with a miotic following an acute attack was another contraindication to peripheral iridectomy. (The result, although suggestive, was not statistically significant.)
4. The state of the optic disc preoperatively did not influence the result.

Chandler series[1]

Chandler, summarizing his indications for peripheral iridectomy in preference to a filtration operation, is in close agreement. However, he believes that peripheral iridectomy is contraindicated in the presence of a cupped disc and loss of visual field. He emphasizes the importance of the degree of angle closure.

Chandler's indications for peripheral iridectomy are the following.

1. The early case with angle capable of opening extensively
2. Good response of intraocular pressure to miotic therapy
3. A good C value with miotic therapy
4. A normal optic disc and full field
5. Patients of advanced age or short life expectancy

Chandler proposes gonioscopy during surgery and an intracameral injection of saline solution to allow an assessment of the degree to which the angle will open. If this is less than one-half of its circumference, a filtration operation should be done.

Chandler has chosen to restrict peripheral iridectomy to those eyes that satisfy a predetermined set of criteria, as Redmond Smith and I did in 1960. These indications are based on clinical experience. One might ask whether these are "failure-proof," that is, if these indications are followed will all the peripheral iridectomies be successful? There are also eyes that do not satisfy these criteria. Is subjecting them to a drainage operation—a major procedure—justified? Would some of these eyes not have done equally well with the smaller procedure of peripheral iridectomy ab externo? Under what circumstances will peripheral iridectomy inevitably fail to control the disease?

1965-67 series

The above questions are ones that neither the 1960 series nor Chandler has answered. In the following, the concepts formed in 1960 will be reviewed and the accepted indications for peripheral iridectomy will be tested by assessing a further series of forty-three patients (60 eyes) from the Glaucoma Clinics of the Department of Ophthalmology, Witwatersrand University, Johannesburg. These patients were seen over the 2 years from 1965 to 1967 (Table 9-2). All of these are cases of angle-closure glaucoma diagnosed as such before operation was advised. The results of operation are compared in relation to a wide range of preoperative tests.

Table 9-2. Analysis of 1965-67 series

Operation	Number of patients	Number of eyes
Peripheral iridectomy	25	34
Filtration operation	15	20
Total number of operations		54
Eyes lost from A.C.G.		6
Total number with A.C.G.	43	60

Method and material. Results are recorded as *failed, controlled,* or *cured.* In the former, ocular tension remains raised (over 21 mm. Hg by applanation) in spite of the operation and the use of medical therapy. Controlled cases are those in which postoperative control of the intraocular pressure depends on the use of medical therapy. Cured cases maintain normal intraocular pressure without drugs. In cured or controlled cases, the visual fields are not affected, and there are no postoperative congestive attacks. Peripheral iridectomy was performed on 34 eyes (twenty-five patients) following the technique described by Barkan and modified by Chandler.[20, 21]

Follow-up. The period between operation and the last follow-up examination is from 1 to 36 years; the average is 5½ years (Table 9-3).

Sex. Sex incidence follows the usual pattern for angle-closure glaucoma—more females than males (Table 9-3).[22]

Age. The average age of onset of the first attack is 55½ years (Table 9-3).

Race. The majority of patients are white; the disease is rare in the South African Negro (Bantu) race (Table 9-3).

Prophylactic iridectomies. There are not enough prophylactic iridectomies in this series to make analysis significant, and these are not included.

Results. The overall results of peripheral iridectomy (Table 9-4) in the 34 eyes studied

Table 9-3. General information concerning 1965-67 series

	Years	Number of patients	Number of eyes
Follow-up	1		15
	3		13
	5		7
	8		13
	10		4
	22		1
	36		1
Sex incidence			
Male		13	
Female		30	

	White	Bantu
Number patients with glaucoma	264	340
Number patients with angle-closure glaucoma	43 (16%)	5 (1.6%)

Age at onset of attack		
Range	34 to 71
Average	55.5

are disappointing and resemble the results of the 1960 series. Only 62% are cured, 18% are controlled, and 20% (7 eyes) failed. Since this is a rather high number of failures, particular attention will be paid to the causes of failure in an attempt to define more closely contraindications to peripheral iridectomy. Some failures are inevitable, such as cases of mixed glaucoma. All our cases of mixed glaucoma, however, are controlled. Occasionally failure may be caused by an unrecognized case of glaucomatocyclitis crisis, but there were no cases of this disease in the series.

Correlation of 1960 and 1965-67 series

Preoperative tests used in both series. The following preoperative tests were used in the 1960 series and the 1965-67 series.

Dark room test. The major criterion used to select the 1965-67 series of cases for surgery was a positive dark room test. In 1960 we were able to show that significantly more eyes were cured if the preoperative dark room test was positive. Dark room tests have been done on 22 eyes, of which 4 were repeatedly negative and were not subjected to peripheral iridectomy. These were fellow eyes

Table 9-4. Overall results of peripheral iridectomy (1965-1967)

Results	Number of eyes	Percent
Cured	21	62
Controlled	6	18
Failed	7	20
	34	

of patients who had had acute attacks of glaucoma in the other eye and had refused prophylactic surgery. Over a period of 4 to 6 years they have remained normal. The operation was performed on 18 eyes with a positive dark room test and of these 22% failed (Table 9-5).

Response of acute attack to miotics. Eight eyes responded well to miotics (Table 9-6). Of these 6 (75%) are cured, 2 (25%) are controlled, and there are no failures. In 12 eyes the response to miotics is poor. Four (33%) are cured, 2 (17%) are controlled, and in 6 (50%) the operation failed.

It is important that one measures the response of the intraocular pressure to miotics only. If it is necessary to use acetazolamide

Table 9-5. Peripheral iridectomy results related to preoperative dark room test

Results	Positive test		Overall results		No test	
	Number of eyes	Percent	Number of eyes	Percent	Number of eyes	Percent
Cured	10	56	19	62	11	69
Controlled	4	22	6	19	2	12.5
Failed	4	22	6	19	3	18.5
	18		31		16	

Table 9-6. Peripheral iridectomy related to response to miotics following acute attack*

Results	Good response		Poor response		Unknown	
	Number of eyes	Percent	Number of eyes	Percent	Number of eyes	Percent
Cured	6	75	4	33	11	79
Controlled	2	25	2	17	2	14
Failed	0	0	6	50	1	7
	8		12		14	

*Correlation of cured and controlled cases vs. failures with reference to miotics is statistically significant at the 5% level.
$x^2_{.95} = 3.84$ (with Yates correction).

Table 9-7. Peripheral iridectomy related to preoperative state of optic disc (22 eyes)

Results	Normal disc		Cupped disc		Not seen	
	Number of eyes	Percent	Number of eyes	Percent	Number of eyes	Percent
Cured	8	61.5	5	55.5	8	68
Controlled	2	15.5	1	11.2	3	25
Failed	3	23	3	33.3	1	8
	13		9		12	

(Diamox) or osmotic diuretics, drug treatment must be stopped as soon as the intraocular pressure reaches normal levels so that the effect of the miotic can be gauged. These agents and the raised intraocular pressure may inhibit ciliary body secretion for some weeks and give false low intraocular pressure readings.

Preoperative state of the optic disc (Table 9-7). The optic disc is normal in 13 eyes and pathologically cupped in 9. In the remaining 12 the disc could not be seen preoperatively, and unfortunately there is no record of it having been seen postoperatively.

Of the 13 eyes with normal discs, 8 (61.5%) are cured, 2 (15.5%) controlled, and 3 (23%) failed. In the 9 eyes with pathologically cupped discs 5 (55.5%) are cured, 1 (11.2%) controlled, and 3 (33.3%) failed.

Comparing the eyes with normal optic discs to those with cupped discs it is obvious that the same proportions fall into the cured or noncured categories.

Gonioscopy—degree of preoperative angle closure (Table 9-8). Gonioscopy was performed as part of the routine examination: In a number of instances it was performed

Table 9-8. Peripheral iridectomy results related to degree of preoperative angle closure

| Results | Closure greater than 75% | | Closure less than 75% | | Angle not seen | |
	Number of eyes	Percent	Number of eyes	Percent	Number of eyes	Percent
Cured	5	36	10	71.5	6	100
Controlled	3	21	3	21.5	0	0
Failed	6	43	1	7	0	0
	14		14		6	

Table 9-9. Peripheral iridectomy results related to duration of acute attack

| Results | Less than 36 hrs. | | More than 36 hrs. | | Unknown | |
	Number of eyes	Percent	Number of eyes	Percent	Number of eyes	Percent
Cured	5	71	1	14	15	75
Controlled	2	29	2	30	2	10
Failed	0	0	4	56	3	15
	7		7		20	

Table 9-10. Peripheral iridectomy related to preoperative tonography combined with dark room test

| Result | Preoperative C value | | | | Tonography not done | |
| | Less than 0.18 µl/min./mm. Hg | | Greater than 0.18 µl/min./mm. Hg | | | |
	Number of eyes	Percent	Number of eyes	Percent	Number of eyes	Percent
Cured	7	75	5	62.5	9	53
Controlled	2	25	3	37.5	1	6
Failed	0	0	0	0	7	41
	9		8		17	

in each eye preoperatively after control of the acute attack. Glycerine drops were used to clear the cornea if necessary. The angle was adequately visualized in 28 eyes, but not in 6. In 14 eyes more than 75% of the angle remained closed, and it is significant that 6 of the 7 failures in the series occurred in this group, compared to only one failure in the group of 14 eyes in which less than 75% of the angle is closed.

It is significant that five patients (36%) with more than 75% of angle closure preoperatively are cured and three (21%) controlled.

Criteria not used in 1960 series. The following criteria were not used in the 1960 series.

Duration of acute attack (Table 9-9). The dividing line is set at 36 hours.[1] Eyes subjected to an acute attack lasting less than 36 hours (7 eyes) are compared to those in which the acute attack lasted more than 36 hours (7 eyes). In 20 eyes, however, the duration of the attack is unknown. Results are inconclusive, but it is of interest that there are 5 cures (71%) and no failures in the first group and only 1 cure with 4 failures (56%) in the second group. There ap-

Table 9-11. Peripheral iridectomy results related to degree angle opens postoperatively

Results	Angle remains over 75% closed		Angle opens over 25%		Angle not seen	
	Number of eyes	Percent	Number of eyes	Percent	Number of eyes	Percent
Cured	0	0	2	50	19	76
Controlled	0	0	2	50	4	16
Failed	5	100	0	0	2	8
	5		4		25	

pears to be a stronger tendency for failure if the acute attack lasts longer than 36 hours.

Preoperative tonography combined with dark room test (Table 9-10). A C value of 0.18 μl/min./mm. Hg or greater is accepted as normal. Becker and Shaffer showed that with an outflow facility of 0.15 μl/min./mm. Hg the failure rate from peripheral iridectomy is negligible.[23] There are 9 eyes with a C value less than 0.18 μl/min./mm. Hg. Of these, 7 (75%) are cured, 2 (25%) are controlled, and there are no failures.

In 8 eyes the C value was greater than 0.18 μl/min./mm. Hg. Five eyes (62.5%) are cured, 3 (37.5%) are controlled, and there are no failures. However, in 17 eyes tonography values are not available, and all 7 failures occurred in this group.

Discussion. An operation was performed on all 18 with a positive dark room test. In this group there were 4 failures (22%). Although a positive dark room test should be accepted as an important indication for surgery, it does not guarantee against failure. Other factors of equal importance must be taken into account; in particular, the degree of preoperative angle closure, the response of the intraocular pressure to miotics, and the duration of the attack before treatment is started. The most important factor is failure of the angle to open in at least 25% of its circumference. This point is well demonstrated in Table 9-11. Of 9 eyes gonioscoped postoperatively the angle remains closed over more than 75% of its circumference in 5 and in all these cases the operation failed. In the

remaining 4 eyes the angle opens over at least 25% of its circumference, and in this group there are no failures. Two eyes (50%) are cured and 2 (50%) controlled.

Another important factor is the response of the acute attack to miotics for control of the intraocular pressure. Chandler and Trotter found this an important factor in subacute cases.[24] In the 1965-67 series, 6 of the 7 failures occurred in eyes that responded poorly to miotics (Table 9-6); there are no failures in eyes that responded well.

The duration of the acute attack before starting treatment appears to be of some importance. If the attack exceeds 36 hours, there is less chance of a successful peripheral iridectomy, although 1 case in this group is cured and 2 cases are controlled (Table 9-9). From the successful operations one finds the success of these is dictated by the ability of the angle to open and the good response to miotics (Table 9-12). Most cured cases are found in the groups in which less than 75% of the circumference of the angle remains closed preoperatively and the acute attack responds well to miotics.

Six of the 7 failures occur in eyes that responded poorly to miotics and the angle remains over 75% closed preoperatively. Chandler reported a similar observation,[12] but even in this group 5 eyes (45%) are cured or controlled.

Some authors maintain that if more than 50% of the angle remains closed, a peripheral iridectomy will fail to control the disease.[1, 25] However, Foulds and Phillips and

Table 9-12. Peripheral iridectomy results related to response to miotics and degree of preoperative angle closure*

Results	Good response				Poor response				Not known	
	Angle more than 75%		Angle less than 75%		Angle more than 75%		Angle less than 75%			
	Number of eyes	Per-cent	Number of eyes	Per-cent	Number of eyes	Per-cent	Number of eyes	Per-cent	Number of eyes	Per-cent
Cured	4	66.6	0	0	1	100	3	27	13	81
Controlled	2	33.4	0	0	0		2	18	2	12.5
Failed	0	0	0	0	0		6	55	1	6.5
	6		0		1		11		16	

*Degree of correlation between response to miotics, degree of angle closure, and response to iridectomy is highly significant (cured and controlled vs. failures).

x^2 with Yates correction and 1 degree of freedom: $x^2_{.995} = 7.88$

Tetrachloric r test: $r = 0.86$

Table 9-13. Overall results of filtration operation

Results	Number of eyes	Percent
Cured	8	40
Controlled	7	35
Failed	5	25
	20	

Forbes and Becker described cases of chronic closed-angle glaucoma with apparently extensively closed angles which were cured by peripheral iridectomy.[26, 27] This has also been my experience (Table 9-12). The preoperative state of the optic disc did not influence the results (Table 9-7). The effect of preoperative tonography on the results is inconclusive because the test was not done in the 7 eyes in which the operation failed. Becker and Thompson pointed out the importance of tonography as an indicator for successful operation.[4] Nevertheless, this criterion is not absolute, since even in their series, 3 eyes (23%) with an outflow facility of less than 0.10 were controlled with peripheral iridectomy.

Reliability of proposed criteria

The questions posed earlier in this paper can now be reconsidered.

Within the limitations of the 1965-67 series the indications for peripheral iridectomy have not proved to be failure-proof. Failures occur in all groups of eyes except those that respond well to miotic therapy and in which more than 25% of the circumference of the angle opened preoperatively. The numbers in this group are very small, so there is no guarantee against failure; however, it is certainly the strongest indication for peripheral iridectomy.

Concerning the question of whether a drainage procedure should be the primary operation, there were eyes that were cured or controlled by peripheral iridectomy in each group in which even more than 75% of the angle is closed preoperatively. Thus there is no preoperative test that positively contraindicates peripheral iridectomy.

An incidental finding during this review of acute-angle closure glaucoma is 10 eyes in which a drainage operation was done on an unselective basis as the first procedure. The results, summarized in Table 9-13, reflect a 25% incidence of failure, not very different from the incidence of failure in peripheral iridectomies.

Goldberg reported an even higher failure rate[28]; thus an initial drainage procedure will not reduce the overall incidence of failure from surgery.

Table 9-11 indicates that the incidence of cure or control is considerably reduced in cases in which the angle remains closed for more than 75% of its circumference postoperatively. The success of peripheral iridectomy will, therefore, depend on recognizing preoperatively the angles that will open over more than 25% of their circumference postoperatively. The question is, however, how is this to be achieved?

Shaffer and, more recently, Chandler have described an ingenious method of assessing whether the closed angle will open postoperatively.[1, 29] The angle is visualized on the operating table with a gonioscope lens and microscope after the aqueous is withdrawn and has been replaced by an intracameral injection of a slightly larger quantity of saline. They argue that by deepening the angle with saline and using a gonioscope lens one can visualize the extent to which the angle can be opened. This determines the choice of operation—if more than 50% of the angle opens, a peripheral iridectomy will be done; if less than 50% opens, a filtration operation will be performed.

There are a number of objections to this maneuver:

1. At very best, a safe and relatively atraumatic operation (peripheral iridectomy) performed without introduction of instruments into the anterior chamber is converted into a traumatic procedure involving the anterior chamber.
2. In inexperienced hands it is not difficult to overfill the anterior chamber with saline and subluxate the lens. Vitreous may pass through the ruptured zonule initiating a series of major complications.
3. Peripheral iridectomy will succeed in an angle which opens to 25% of its circumference (Table 9-11).[26, 27, 30, 31]
4. Even in the best hands instrumentation of the anterior chamber combined with precipitate and forcible breaking of granulation tissue in the angle will, in some cases, result in postoperative iritis

and chronic closure of an angle which was only partly closed at the time of the maneuver.

The last objection to this procedure is illustrated in the following case report.

Case report. Mrs. Y. M., aged 70 years, was seen in June 1967 with an acute attack of angle-closure glaucoma in the right eye. She had had angle-closure glaucoma in the left eye in 1959.

On examination: The right eye showed the features of a typical acute angle-closure attack with intense congestion, corneal edema, a shallow anterior chamber, and a fixed, semidilated pupil. Vision was recorded as perception of hand movements and good light projection. Intraocular pressure with applanation tonometry was 60 mm. Hg. Response to intensive miotic therapy was poor, and tension was finally controlled with the addition of a mannitol 20% intravenous drip (1 liter) and acetazolamide (Diamox), 250 mg., orally every 6 hours. Gonioscopy at this stage showed that the angle had opened by approximately one-third (66% of the angle remained closed).

Anterior chamber. There were a few cells and fine pigmented keratic precipitates. There were no posterior synechiae.

The eye was gonioscoped in theater following the chamber-deepening technique described by Chandler[1] and the angle was seen to open by two-thirds of its circumference. Peripheral iridectomy was then executed uneventfully.

Status at discharge, June 1967

Intraocular pressure: This remained well controlled with no further treatment (approximately 16 mm. Hg by applanation).

Gonioscopy: The angle at discharge was two-thirds open, the remaining one-third closed by peripheral anterior synechiae.

Anterior chamber: Cells + and flare + and fine pigmented keratic precipitates. The iritis was more severe than preoperatively and than would be expected after an uneventful peripheral iridectomy. Controlled with 10% phenylephrine drops at bedtime and Sofradex drops 4 times daily.

The optic disc was normal.

August 1967. At a follow-up examination in August 1967 it was noted that intraocular pressure was 25 to 27 mm. Hg by applanation and controlled only with 4% pilocarpine drops 3 times a day and acetazolamide (Diamox), 125 mg. twice daily. Gonioscopy revealed the angle almost completely closed with peripheral anterior synechiae (approximately 15% of the angle open). The anterior chamber still harbored the occasional cell but there were no fresh keratic precipitates.

Comment. Nearly two-thirds of the angle closed with P.A.S. within 2 months after operation in the presence of a mild chronic iritis which appeared to be related to the surgery. This is an unusual experience following peripheral iridectomy, and in my view is related to the angle deepening maneuver. I, therefore, prefer not to use this maneuver. When, however, this maneuver is used, I introduce saline after the iridectomy has been performed and before the scleral wound is sutured. Saline is forcibly injected from a 5 ml. syringe through a thin cannula held just outside the wound. The stream of saline is directed at the wound edges and away from the iridectomy. In this way the anterior chamber can be deepened without introducing instruments.

Conclusion

Our present criteria do not accurately separate eyes that can be successfully treated with peripheral iridectomy from those that will fail. Therefore it is suggested that peripheral iridectomy be done in all cases of acute angle-closure glaucoma. The iridectomy is made eccentric to the 12 o'clock meridian. In cases that respond poorly to miotics and in which more than 75% of the angle remains closed preoperatively, a failure rate of approximately 56% must be anticipated because of the inability of the angle to open. In this type of case some surgeons would combine peripheral iridectomy with the separation of peripheral anterior synechiae by sweeping an iris repositor on each side of the iridectomy. However, the same objections apply here as to the chamber-deepening maneuver of Chandler. An initial peripheral iridectomy does not alter the chances for success of a subsequent drainage operation, nor does a drainage operation guarantee a successful outcome.[24] Six eyes in which peripheral iridectomy failed subsequently underwent filtration operation (Table 9-14); three were cured, 2 were controlled, and 1 failed (17%).

This approach is preferred to the alternative of attempting selection on the basis of recognized indications which are not sufficiently selective. Faulty selection may expose eyes to a major surgical procedure (drainage operation) with the possibility of serious complications when a minor operation (peripheral iridectomy) would have sufficed.

In discussing controversial aspects of glaucoma surgery I have, no doubt, added to the controversy!

Summary

Apart from a few exceptions all cases of angle-closure glaucoma should be treated surgically. The choice of operation may present difficulty and is the cause of controversy. The indications for peripheral iridectomy or drainage operation have been discussed, but two questions remain unanswered:

1. Are the indications for peripheral iridectomy sufficiently relative to ensure that all are successful?
2. Are the indications for peripheral iridectomy accurate enough to include all those eyes that will respond to peripheral iridectomy, or are some eyes unnecessarily subjected to a drainage operation?

It is concluded from our studies that the present criteria do not adequately separate eyes that can do well with peripheral iridectomy from those in which the operation will fail. All eyes with primary angle-closure glaucoma should, therefore, be treated by peripheral iridectomy; the failures are then treated by a drainage operation. It is considered preferable to do a peripheral iridectomy and to accept some failures rather than to unnecessarily subject eyes to a drainage operation.

Table 9-14. Filtration operation after failure of peripheral iridectomy (poor response; angle closure greater than 75% pre- and postoperatively)

Results	Number of eyes	Percent
Cured	3	50
Controlled	2	33
Failed	1	17
	6	

REFERENCES

1. Chandler, P. A., and Grant, W. M.: Lectures on glaucoma, Philadelphia, 1965, Lea & Febiger.
2. Smith, R. J. H.: Clinical glaucoma, London, 1965, Cassell & Company.
3. Lowe, R. F.: Primary angle-closure glaucoma. A review of provocative tests, Brit. J. Ophthal. **51**:727, 1967.
4. Becker, B., and Thompson, H. E.: Tonography and angle-closure glaucoma: diagnosis and therapy, Amer. J. Ophthal. **46**:(1) 305, 1958.
5. Hildreth, R. H.: Prevention of angle-closure glaucoma, Amer. J. Ophthal. **46**:(4) 600, 1958.
6. Bain, W. E. S.: The fellow eye in acute closed-angle glaucoma, Brit. J. Ophthal. **47**: 193, 1957.
7. Adams, S. T.: Indications for and results of peripheral iridectomy in angle-closure glaucoma, Trans. Canad. Ophthal. Soc. **7**:227, 1954-55.
8. Kronfeld, P. C.: Glaucoma. In Newell, F. W., editor: Transactions of First Conference, 1955, New York, 1955, Josiah Macy, Jr. Foundation.
9. Phillips, C. I., and Snow, J. T.: Peripheral iridectomy in angle-closure glaucoma: a common complication, Brit. J. Ophthal. **51**:733, 1967.
10. Lowe, R. F.: Acute angle-closure glaucoma. The second eye: an analysis of 200 cases, Brit. J. Ophthal. **46**:641, 1962.
11. Luntz, M. H.: A possible aetiology for glaucoma in Negroes, Brit. J. Ophthal. **44**:60, 1960.
12. Chandler, P. A.: Narrow-angle glaucoma, Arch. Ophthal. **47**:695, 1952.
13. Douglas, W. H. G., and Strachan, I. M.: Surgical safety of prophylactic peripheral iridectomy, Brit. J. Ophthal. **51**:459, 1967.
14. Kirsch, R. E.: A study of provocative tests for angle-closure glaucoma, Arch. Ophthal. **74**:770, 1965.
15. Von Graefe, A.: A new method for surgical treatment of glaucoma, Arch. Ophthal. **3**(2): 456, 1876.
16. Curran, E. J.: A new operation for glaucoma involving a new principle in the aetiology and treatment of chronic primary glaucoma, Arch. Ophthal. **49**:131, 1920.
17. Banziger, T.: Ber. Deutsch. Ophth. Ges. **43**: 43, 1922.
18. Haas, J., and Scheie, H. G.: Peripheral iridectomy in narrow angle glaucoma, Trans. Amer. Acad. Ophthal. **56**:589, 1952.
19. Sugar, H. S.: Late refractive changes following various operations for angle-closure glaucoma, Amer. J. Ophthal. **53**:43, 1962.
20. Barkan, O.: Peripheral iridectomy with retention of anterior chamber, Amer. J. Ophthal. **41**:964, 1956.
21. Chandler, P. A.: Peripheral iridectomy, Arch. Ophthal. **72**:804, 1964.
22. Smith, R. J. H.: Trans. Ophthal. Soc. U. K. **78**:254, 1958; Brit. J. Ophthal. **42**:447, 1958.
23. Becker, B., and Shaffer, R. N.: Diagnosis and therapy of the glaucomas, St. Louis, 1961, The C. V. Mosby Co.
24. Chandler, P. A., and Trotter, R. R.: Angle-closure glaucoma; subacute types, Arch. Ophthal. **53**:305, 1955.
25. Graham, M. V.: Surgical aspects of glaucoma, Trans. Ophthal. Soc. U. K. **86**:224, 1966.
26. Foulds, W. S., and Phillips, C. I.: Some observations on chronic closed-angle glaucoma, Brit. J. Ophthal. **41**:208, 1957.
27. Forbes, M., and Becker, B.: Iridectomy in advanced angle-closure glaucoma, Amer. J. Ophthal. **57**:57, 1964.
28. Goldberg, H. K.: Results of various operative procedures in acute congestive glaucoma, Amer. J. Ophthal. **34**:1376, 1951.
29. Shaffer, R. N.: Operating room gonioscopy in angle-closure glaucoma surgery, Trans. Amer. Ophthal. Soc. **55**:59, 1957.
30. Gorin, G.: The value of gonioscopy in diagnosis and treatment of angle-closure glaucoma, Eye, Ear, Nose, Throat Monthly **40**:469, 1961.
31. Sugar, S.: The glaucomas, ed. 2, London, 1957, Cassell & Company.

Cataract and glaucoma

Adolph Posner

Glaucoma and cataract can be divided into two headings—cataract as a cause of angle-closure glaucoma, and cataract as a cause of open-angle glaucoma.

Cataract as the cause of angle-closure glaucoma

At one stage in the development of cataract, the angle may become closed; the patient then suffers an acute or subacute attack of glaucoma. The obvious explanation would seem to be that the swollen intumescent lens, by its mere presence, causes the angle to become narrow and eventually to close. The progressive shallowing of the anterior chamber can be attributed to intumescence of the cataract, but closure of the angle cannot be caused directly by crowding of the angle structures by the lens.

The equatorial region of the lens always remains a safe distance away from the angle. The narrowing and eventual closure of the angle is either caused by a change in character of the surface of the cataractous lens or to the deposition of a gelatinous mucoid material between the lens and the iris. Both factors tend to increase the pupillary block and cause the periphery of the iris to bulge forward. Miotics in these cases act as a two-edged sword. They may stretch the iris sufficiently to open the angle, but they also tend to increase pupillary block. Miotics, in fact, contribute to the pupillary block by immobilizing the pupil and preventing the circulating aqueous from flushing the mucoid material through the pupil into the anterior chamber.

Dr. Robert Newhouse and I studied a number of such cases and were able to demonstrate the relationship between this mucoid material in the posterior chamber and pupillary block, or retroiridic block, as we prefer to call it. When the pupil is dilated, the viscous material herniates into the anterior chamber. Sometimes the angle subsequently reopens and remains open. In other cases the angle remains closed and a peripheral iridectomy has to be performed. One or 2 days after surgery the viscous material is seen to herniate through the coloboma into the anterior chamber, where it forms a lenticular-shaped mass, almost filling the chamber. It resembles either a knuckle of vitreous or a dislocated lens. This material becomes absorbed within 1 to 2 weeks.

One predisposing factor in this form of glaucoma is, of course, a previously narrow angle. Another predisposing factor is the presence of capsular exfoliation. In capsular exfoliation, when the pupil is dilated, even in the course of a routine examination, a cloud of pigment dust is frequently observed embedded in a vitreous-like matrix, entering the anterior chamber through the pupil at one or two points. If this material is allowed to accumulate in the posterior chamber, it becomes inspissated and then acts as a barrier to the circulating aqueous. Prophylaxis consists of dilating the pupil frequently during the course of miotic therapy. To do this safely, a diagnosis must be established by gonioscopic study. Also, the course of the mydriasis should be followed by gonioscopy so that any tendency to angle closure can be detected before an acute attack.

Once an acute angle-closure glaucoma develops, either spontaneously or precipitated by mydriasis, there are two choices open—iridectomy or lens extraction. If the vision is reduced by lens opacities, lens extraction is preferable.

Cataract as a cause of open-angle glaucoma

In the following, a group of conditions will be discussed, which I prefer to designate by the more general term "phakogenic glaucoma," rather than by the terms phaco-anaphylactic, phacotoxic, and phacolytic glaucoma. This group includes some of the most difficult problems in clinical management.

Hypermature cataract is known to sometimes produce a type of hypertensive uveitis that is resistant to all forms of medical therapy, but which responds miraculously to cataract extraction. The problem is to make the diagnosis. My attitude is that if the doubt cannot be resolved, both the uveitis and the glaucoma should be considered as phakogenic.

At least this approach leads to a positive plan of action, and if proved correct, an eye can be saved that would otherwise be lost. Sometimes the signs of uveitis dominate the picture. There are large keratic precipitates, aqueous flare, peripheral anterior synechiae extending onto the cornea, and glaucoma. In other cases, the uveitis is hardly discernible, with only occasional cells, faint aqueous flare, plus filamentary or conical anterior synechiae. The glaucoma is very much in evidence, for glaucoma is an essential feature of phakogenic uveitis. In fact, I believe that any uveitis of undetermined etiology that is accompanied by open-angle glaucoma may be presumed to be phakogenic glaucoma. Another characteristic of phakogenic glaucoma is the great variability of the ocular tension. It may be normal for days or weeks, then rather suddenly become elevated without apparent cause, only to return to a lower level without any change in the treatment. The tension responds only to carbonic anhydrase inhibitors.

In the case of hypermature cataract the leakage of lens material is assumed to be the cause of the uveitis and the glaucoma. The leakage of lens material or soluble products of lens metabolism, is probably also the cause of phakogenic glaucoma associated with some intumescent cataracts. When these cataracts are removed, the glaucoma subsides. The chemicals derived from the lens flow with the aqueous toward Schlemm's canal, and they apparently have a toxic action on the membranes and cells concerned with the transfer of aqueous.

By extrapolation I would like to propose the following hypothesis. Certain cases of open-angle glaucoma diagnosed as chronic simple glaucoma may, in fact, be phakogenic in nature, even though the lens is still transparent and vision is normal. The transparency of a lens is an optical phenomenon, not a biochemical fact. Every normal lens is opaque to the short ultraviolet rays, and some cataractous lenses will transmit infrared rays. We do not know when the abnormal biochemical processes that lead to the formation of cataracts begin, but that they are present before vision fails is a reasonable assumption.

We are unable as yet to distinguish those cases of open-angle glaucoma that will respond favorably to lens extraction from those that will not. It is my practice to carry every early case of chronic simple glaucoma on medical therapy (including the use of small doses of carbonic anhydrase inhibitors) as long as possible, even if the tension cannot be fully controlled. If the glaucoma is phakogenic, it will usually become evident in 1 or 2 years when a cataract begins to develop. At this point I perform intracapsular cataract extraction.

In the majority of cases this plan of management has proved successful in controlling the glaucoma. After the cataract surgery the patient requires either no medication or a minimum dose of carbonic anhydrase inhibitors with or without epinephrine. Echothiophate (Phospholine) iodide may have to be used for a short time if there is a transient phase of increased tension caused by contact between the iris and the trabecular band. In those cases in which the glaucoma fails to respond to cataract extraction despite the postoperative use of echothiophate iodide, cyclodialysis usually restores the intraocular pressure to normal. The question as to how a "normal" lens produces glaucoma cannot be answered; nevertheless it is a provocative one. In most instances, certain soluble constituents of the lens that leak through the capsule probably cause the glaucoma. In some cases, the process may be even more elusive. I would like to mention one case that still remains unique in my experience.

A 65-year-old woman gave a history of recurrent acute attacks of glaucoma in her right eye. The angles were narrow. The tensions were normal under repeated examination, but the dark room test was positive in the right eye. Influenced largely by the history, I performed a peripheral iridectomy on the right eye. Postoperatively the patient experienced severe attacks of acute glaucoma in this eye once or twice each day. These could be controlled only by oral administration of acetazolamide (Diamox) or glycerine. The angle remained open during the attacks, and no peripheral anterior synechiae were present.

After a week, slight flare and a few cells appeared in the aqueous and faint opacities were discernible in the lens behind the anterior capsule. Vision had dropped from 20/20 to 20/30. Lacking any other positive plan of action, I felt that the lens should be extracted.

Dr. Herbert Katzin, who saw the patient in consultation, was in essential agreement. An intracapsular cataract extraction was attempted, but the capsule ruptured, and about half of the lens cortex remained within the eye. The anterior lens capsule was stripped off. The posterior capsule remained in place. What is remarkable is that despite the retention of this large amount of lens matter, the patient suffered no further attacks of glaucoma, and the intraocular pressure has remained normal.

The unexpected dramatic success that cataract surgery had in this patient suggests that it was not the lens substance as such that caused the acute attacks of glaucoma, but a chemical derived either from the epithelium of the anterior lens capsule or from the metabolism of the lens, which was not produced once the subcapsular epithelium had been removed. Cases such as this should be carefully studied for their possible implication. They contain clues that may lead to fruitful biochemical investigation.

This brings me to the question of a possible relationship between pigmentary glaucoma and cataract. Patients with Krükenberg spindles do not always develop glaucoma, of course, but they should all be followed carefully. Many of them, indeed, develop cataracts within 10 years. Another question difficult to answer categorically is what effect lens extraction may have in arresting a case of glaucoma capsulare. It has been my practice to extract the cataract, in the presence of uncontrolled glaucoma (with capsular exfoliation), before the cataract becomes mature, if it can be demonstrated that the cataract is progressive. In several such cases I found that both the glaucoma and the exfoliation were arrested by the surgery.

In conclusion, under certain circumstances, cataract extraction is a specific treatment for glaucoma. Cataract extraction today is safer and more predictable than a fistulizing operation.

Secondary glaucoma

Rudolf Witmer

The basic indication for surgery in secondary glaucoma cannot be different from the one in primary glaucoma: if the tension can no longer be lowered to values below 25, and preferably to 20, by means of miotics, epinephrine and diuretics, surgery becomes necessary. There is only the question of duration of intraocular hypertension. It is often hoped that in secondary glaucoma the cause of hypertension may slowly disappear under the influence of an anti-inflammatory or other medication. In many cases it can be assumed that a formerly normal eye may stand a tension above 30 mm. for a few days or even weeks without too much damage. Therefore, except for the very acute forms of iris bombé with blocking of the angle, surgery is usually not very urgent.

Since there are many different causes for hypertension in the eye, the indication for surgery varies a great deal and the operative procedure has to be adjusted to the cause of the secondary glaucoma. I will discuss, therefore, the different forms of secondary glaucoma and the surgical procedure to be chosen in each case. I will base my considerations on an analysis of 81 cases, all operated upon for secondary glaucoma during the last few years.

Classifications

There are at least six etiologically different classifications of secondary glaucoma (see listing below). The largest group is formed by the postinflammatory cases. They can be differentiated into hypertensive uveitis and keratitis; the latter is very often metaherpetic. The second largest group in the study is made up of traumatic secondary glaucoma after contusion of the globe (with or without luxation of the lens) and after penetrating injury, combined with traumatic cataract. An important group consists of all cases with aphakic glaucoma. Hypertension caused by vascular disorders is less common, but usually severe. There is a small group of degenerative diseases, and finally intraocular tumors or drug-induced glaucomas have to be included in this series. With a few exceptions I have taken into consideration only those cases which had to undergo surgery.

Classification of secondary glaucoma
1. Inflammatory
   a. Keratitis (metaherpetic)
   b. Uveitis (sarcoidosis, ankylosing spondylitis, Behçet, heterochromia, Posner-Schlossmann, undetermined)
2. Vascular
   a. Extraocular venous congestion
   b. Diabetic rubeosis iridis, central venous thrombosis, Sturge-Weber
3. Degenerative
   a. Marfan, Marchesani syndrome
   b. Aniridia, essential iris atrophy
4. Tumor
   a. Melanoma of choroid and ciliary body
   b. Diktyoma of ciliary body
5. Traumatic
   a. Perforating injury
   b. Rupture of globe
   c. Contusion of globe
6. Aphakic
   a. Congenital
   b. Heterochromic cyclitis
   c. Vitreous loss, postoperative wound rupture
   d. Epithelial ingrowth
7. Phacolytic
8. Iatrogenic (cortisone, α chymotrypsin)

Operative procedures

The different operative procedures used are listed below:

1. Improvement of outflow
   a. Filtering
      (1) Scheie
      (2) Preziosi
      (3) Elliott
      (4) Iridencleisis
   b. Nonfiltering
      (1) Goniolysis
      (2) Trabeculotomy
      (3) Goniotomy
      (4) Iridectomy peripheral (total)
      (5) Transfixion of iris
      (6) Cyclodialysis
2. Decreasing aqueous humor formation
   Vascular
      (1) Cyclodiathermy
      (2) Cyclocryotherapy

The technique of well-known operations will not be discussed, but the terms "goniolysis" and "trabeculotomy" should be mentioned. Goniolysis is an opening of the chamber angle from behind (Fig. 9-1). After a scleral incision 2 to 3 mm. from the limbus, and parallel to it, a modified cyclodialysis spatula is pushed forward parallel to the limbus and then rotated into the anterior chamber. With this maneuver only the angle is opened. The ciliary body is not detached from the sclera, as is the case in cyclodialysis.

In trabeculotomy the canal of Schlemm is prepared by dissecting the overlying sclera under the operating microscope. Then a

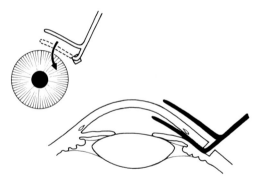

Fig. 9-1. Goniolysis.

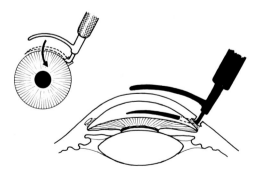

Fig. 9-2. Trabeculotomy.

Table 9-15. Surgery in eighty-one patients with secondary glaucoma

Disease	Operations performed	Repetition of operations			Results	Enucle-ation
		1	*2*	*3*		
Inflammatory (31 eyes)						
Keratitis (5 eyes)	4 filtering procedures	3	2	–	Tension normal in all	0
5 metaherpetic	1 total iridectomy				eyes; 4 have compli-	
	1 cyclodialysis				cated cataract	
	1 cyclodiathermy					
Uveitis (26 eyes)						
2 sarcoidosis	9 filtering procedures	21	4	1	Tension normalized in	0
1 ankylosing spondy-	2 peripheral iridect.				23 eyes; hypotony 3	
litis					eyes; useful vision in	
1 Behçet's syndrome	13 total iridectomy*				22 eyes; poor in 2 eyes	
1 heterochromic cy-	4 cyclodia-(gonio)lysis					
clitis						
1 glaucoma cyclitis	1 trabeculotomy					
18 undetermined	1 goniotomy					
7 pupillary seclu-	3 cyclodiathermy					
sion (iris bombé)						
Vascular (11 eyes)						
1 extraocular venous	1 filtering procedure	1			Tension normal; vision	
congestion					= 0.2	
4 diabetic rubeosis	3 cyclodiathermy	1	1		Tension high†	
iridis	1 light coagulation	1			No pain	
	1 iridencleisis	1			Blind	
6 hemorrhagic glau-	1 filtering procedure	1			Tension high	2
coma, central venous	1 iridectomy	1			Blind	
thrombosis						
Degenerative (4 eyes)						
2 Marfan's syndrome‡						
1 Marchesani syn-	1 iridencleisis	1			Tension normal	
drome (Sphaeroph-						
aky)						
1 Aniridia‡						
Tumor (2 eyes)						
1 Melanoma of the	1 posterior sclerectomy	1				1
choroid§						
1 Diktyoma of the						1
ciliary body‖						
Traumatic (15 eyes)						
6 perforating injuries	7 cyclodialysis	3	2		3 good	
traumatic cataract	(4 goniolysis)				3 poor	
2 intraocular foreign	1 cyclodialysis	2			2 good	
body	1 filtering procedure					
2 rupture of the globe	1 cyclodialysis					
	3 cyclodiathermy	1		1	1 fair	1
5 contusion of the	4 cyclodialysis	4		1	4 good	
globe	3 cyclodiathermy					
Aphakic (21 eyes)						
1 congenital (bilat-	1 transfixion	1			Hypotony	
eral)	3 cyclodialysis			1	Vision good	

*On both eyes in one patient.
†Three of these patients died within 2 years postoperatively.
‡Not operated upon; tension controlled medically.
§Patient died from liver metastases 2 years after enucleation.
‖Eight-month-old boy.

Table 9-15. Surgery in eighty-one patients with secondary glaucoma—cont'd

Disease	Operations performed	Repetition of operations			Results	Enucle-ation
		1	*2*	*3*		
Aphakic (21 eyes)— cont'd						
2 heterochromic cyclitis	3 cyclodialysis	1	1		Hypotony V-good	
4 loss of vitreous during cataract surgery	3 cyclodialysis 1 trabeculotomy 1 cyclodiathermy	2 1	1		Good Good	
2 rupture of wound postoperatively	2 cyclodialysis 2 cyclodiathermy		2		Good	
7 epithelial ingrowth	4 cyclodialysis 5 removal of epithelium 3 x-ray	5	2		2 good 1 fair 4 poor	1
1 plastic lens in ant. chamber	1 removal of lens				Poor corneal dystrophy	
3 no obvious reasons	5 cyclodialysis	1	2		Fair	

small probe is introduced into the canal and is rotated into the anterior chamber (Fig. 9-2).

Results (Table 9-15)

The group of *inflammatory secondary glaucoma* consists of 5 cases of metaherpetic keratitis. In most of them a filtering operation controlled the tension despite marked exudation in the anterior chamber and thickening of the cornea; however, 4 eyes developed a complicated cataract.

In *hypertensive uveitis* (26 eyes) with a rather chronic course, filtering procedures are quite successful. In acute cases with iris bombé a total iridectomy controlled the tension and preserved useful vision in almost all cases. Only 3 cases developed hypotony after glaucoma surgery. Most cases were operated upon only once; 4 needed a second procedure and in one case there were 3 interventions. In this group, filtering procedures and iridectomies are indicated, and seem to be very effective.

The second group, *vascular secondary glaucoma* (11 cases) caused by rubeosis with diabetic or post-thrombotic retinopathy, is the worst one. Filtering procedures were tried 3 times but were complete failures.

Cyclodiathermy never was able to control the tension, but in some cases, it at least relieved severe pain. One case with extraocular venous congestion caused by an arteriovenous aneurysm of the cavernous sinus was improved. Useful vision was retained following a filtering procedure, although there was some bleeding after the operation.

I would like to mention the *degenerative* forms very briefly; it is seen from Table 9-15 that we only operated upon one case of spherophakia. Both eyes with hypertension caused by intraocular tumors had to be enucleated.

The important group of *posttraumatic secondary glaucoma* (15 cases) shows that most cases had a partially blocked angle caused by goniosynechiae. Therefore, mainly cyclodialysis and goniolysis were chosen as operative techniques. The results are not splendid, but are often related to severe damage to other parts of the injured eye.

Aphakic glaucoma made up the second largest group in our series (21 eyes). Except for 3 cases which had apparently no surgical or postoperative complications, a reason for the intraocular hypertension was always found. It was caused by heterochromic cyclitis, vitreous loss, wound rupture, and epithelial ingrowth. Cyclodialysis is a most useful operation, but it has to be done at the site where the angle is still open. It will not work if there is a complete goniosynechia all around. Epithelial ingrowth is a very serious problem. Diagnosis can be facilitated by cytologic examination of the aqueous humor. Irradiation with x-rays does not inhibit further growth of the epithelium in the anterior chamber and, therefore, is not able to lower the tension. Complete surgical removal of the epithelial layer covering the posterior surface of the cornea (and often great parts of the iris) is very difficult, even with the use of the microscope. Among our 7 cases, we tried it 4 times, twice with apparently good result. The 2 other cases are still questionable.

Summary

In summary, surgery in inflammatory secondary glaucoma is usually successful. Despite irritation of the anterior segment, filtering procedures seem to work. In iris bombé, iridectomy is very helpful. Post-traumatic secondary glaucoma very often requires cyclodialysis or goniolysis. The same is true for uncomplicated aphakic glaucoma. In cases of epithelial ingrowth, surgical removal of the epithelium should be tried at an early stage.

Vascular glaucoma has a very poor prognosis; all surgical techniques seem to fail, and most eyes become blind. Cyclodiathermy seems to be a rather worthless technique. It lowers the tension, if at all, only for a short time.

Discussion

Moderator:
Raymond Harrison

Dr. Harrison: We have a number of questions that have been submitted to the panel. Can the use of carbonic anhydrase inhibitors for uncontrolled glaucoma in one eye jeopardize the integrity of a functioning filtering bleb in the other eye, where the pressure is 12 to 15 mm. Hg without medication? If the answer is yes, does this constitute an indication for surgery on the second eye? Professor Luntz, would you care to answer that question?

Prof. Luntz: My answer to that question is that I don't know the answer. It has been said that carbonic anhydrase inhibitors may embarrass the function of a filtering bleb. In my experience and in our own work, it seems as though these drugs tend to inhibit the formation of a good bleb, rather than actually embarrass the function of a well-formed functioning bleb.

I would answer the question by saying that I would certainly not undertake surgery in the second eye of an open-angle glaucoma,

merely because I am forced to use Diamox in order to control the intraocular pressure. I don't think that we really are certain that Diamox inhibits the function of a fully formed bleb.

Dr. Posner: I would not be influenced by the low tension of the other eye, simply because we don't know enough about the mechanism of the action of Diamox.

Dr. Sugar: I would not be influenced by the use of Diamox. I certainly would never consider surgery on the basis of the need for the use of Diamox.

Dr. Harrison: Thank you. There doesn't seem to be a great difference of opinion on this topic. Dr. Sugar, does the age of your patient influence you in starting Diamox? For example, in young adults or juveniles, do you alter your criteria for surgery because of the age?

Dr. Sugar: My criteria for the use of Diamox would not be influenced in any way by the possibility of long-term use. Most of the problems in the use of Diamox have had to do with side effects, not uncommonly resulting in abandonment, but I have used Diamox in some patients for as long as it has been available, without any problem whatever. The number of patients who have had to give it up over this period of time has increased linearly.

Dr. Harrison: Now, there are several questions on the matter of combined lens extraction and filtering procedure. First, what are the indications for combined lens extraction and filtering procedure?

Dr. Posner: In my hands, none.

Dr. Harrison: I agree. Dr. Sugar?

Dr. Sugar: I prefer not to do combined operations.

Prof. Witmer: I agree with both Dr. Sugar and Dr. Posner. I had to take over a series of such cases operated on by my predecessor, who was very fond of the "La Grange" procedure. We surveyed these cases and it showed that actually only about 5% of all these cases had a real filtering wound. In most cases, there was no filtering at all, but the tension was still controlled. I think that cataract extraction alone would have done the same thing, as Dr. Posner mentioned, therefore we do not perform the combined operation anymore.

Dr. Harrison: Professor Luntz, do you agree?

Prof. Luntz: Yes, I agree with that. I get enough complications from one procedure without bothering to combine them.

Dr. Harrison: There are several questions on technique with regard to peripheral iridectomy for acute angle-closure glaucoma that has failed to respond to medical measures. First, should the incision be made through clear cornea with the idea that in these cases a filtering procedure may well be needed, and therefore, the intact conjunctiva would be desirable?

Dr. Sugar: I think it makes no difference really. It depends on what you prefer to do. Some people go through clear cornea and have the advantage that there is no bleeding. I prefer to go through the limbus under a small conjunctival flap because this is the way that I have found it to be easy and successful.

Dr. Harrison: Thank you. Dr. Posner, do you ever go through clear cornea?

Dr. Posner: I have never done it. I imagine that when the iridectomy is performed on a quiet eye, prophylactically, it can be done through clear cornea, but when it is performed on an eye that has just undergone an acute attack, I have seen postoperative tension rise as high as 40 and over, and I think for that reason it is good to have a conjunctival flap, to prevent any mishaps or infections.

Dr. Harrison: Professor Witmer, are you a clear cornea proponent?

Prof. Witmer: No, I am not. In Berne, with Professor Goldmann, we tried this procedure quite a number of times. The iridectomy is not really basal, unless you pull so very hard on the iris that you make a sort of dialysis as well. I think Professor Goldmann does not do it anymore, and we prefer a small flap.

Dr. Harrison: Professor Luntz?

Prof. Luntz: I think there are distinct advantages to gain through the clear cornea as has already been stated in your question. One leaves the conjunctiva unscarred, and also, there is very little bleeding. One must point out that technically it is more difficult to operate through clear cornea, and I think this is why perhaps it is not so widely accepted.

One has to be sure that the incision is actually vertical and near the limbus. If it is beveled forward, it is difficult to get a basal iridectomy, as Professor Witmer has already said. If it is beveled too far backward, one gets into the angle and into the canal of Schlemm; and you run into difficulties there. I don't oppose the method and I think there are some advantages, but it is certainly more difficult technically. I personally incise through the limbus under the conjunctiva.

Dr. Harrison: Do you ever prefer a sector iridectomy over a peripheral iridectomy in angle-closure glaucoma?

Prof. Luntz: By sector iridectomy you mean iridectomy through the sphincter.

No, I see no advantage in a full iridectomy at all. Mechanically this should have no better effect than peripheral iridectomy, as was shown early in the century by Curran and other workers. In fact, there are many disadvantages to sector iridectomy. One is destroying the sphincter, which is quite unnecessary. I never do sector iridectomy for angle-closure glaucoma.

Dr. Harrison: Do those remarks still hold when you have sufficient rise of pressure to paralyze the sphincter, resulting in pupillary dilatation?

Prof. Luntz: Even then, I think that it is difficult to be sure at the early stage immediately after the acute attack that this sphincter paralysis is permanent; many of these, as you know, do recover partially. I would still prefer to maintain a round pupil and an even partially functioning sphincter.

Prof. Witmer: I agree, with the exception of the paralyzed pupil; there we perform a total iridectomy.

Dr. Posner: I agree with Professor Witmer.

Dr. Sugar: I prefer the peripheral iridectomy.

Dr. Harrison: Professor Witmer, does the first episode of acute angle-closure glaucoma in an elderly patient suggest to you that perhaps you are dealing not with a primary glaucoma?

Prof. Witmer: I think that you always have to consider the condition of the lens in these cases. Maybe it is due to intumescent cataract, as Dr. Posner pointed out, but I do agree with him that this is never the only reason.

Dr. Harrison: I think the reason for this question was probably a suggestion made recently at our hospital rounds that if you are going to get primary angle-closure glaucoma, you get it in an earlier age group in general than open-angle glaucoma.

Now a question on plateau iris configuration. In known angle-closure glaucoma in which gonioscopy reveals the angle to be of the plateau iris type, do you feel that peripheral iridectomy or a filtering operation would be preferable?

Dr. Posner: In the plateau iris, peripheral iridectomy is just as effective as in any other kind of angle-closure glaucoma. However, it may be necessary subsequently to continue the use of miotics, because there is a tendency for the rest of the iris to come into apposition with the trabecular band and in this way interfere with outflow.

Dr. Sugar: I would like to point out that I have never been sure that there is such an entity. I have found so few cases that there is still a question in my mind concerning this diagnosis.

Dr. Harrison: Professor Witmer, several people have asked about a useful alternative to cyclodiathermy. You did mention the disappointing features of cyclodiathermy in secondary glaucoma, and particularly in hemorrhagic glaucoma. Have you explored the use of cyclocryo applications?

Prof. Witmer: We have started using it and it seems to have a similar effect. It does not lower the tension very much, unless you go to dosage which is close to producing phthisis bulbi. I think it may relieve the pain if you destroy the long ciliary nerve, and this is often quite useful for eyes which are blind.

Dr. Harrison: Thank you. This is a rather unfortunate note on which to stop, but our time is now up. Thank you very much, members of the panel.

PEDIATRIC OPHTHALMOLOGIC PROBLEMS

Presiding Chairman: **Algernon B. Reese**

Chapter 10

Surgical treatment of soft cataracts (congenital and other causes)

Harold G. Scheie

Surgical techniques

Several different techniques are available for operating upon congenital or soft cataracts: (1) optical iridectomy, (2) discission, (3) linear extraction, (4) Ziegler through-and-through discission, (5) intracapsular extraction, and (6) aspiration. Nearly all of these methods date back to antiquity, although changes and refinements are still being made.

Optical iridectomy. Optical iridectomy has been more widely used in Europe than in the United States. It possesses the virtues of simplicity and safety, but the visual results are not as good as through a clear pupillary space following removal of the lens. It is useful for nuclear (central) cataracts, especially in retarded children who do not require maximum visual acuity.

Discission. Discission (needling) of the lens is widely used and is advocated by many ophthalmologists. I was taught this method during my training and employed it for several years in practice. Multiple operations usually are necessary and considerable time is usually required. The results are good, and the procedure is safe and simple to perform. Repeated needling, however, may lead to adhesion of the iris to lens remnants with subsequent dense pupillary membrane or pupillary block. Wound complications are avoided.

Linear extraction. Linear extraction also has many advocates. An incision of approx-

imately 5 mm., however, is required, which, in my experience, can lead to wound complications in children. Furthermore, vitreous loss is a real hazard and not infrequently involves loss of the eye.

Ziegler through-and-through discission. The Ziegler through-and-through discission of the lens is not looked upon with great favor. It is, however, useful in the management of membranous cataract.

Intracapsular extraction. Intracapsular extraction of cataracts, particularly the congenital types, is contraindicated in young individuals. A large incision must be made and vitreous loss usually occurs. Even with the use of alpha-chymotrypsin, which dissolves the zonule, the ligamentum-hyaloideo-capsulare, which attaches the lens to the face of the vitreous, remains intact. Vitreous, therefore, is literally withdrawn from the eye with the lens.

Aspiration. I began to use the aspiration method, a principle that is very old, in 1950.[1] The suction tips that were used at that time were rather large and cumbersome, and required an incision as large as for linear extraction (usually 4 or 5 mm. in length). Wound complications and vitreous loss, therefore, were not uncommon. I evolved a technique in which the lens was aspirated by inserting a thin-walled No. 19 needle with a blunt tip through a puncture in the corneoscleral wall beneath a small conjunctival flap. Such a small opening avoided practically all danger of wound complications and vitreous loss, and the results have been most encouraging.

Aspiration technique

Aspiration is done under general anesthesia in infants and children and with local anesthesia in older individuals. Atropine sulfate 1% and phenylephrine hydrochloride 10% are used to obtain maximum pupillary dilatation. The procedure varies slightly depending upon whether or not the cataract is complete and if good pupillary dilatation can be obtained preoperatively by mydriatics.

Complete cataract

An eye speculum is inserted and a superior rectus suture is placed. A small conjunctival flap is dissected superiorly toward the limbus. The eye is fixed at the 6 o'clock position and a Ziegler type knife-needle or Barkan goniotomy knife is inserted into the anterior chamber 1.5 to 2.0 mm. behind the limbus. A wide cruciate incision is made through the lens capsule and, as the knife-needle is withdrawn, the scleral opening is enlarged very slightly to create a puncture just large enough for suction and to admit the aspiration needle.

The needle is a specially made thin-walled No. 19 needle with an oval and rather blunt tip. The aperture is equivalent to that of a No. 18 needle because of the thin wall. The needle is inserted, bevel down, through the knife-needle incision at the 12 o'clock position. It is attached to a 2 ml. syringe containing approximately 0.25 ml. of saline solution. When the tip of the needle is at the lower pupillary border, the needle is rotated so that the bevel is turned forward with the aperture facing the cornea. In this position, the tip of the needle is less prone to injure the face of the vitreous when suction is applied. Care should be taken to avoid sucking upon the iris which would promote traumatic iritis and posterior synechia.

Suction is created by withdrawing the plunger of the syringe with the needle in place. If the lens does not aspirate completely, fluid can be forced into the anterior chamber and sucked out several times. This helps to break up and remove the lens material, but there is usually no difficulty in removing the lens material when the cataract is complete. The tip of the needle can be directed to various positions in the anterior chamber to gather up any residual lens material. Even dense central nuclear plaques can be sucked into the lumen of the needle and removed. The needle is withdrawn when the chamber is clear; if any lens material remains, the needle can be reinserted. Saline is injected into the chamber to deepen it and to protect the face of the vitreous as the needle re-enters the eye. On occasion, the pupillary border is displaced as the needle is withdrawn, indicating that the iris is caught in the scleral puncture. A stream of saline directed into the opening by an anterior chamber irrigator is usually effective in freeing the iris. Finally, a 7-0 mild chromic catgut appositional suture is placed across the knife-needle incision with an atraumatic needle and the conjunctiva is closed. Atropine sulfate 1% and phenylephrine 10% are instilled to maintain pupillary dilatation.

Incomplete cataract

If the cataract is incomplete, a preliminary needling or ripening procedure is done, using a Ziegler knife-needle or Barkan goniotomy knife. It is inserted as in making the puncture for aspiration. A wide cruciate incision is made through the anterior lens capsule. No attempt is made to stir up the cortex because of possible injury to the posterior capsule. The lens usually is completely cataractous and becomes semiliquefied in several days to 2 to 3 weeks and can then be readily aspirated. To help prevent secondary glaucoma from lens material in the anterior chamber, acetazolamide (Diamox) is given prophylactically. If the pressure should rise, prompt relief is given by aspiration. Pupillary dilatation is maintained postoperatively with atropine sulfate 1% and phenylephrine 10%.

Conclusion

Regardless of the technique that is employed for operating upon congenital cataracts, wide pupillary dilatation is essential to prevent occluded pupil or pupillary block and secondary glaucoma. The pupils of all patients should be dilated preoperatively. If they do not dilate well, a broad sector iridectomy should be done. This can be done as a separate procedure, which I prefer, or it can be combined with the congenital cataract surgery. The dangers of pupillary block and occluded pupil were first mentioned by Haskett Derby in 1885. His reasons for doing sector iridectomy were the same as those I have advocated, and which have been emphasized by Chandler, Cordes, Barkan and others.[2-4]

Good pupillary dilatation can be maintained postoperatively by the instillation of atropine sulfate ointment 1% and phenylephrine 10%, each instilled twice daily. Upon dismissal of the child from the hospital, the importance of faithful instillation of the medication should be emphasized to the mother, and she should be given specific instructions as to how to instill it. Failure to continue medication can result in a lost eye.

The results obtained in operating upon congenital cataracts not caused by maternal rubella were excellent.[1] In a comparison of uncomplicated nonrubella cataracts and a series of rubella cataracts, the difference was astounding. In 84 eyes studied of the nonrubella type, there was an incidence of complications of about 5%. However, in the rubella cataracts, 43% had severe complications.[5] In another study of 61 eyes, sector iridectomies were done as a preliminary procedure at any time after 6 months of age. The incidence of complications from iridectomy was very low. The difference was probably explained by the presence of rubella virus in the lens. Positive cultures were obtained from many lenses. Of 17 lens aspirates that were cultured, 47% were positive. Of 16 iris cultures taken at the time of iridectomy,

a very few were positive. This was surprising because cultures, other body tissues, and secretions become negative by 6 months to 1 year of age. In the lens, however, cultures remain positive for as long as 22 months and a positive culture has now been reported from Australia in a patient 35 months of age. It is felt that the virus probably is contained and maintains its viability within the lens, which is isolated by the lens capsule. For this reason, a preliminary iridectomy can be done safely and is advised as a preliminary procedure for rubella cataract. We defer cataract surgery in rubella patients until 2 years of age or older, hoping that the virus will disappear by that time. Furthermore, since the children are often retarded and because the cataract tends to be central, sufficient vision for relatively normal development is provided by the iridectomy.

Aspiration is effective for any type of cataract in patients up to 30 years of age. The most common types encountered are metabolic, developmental, and traumatic. Rarely, one encounters a rather dense sclerotic type of lens which cannot be removed through the aspiration needle. The opening in the corneal scleral wall can then be enlarged and a routine extracapsular extraction done.

Summary

I prefer the aspiration technique for the removal of all types of cataract in patients under 30 years of age. Wide pupillary dilatation is essential to prevent pupillary block, and if the pupil does not dilate well preoperatively, a sector iridectomy should be done. The incidence of serious complications caused by postoperative iridocyclitis is high in operating upon rubella cataracts and probably results from live virus which persists within the lens.

REFERENCES

1. Scheie, H. G., Rubenstein, R. A., and Kent, R. B.: Aspiration of congenital or soft cataracts; further experience, Trans. Amer. Ophthal. Soc. **64:**319, 1966; Amer. J. Ophthal. **63**(1):3, 1967.

2. Chandler, P. A.: Surgery of the lens in infancy and childhood, Arch. Ophthal. **45:**125, 1951.

3. Cordes, F. C.: Surgery of congenital cataract, Amer. J. Ophthal. **31:**1073, 1948.

4. Barkan, O.: A procedure for the extraction of congenital, soft, and membranous cataracts, Amer. J. Ophthal. **15:**117, 1932.

5. Scheie, H. G., Schaffer, D. B., Plotkin, S. A., and Kertesz, E. D.: Congenital rubella cataracts; surgical results and virus recovery from intraocular tissue, Arch. Ophthal. **77:**440, 1967.

Chapter 11

Surgical tricks for strabismus

Philip Knapp

The title of this article may make one think of legerdemain or pulling rabbits out of a silk hat. Unfortunately, I have no such ability in dealing with squint operations. However, there are a few variations of the usual procedures that I have found helpful.

The first procedure is what I call surgical orthoptics.[1] By this I mean that although surgery is considered primarily to affect the motor apparatus of the eye, it certainly has definite effects on the sensory apparatus also. The salutary effect of surgery on abnormal correspondence was first reported by Travers.[2] In young children with amblyopia in whom conventional occlusion of the good eye has not succeeded, an operation to correct the strabismus is performed. Irrespective of whether one or both eyes were operated upon the nonamblyopic eye is patched in the operating room and the patching is continued postoperatively. Frequently, the fixation becomes centric, and there have been many cases in which this has been successful. The most dramatic case in which centric fixation was successful was a little boy with congenital cataracts and esotropia. We were fortunate to obtain a good result in the first eye. We operated upon the second eye a few months later, but the visual acuity was less than 20/400. We went ahead and did a squint operation on him and patched the 20/20 eye. In a matter of 2 months, this 3½-year-old had 20/20 with the illiterate E in the formerly amblyopic eye. At the present time, we have switched his fixation over so that we are actually using mild lens occlusion

on the formerly nonamblyopic eye. I certainly recommend this procedure.

I feel strongly that to cure intermittent exotropia one must secure an immediate, and of not too short duration, over-correction. This is for sensory reasons of antisuppression.

Comitancy, as Berke showed, is one of the important factors in securing a functional result.[3] If there is a residual vertical imbalance, there is almost no chance for a functional cure. Similarly an A or V pattern cannot be ignored or overlooked. It must be corrected or the result will be poor. However, the main part of surgical orthoptics is prophylaxis against recurring amblyopia. Formerly, at the Muscle Clinic children would be patched until either the visual acuity was equalized or the original fixation preference was reduced to where the child preferred only one eye. In other words, fixation was held with the formerly amblyopic or nonused eye through a blink. The patient would then go to the regular clinic and have an operation, usually a recession-resection on the nondominant eye. By the time the patient came back to the Muscle Clinic the amblyopia had frequently recurred. Parents dislike the idea of resuming the patching after the eyes have been straightened. Usually they never bother to bring the child back, because they think that since the child's eyes are straight, their troubles are over. We learned empirically that if, by mistake, the surgeon operated on the dominant eye, there was much less of a problem in dealing with the amblyopia postoperatively. In 60 cases of esotropia in which an operation was performed on the dominant

127

eye there were only 3 cases with two or more lines of amblyopia. On the other hand, out of 70 operations on the nondominant eye, there were 24 cases of amblyopia.

By the term double elevator paresis, I do not mean paired bilateral paresis. In double elevator paresis both elevators or depressors of one eye do not work. Spontaneous double elevator paresis is usually thought to be caused by a nuclear lesion involving the superior rectus and the inferior oblique. The paresis is frequently associated with a true or a pseud-optosis. I have never been able to distinguish between the true and pseudoptosis preopera-tively, but in the procedure that we advocate, if there is a true ptosis, it is aggravated; if pseudoptosis, it is corrected. Passive duc-tion testing is important because if the duc-tion test is positive, our procedure will not work. The causes of positive duction tests are fibrosis of the inferior rectus, fracture of the floor of the orbit with incarceration of the inferior rectus, and the superior oblique sheath syndrome of Brown. Although this syndrome shows primarily a restriction of elevation in adduction, many of these eyes do not go up well in abduction either. When the traction test is negative (and the full arc of rotation should be followed) the cases are either secondary to a Berke-Motais or are primary. The operation of choice is the transplantation of the entire medial rectus and lateral rectus up across the corners of the superior rectus. The results using this procedure have been almost unbelievably good. There has been only one failure in 12 operations—one over-correction. The pro-cedure is very simple. The medial and lateral recti are freed up as though they were going to be recessed and then they are moved up to the corners of the superior rectus. In a double depressor paralysis, the problem is different, because it is almost inconceivable that a lesion could involve the inferior rectus supply of the third nerve and the fourth nerve. I follow the theory of Harold Brown that these cases probably start out as paraly-sis of the superior oblique. In time the in-

ferior rectus can no longer pull the eye down, and the deviation spreads across the lower field into a deviation in which the eye does not depress. In the past I tucked the superior oblique and resected the ipsilateral inferior rectus. This worked fairly well in the primary position, but most of the patients still showed substantial hyper in the eyes down position. We, therefore, now advocate tucking the superior oblique of the affected eye and an intrasheath tenotomy on the opposite su-perior oblique.

The trick in superior oblique surgery is good technique. I use John McLean's No. 3 technique on the superior oblique tuck.[5] In other words, the tendon is picked up tem-poral to the superior rectus, which is dis-turbed as little as possible. Any wild sweeping movements are avoided and it is picked up under direct vision. If you cannot find the tendon, an alternative procedure should be done, rather than causing a lot of scar tissue under the upper lid. The scar tissue can cause a malignant hypertropia in which the eye is frozen in the eyes up position.

There are three tricks that can be used with the superior oblique intrasheath tenot-omy of Berke.[6] When the superior oblique is picked up, the eye should be looking straight ahead. This moves the tendon anteriorly until it is almost at the nasal corner of the superior rectus. A miniature muscle hook should be used to pick up only the tendon. In this procedure the nasal extension of the elevator does not go over to the trochlea and all the other tissues, which produce complications. After intrasheath tenotomy has been done it should be done over again. In approximately 4 cases we picked up another tendon. Whether the first band that was picked up was or was not the ten-don, I do not know, but the second one is cut in the same way. Approximately 11 tenotomies have been done in which surgeons have thought they cut the tendon; however the tendon was subsequently found to be intact. As to what this band is that is first cut, I do not know, but I had been guilty of cutting it three times, before I thought of going back and looking for another one.

In long-standing cases with deficient motility there is frequently a shortage or contracture of the tissues. This can be compensated for by the recession of the conjunctiva as described by Cole.[7] I have found this maneuver most useful as a barrier to the regrowth of scar tissue. I prefer to call the procedure a bare sclera closure (as utilized by Boechmann[8, 9]). Another trick is useful if there is a large residual deviation after maximal recessions. A re-recession frequently cripples the duction of the involved muscle. I have found a marginal myotomy to be most helpful, for it lengthens the tendon simulating the effect of a recession, but full duction power is retained since the arc of contact is maintained.

Another helpful trick is the insertion of sheets of Supramid Extra* to separate the two surfaces and prevent scar tissue from restricting ocular rotations. We use the 0.05 mm. thickness and anchor the suture with 6-0 Mersilene† sutures.

In cases of third and fourth nerve paralysis, the fixation suture described by Callahan has been most helpful.[10] In third nerve paralysis in which the fourth nerve is functioning, transplanting of the superior oblique to the medial rectus gives better motility. The trick is in getting the superior oblique out of the trochlea. I place my finger on the trochlea and follow the isolated superior oblique tendon up to it with the tip of a pair of Stevens scissors. Once the tip is in the trochlea, the trochlea is cut with the scissors. This maneuver does not always succeed. When it fails I use Callahan's method.

A final trick is the treatment for the superior oblique sheath syndrome that was

described by Harold Brown.[11] In the past, everything was fine during the operation; however, within two weeks, the condition had recurred because of the readherence of the sheath. Two years ago Alan Scott discovered that if the eye was anchored up in adduction so that the insertion of the superior oblique was maximally distant from the trochlea, the sheath would not readhere. The trick is in getting the sutures deep enough into the sclera so that they do not pull out immediately. With a 4-0 Mersilene suture on a spatula needle, the suture can be placed deep in the sclera without entering the globe. A large curved needle is then threaded onto the sutures to anchor the eye up in adduction to the brow. These sutures should be removed after 4 days. We have had 3 successes using this method.

REFERENCES

1. Knapp, P.: Surgical orthoptics in strabismus, Symposium, Giessen, Aug. 1966, New York, 1968, Karger.
2. Travers, T. A. B.: The practical importance of abnormal retinal correspondence, Trans. Amer. Acad. Ophthal. Otolaryng. **54:**565, 1950.
3. Berke, R. N.: Requisites for post-operative third degree fusion, Trans. Amer. Acad. Ophthal. Otolaryng. **62:**38, 1958.
4. Brown, H. W.: Personal communication.
5. McLean, J. M.: Direct surgery of underacting oblique muscles, Trans. Amer. Ophthal. Soc. **46:**633, 1948.
6. Berke, R. N.: Tenotomy of the superior oblique for hypertropia, Trans. Amer. Ophthal. Soc. **44:**304, 1946.
7. Cole, J. G., and Cole, H. G.: Recession of the conjunctiva, Amer. J. Ophthal. **53:**618, 1962.
8. Knapp, P.: The surgical treatment of persistent horizontal strabismus, Trans. Amer. Ophthal. Soc. **63:**75, 1965.
9. Boechmann, E. J.: The operative treatment of recurrent pterygia, J.A.M.A. **28:**97, 1897.
10. Callahan, A.: The arrangement of the conjunctiva in surgery for oculomotor paralysis and strabismus, Arch. Ophthal. **66:**241, 1961.
11. Brown, H. W.: Surgery of the oblique muscles. In Allen, J. H., editor: Strabismus ophthalmic symposium, St. Louis, 1950, The C. V. Mosby Co.
12. Scott, A. B.: Personal communication.

---

*Available from Dr. S. Jackson, 7801 Woodmont Avenue, Washington, D. C. 20014.
†Available from Ethicon, Inc., Somerville, New Jersey 08876.

Chapter 12

Corneal disease in children

Arthur Gerard DeVoe

Congenital abnormalities

Although the disorders that affect the cornea of children are basically those that affect the adult, there are a number of situations in which corneal aberrations occur only in children or in which their manifestations are significantly different from the same disease in adults. In many cases management of these problems in the child presents a formidable, if not hopeless, problem.

Variations in size, shape, and anterior and posterior curvature are almost limitless, but a descriptive name can usually be found for them in the major treatises on ocular development. It is important to differentiate between macrocornea and congenital glaucoma. Sometimes referred to as anterior megalophthalmos, enlarged corneas occur familially and almost invariably in males. They are bilaterally symmetrical, without opacities, and with little or no functional defect in the early stages other than a relatively high astigmatism. In adult life, however, these eyes are subject to subluxation and opacification of the lens with subsequent glaucoma. Most surgeons have encountered complications when removing these lenses.

The occurrence of corneal opacities in the newborn is most distressing to the parents and nearly equally so to the ophthalmologist who, in most instances, can do little of a remedial nature. It is usually impossible to differentiate between a developmental anomaly and one that is perhaps secondary to intrauterine inflammation. The corneal dermoid, which may vary from a small limbal deformity to a mass completely replacing the entire cornea, is not technically a neoplasm; ordinarily it does not progress. Small lesions need no treatment, and the larger ones are usually not amenable to medical or surgical therapy.

In recent years a number of seemingly unrelated conditions, such as prominent Schwalbe's ring, posterior embryotoxon, persistent mesenchymal tissue in the form of a "glass membrane," congenital anterior synechia (both central and paracentral), congenital corneal leukomata, sclerocornea or scleralization (both segmental or total), and keratoconus posticus, have been classified by Reese and Ellsworth as the anterior chamber cleavage syndrome.[1] It is postulated that the three waves of mesothelial ingrowth from the margin of the optic cup (which in the normal course of events form Descemet's mesothelium, corneal stroma, and iris stroma) are in some manner disturbed from following their usual pattern. The result is that various elements of the anterior segment differentiate improperly or show aberrant adhesions to each other. In its milder degree, such as persistent glass membranes, enlarged Schwalbe's line, and minor anterior synechiae, there may be little or no alteration in function and no treatment required. In the more advanced state, with adhesion of the iris collarette to an opaque cornea, little, if anything, can be done. Many such eyes develop an uncontrollable glaucoma. The causes of these aberrations are unknown. Since the anterior segment, including the anterior chamber, is most actively formed from the seventh to the tenth week, any maternal toxic process during this period could be a factor. I have seen one case, however, in which a mother and child had the identical syndrome suggesting the possibility of a hereditary nature. Others have reported different genetic patterns.

The major complicating factor in advanced anterior cleavage syndrome has been a development of an intractable glaucoma. Filtering surgery, although not offered with much enthusiasm, probably presents the best hope of salvaging the eye. Corneal surgery has not been notably successful in restoring useful vision. It is important to note that in 5 of Reese's 21 cases the mothers had had a viral infection during the first trimester of pregnancy. Goldstein and Cogan have reported extraocular abnormalities associated with sclerocornea in several of their cases (skin, facies, ears, testes, and cerebellum).[2] In one of our cases, a premature retarded infant, spontaneous perforation occurred in the center of the opaque cornea, which required a conjunctival flap to close it.

Injuries

With few exceptions, corneal injuries seen in children do not vary greatly from those in the adult. Notoriously, however, an injury in a child must be approached cautiously. Not infrequently the child was injured while doing something he had been told not to do, with the result that the history may be totally inaccurate. X-rays for foreign bodies and bony injury are mandatory even though the history may not suggest their need.

Stellate injuries to the cornea present a serious problem in repair. If there has not been gross loss of substance, it is possible to suture the major fragments into place and to cover the entire area with a conjunctival flap. In most instances a purse-string flap, which will retract spontaneously in 8 to 10 days, will provide sufficient support during the immediate reparative procedure. If, on the other hand, there has been sufficient loss of substance so that it seems unlikely that

the tissues will adhere properly, a more permanent type of flap, such as that advocated by Gundersen, may be required.[3] Although we have had no experience with the "tire patch" lamellar keratoplasty described by Dohlman it seems a reasonable procedure worth a trial in selected cases.[4] In several instances we have elected to trephine out the entire shattered mass and replace it with a free penetrating keratoplasty. These corneas have not remained clear but have retained the integrity of the globe to preserve it for later reparative surgery. In such instances it is, of course, not possible to trephine the entire button from the host eye. All that is needed is to outline the area to be removed, which is then excised by scissors through the already perforated cornea.

In addition to the usual penetrating injuries from sharp instruments, twigs, sticks, toy bows and arrows, improvised swords, and the like, the child's eye is exposed to chemicals commonly found in the house. Of these, lye and ammonia are probably the most serious offenders. Mothers should be warned to keep these strong chemicals far from investigating fingers. The adage that "if something can go wrong it will go wrong" is quite applicable to the toy chemistry sets that have always intrigued older children. Not content with following the experimental procedure outlined in instruction booklets, sooner or later the child attempts to produce some type of explosive by adding additional ingredients. In many cases a highly successful explosion is obtained at the cost of one or more eyes. There is little that can be done for any severe burn produced by the common strong alkalis or acids. To be successful, copious irrigation must be performed within seconds. This is ordinarily not possible. Forethought and prevention are our most effective weapons against injuries of all kinds.

Dystrophies

Most of the classical dystrophies, such as the granular, macular, lattice, and keratoconus do not show much in the way of objective changes until adolescent years. However if they are detected in a family, all children as well as adults should be examined periodically. We have one family of five girls all with keratoconus in various stages of advancement. We have recently seen a father aged 34 and two sons aged 5 and 7 with exactly comparable deep opacifications in both corneas, none of which have shown any change in a year's time. They may well represent a stationary type of hereditary deep dystrophy of the cornea originally described by Theodore.[5] It seems possible that the children may follow the same course as their father and not suffer significant visual loss.

With regard to corneal dystrophies in general, we are seeing with increasing frequency eyes that do not fit any of the classical or more recently described patterns; it is necessary to describe these lesions anatomically without specifically categorizing them. Many of these do not appreciably decrease vision and do not appear to be progressive in nature.

Infectious processes

Although the usual adult bacterial infections can occur in childhood, they are not common in normal healthy individuals who are not debilitated from one cause or another. In the acute exanthematous diseases, such as measles, chicken pox, and German measles, corneal changes may occur. A superficial punctate keratitis is common and, if searched for, will probably be seen in nearly all cases of measles. It does not ordinarily cause permanent visual loss. However, virulent strains (which are said to commonly produce a phthisical eye in African natives) can also bring about corneal scarring severe enough to effectively reduce vision in Caucasians. German measles, on the other hand, usually produces a superficial keratitis without serious sequelae. In chicken pox, although serious forms of interstitial keratitis have been reported late in the disease, the average case shows little corneal involvement.

Herpes zoster, although uncommon in chil-

dren, has been described. Serious corneal complications are rare. However, herpes simplex can be a most troublesome condition in children and can easily lead to serious and permanent visual loss. I have seen bilateral severe herpes simplex in a 6-weeks-old premature infant which was completely cured by curettage of the epithelium and application of $3\frac{1}{2}\%$ iodine and alcohol to both corneas. Once a herpetic keratitis has appeared, children seem unusually prone to recurrences, frequently with associated stromal involvement and a prolonged course. In our experience, treatment with idoxuridine (IDU) has not been spectacularly successful. However, since the disease is ordinarily self-limiting, it has been our practice to use IDU drops every hour during the day and the ointment at night. If there has not been significant improvement by the third day we proceed to curettage of the corneal epithelium and an ether scrub. In adults who have had repeated and prolonged episodes of stromal herpes we have resorted to lamellar keratoplasty, either full-thickness or split-thickness. However, we have not been sufficiently impressed by the results to advocate this in children. We prefer to wait until the disease has exhausted itself and then perform a penetrating keratoplasty for visual purposes, if necessary.

Phlyctenular disease, largely associated with poor nutrition and environment, was formerly a common cause of corneal opacification. We no longer see it frequently, but when we do treatment with local steroids and attention to vitamins, nutrition, and general surroundings has been usually quite satisfactory.

Erythema multiforme, commonly known in the United States as the Stevens-Johnson syndrome, appears idiopathically as well as secondarily to various infections and drug sensitivities. The sulfonamides and antibiotics have been particularly notorious offenders. Ocular complications are frequent and may in fact present the most serious of the permanent sequelae. Since children and young men are those most frequently afflicted, the disease is a most serious one. Unfortunately there has been no really effective therapy. Xerophthalmia, associated with the mucous membrane shrinkage, is the most serious factor with regard to corneal transplantation. Attempts to remedy this by transplantation of the parotid duct have not been significantly helpful in our experience. In some instances it is possible to install a flush-fitting contact lens under careful supervision.

In 1949 Riley and Day presented 5 cases of a clinical syndrome predominant in the Jewish race that is characterized by alacrima, sweating, drooling, erythematous patches on the skin, intermittent vascular hypertension, vomiting, decreased reflexes, muscular hypotonia, and extreme emotional instability.[6] The ophthalmic problem, chiefly corneal, may be one of the major incapacitating features of the condition. The cornea, usually anesthetic, develops an infiltrative lesion quite suggestive of neuroparalytic keratitis; the eye is usually not very inflamed. Ulceration occurs and may proceed to the point of perforation. Treatment is most difficult, but the frequent instillation of artificial tears combined with moist-chamber spectacles may be helpful. The use of scleral contact lenses is hazardous unless the child is in a position to be followed with great regularity. Although corneal anesthesia permits wearing lenses for a long time, it also makes it possible for an ulcer and secondary infection to develop rather rapidly without the patient's being aware of it. In severe cases permanent lid adhesions may be required.

Luetic interstitial keratitis, in the past a formidable cause of corneal opacification, is so rare these days that most residents go through their entire training period without seeing an active case. However, classically at least 90% of cases of diffuse interstitial keratitis have been considered luetic in origin and of these some 97% have been congenital in origin. Although the disease has been noted at birth, the more usual history is for it to appear some 5 to 10 years after birth. Ordinarily the inherited form is bilateral and

the acquired form is unilateral. Previously, treatment had been notoriously unsuccessful; however, systemic and local cortisone has proved most effective. Since spontaneous clearing is a prominent feature of the condition, active surgical treatment should be postponed until all possible resorption has occurred. These eyes are good candidates for penetrating keratoplasty.

Thesauroses

The thesauroses include a group of diverse conditions characterized by the storage in various tissues of one or more products of metabolism, usually due to the absence of an enzyme normally present in a chain of metabolic events. The absence of this enzyme prevents complete progress to the normal end-product, and results in retention of partially metabolized products. These are frequently inborn errors of metabolism; 123 have been detected and studied.

Cystinosis, a rare disorder of infants and children, is characterized by a deposition of cystine throughout the body. The cornea may present such characteristic deposition of fine, needlelike crystals in its anterior stroma as to be pathognomonic. Systemic manifestations of the disease include dwarfism, renal rickets, acidosis, hypophosphatema, glycosuria, and aminoaciduria. Death usually occurs before the age of 10 because of progressive kidney damage. A prerenal disturbance of the whole amino acid metabolism involves many amino acids, but cystine, because of poor solubility, is deposited in the tissues. A related condition, the oculocerebrorenal syndrome of Lowe, occurs only in males and may present a corneal dystrophy in association with cataract, buphthalmos, and the accompanying systemic signs and symptoms as noted in cystinosis.

In recent years considerable attention has been paid to the mucopolysaccharidoses. These are now generally classified as follows:

MPS I. The true Hurler's syndrome is an autosomal recessive with death occurring before adolescence. Gargoylism and skeletal deformities occur. There is an excess of chondroitin sulfate B and heparatin sulfate in the urine. Corneal clouding occurs and is progressive.

MPS II. Hunter's syndrome is an X-linked recessive Hurler's syndrome. It is a milder form of MPS I with little, if any, corneal clouding.

MPS III. Sanfilippo's syndrome is an autosomal recessive in which heparatin sulfate is found in excess. Mental deficiency is severe. There are no macroscopic corneal findings.

MPS IV. Morquio-Brailsford syndrome is an autosomal recessive with excess keratosulfate in the urine. There is dwarfism, skeletal deformity, lax joints, aortic valve disease, and occasional hazy cornea.

MPS V. Scheie's syndrome is an autosomal recessive with normal intelligence and no gargoylism. There may be thickening of the joints, limitation of motion, and aortic valve disease with marked progressive corneal clouding.

There is nothing pathognomonic about the appearance of the cornea in any of these conditions and it may be clinically difficult to differentiate from the condition described by Maumenee as congenital hereditary corneal dystrophy.

In the few cases in which we have had surgical experience, Hurler's disease has not responded well to penetrating keratoplasty.

Fabry's disease, a hereditary lipoid storage disease in which lipid material accumulates in the myocardium, smooth muscle, kidney, and cornea, and central nervous system, is rare. It might be suspected when a diffuse epithelial haze is noted in early youth that advances to the bronze-colored whorl-like streaks, such as those noted in Fleischer's dominant hereditary whirlpool dystrophy. Similarly, in Tay-Sach's amaurotic familial idiocy, a diffuse haze may occasionally be noted in the corneal stroma. This is thought to be an accumulation of glycolipids.

Although calcium storage diseases do not commonly show much in the way of corneal deposits in childhood, band keratopathy frequently occurs in children with the severe uveitis of Still's disease. These respond quite well to chelation with EDTA.

REFERENCES

1. Reese, A. B., and Ellsworth, R. M.: The anterior chamber cleavage syndrome, Arch. Ophthal. 75:307, 1966.
2. Goldstein, J. E., and Cogan, D. G.: Sclerocornea and associated congenital anomalies, Arch. Ophthal. 67:99, 1962.
3. Gundersen, T.: Conjunctival flaps in the treatment of corneal disease with reference to a new technique of application, Arch. Ophthal. 60:880, 1958.
4. Dohlman, C. H., Boruchoff, A., and Sullivan, G. L.: A technique for the repair of perforated corneal ulcers, Arch. Ophthal. 77:519, 1967.
5. Theodore, F. H.: Congenital type of endothelial dystrophy, Arch. Ophthal. 21:626, 1939.
6. Riley, C. M., Day, R. L., Greeley, D. M., and Langford, W. S.: Central autonomic dysfunction with defective lacrimation, report of 5 cases, Pediatrics 5:468, 1949.

Chapter 13

Clinical experience with the epikeratoprosthesis*

Herbert E. Kaufman and Antonio R. Gasset

In April, 1968, we described experiments in rabbits and monkeys in which a methacrylate covering was bonded to the anterior surface of the cornea by octyl cyanoacrylate monomer.[1] The excellent tolerance of these lenses by the animals suggested the possibility that they might be used in man for the protection of the cornea, as well as for optical improvement. In some cases they would obviate the need for flush-fitting contact lenses; in others, they would permit the optical correction of patients who require the optical benefit of a contact lens but do not have tolerance for such a lens. In still another group, they would perhaps permit the medical protection of the globe in a variety of conditions in which no other sight-preserving technique could be expected to give satisfactory results. Although the technique of epikeratoprosthesis (EKP) is simple and easily adapted to an office procedure, meticulous attention to detail is important. This discussion will outline our present technique for the application of the epikeratoprosthesis and will summarize our clinical results to date.

Material and methods

The prosthesis. The prosthesis is basically an ordinary methyl methacrylate lens similar in many ways to the common corneal contact lens. Any diameter EKP can be employed, but larger diameters seem most useful. Most patients require protection of the cornea and it is desirable for the EKP to be large enough so that the adhesive can remain at the periphery of the lens with the central part of the EKP clear. For these reasons, a 9.5 mm. prosthesis is most commonly used. With an EKP of this size, care must be taken to center the prosthesis on the cornea and not to overlap the limbus.

The normal corneal contact lens has intermediate and secondary curves, which lift the edge away from the cornea to facilitate tear flow. With the EKP, the epithelium of the cornea is removed, and the lens must abut tightly against Bowman's membrane in such a way that epithelium does not grow under it. We use EKP's with a single curve and no intermediate peripheral curves. This brings the edge of the lens tight against Bowman's membrane.

The usual corneal contact lens has a somewhat rounded edge so that it does not abrade the epithelium as it moves. Since there is no movement, EKP lenses are made with a sharp edge angled down to the cornea at an angle of about 45° (Fig. 13-1). Of course, any optical correction can be incorporated into the lens and either a full cut or lenticular anterior surface can be used. It is relatively easy and inexpensive to purchase single curve lens blanks and edge them down at the time that the prosthesis is being applied, cutting the diameter to any which is desired. Even for aphakes, single cut lenses seem as useful as lenticulars, since the weight of the lens

*This work was supported in part by Research and Training Grants from the National Institute of Neurological Diseases and Blindness, National Institutes of Health, U. S. Public Health Service, Bethesda, Maryland. The tissue adhesive was kindly supplied by the Ethicon Company. Mr. Malcolm Dunn fitted and modified the methacrylate lenses used in this study.

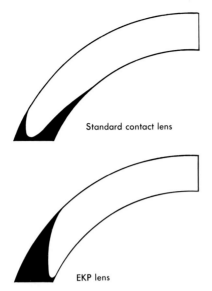

Standard contact lens

EKP lens

Fig. 13-1. The EKP must be tight against the cornea and no epithelium must grow under it. It has a single posterior curve and an edge which slopes at a 30 to 45 degree angle to the corneal surface making a knife edge at the corneal margin. The standard corneal contact lens has peripheral curves, which elevate it from the cornea and facilitate the tear flow required to maintain the epithelium intact. The edge is rounded to minimize epithelial trauma from movement.

is not important because the lens is glued onto the surface of the cornea. The prosthesis can be fitted from a keratometer reading, if one can easily be taken. If not, it is possible to obtain a general fit of the cornea with an ordinary contact lens fitting set, or with an EKP fitting set either before or after removal of the epithelium. The fit seems less critical than that required for fitting ordinary contact lenses, but when in doubt, it seems preferable to use a prosthesis which is slightly steep. The prosthesis must be meticulously cleaned of debris and skin oils and must be lint free.

Since infection can develop between the cornea and Bowman's membrane, it is essential that the prosthesis be absolutely sterile when it is applied and that it be applied under aseptic conditions. We soak the EKP

lenses in glutaraldehyde (Cidex) for at least 20 minutes and wash them 3 times in sterile saline before use; ethylene oxide sterilization may also be used.

Preparing the cornea. The corneal bed should be prepared by removing as much superficial corneal tissue as desired, but *all epithelium must be removed.* In most of our cases, this was done by scraping with a No. 15 Bard-Parker blade. It is important to be certain that no epithelium remains. Animal experiments with denaturing chemicals to aid in removal of epithelium have revealed such significant toxicity that these have not been used.[2]

Patients with bullous keratopathy often have a thin layer of hazy fibrous overgrowth above the original Bowman's membrane. This can be scraped off along with the epithelium, and in some patients, a superficial keratectomy may be desirable before the EKP is applied. It is not necessary for the bed to be absolutely even, but it must be clean. Blood should be irrigated from the surface before the lens is attached.

The surface of the cornea must be absolutely dry or the lens will not adhere properly. Since the bonding takes more than a minute to become firm, dryness after the application of the prosthesis is desirable, and this is facilitated by putting a small amount of cotton in the upper temporal fornix to absorb any tear flow.

The adhesive. Cyanoacrylate adhesives bond biological tissues and adhere by polymerization, not by evaporation. The methyl cyanoacrylate (Eastman 910) is the most familiar and the oldest of the cyanoacrylate monomers used as a tissue adhesive, but is quite irritating to the eye. In our studies, the octyl cyanoacrylate was used exclusively. This seems to be quite nonirritating and is extremely well tolerated under the EKP. The adhesive itself is liquid and sterile. It remains liquid as long as it is in the tube, or in a pool on a plastic surface. It polymerizes only when squeezed into a thin layer between two surfaces, or when exposed to water.

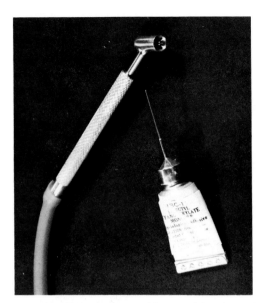

Fig. 13-2. This applicator (designed by Gasset) is attached to a motorized suction pump. It is easily sterilized and facilitates both holding of the EKP during application of the adhesive and the application of the pressure on the EKP during bonding to the cornea. Other sterilizable contact lens applicators that can hold the EKP are also usable.

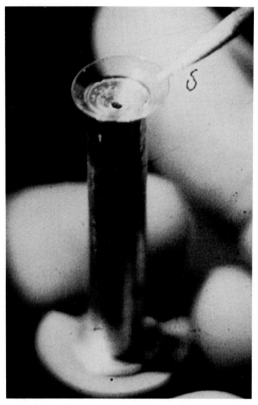

Fig. 13-3. EKP with adhesive. Adhesive is applied around the total circumference of the EKP so that the lens is completely bonded to the cornea and epithelium cannot grow under it. An excess of adhesive in the center can cause optical interference and adhesive on the outside can be irritating.

Application of the adhesive. After removing the corneal epithelium, drying the cornea and inserting a small piece of cotton into the temporal upper fornix, the surgeon holds the lens on a suction device. Any suction used for contact lenses is suitable but we prefer the metal instrument shown in Fig. 13-2, which is attached to a suction pump such as a motor driven erysiphake pump. A small amount of adhesive is squeezed into a sterile polyethylene cup (the top of the container of a disposable syringe is well suited for this). Then, using loupes or a surgical microscope, a sterile toothpick is dipped into the glue and touched to the inside of the EKP at its peripheral margin. The glue is then spread around the edge, care being taken not to spread it to the center of the lens. *Very little adhesive* should be used, although the inside circumference adjacent to the edge of the

EKP should be completely covered all the way around (Fig. 13-3). If too much adhesive is used, it will be squeezed into the center of the lens, causing some optical interference, and may be squeezed outside the EKP, producing some irritation. If it appears that there is too much adhesive on the rim of the EKP before it is placed on the eye, a sterile toothpick which has not been immersed in adhesive can be moved around the rim to remove some of the material. There is no need to hurry during this procedure since the adhesive will not dry.

The EKP is retained on the suction applicator with glue spread around the inside rim while the cornea, with its epithelium previously removed, is dried and cleaned a final time. The EKP is centered over the cornea while the eye is held stationary, and when centering appears perfect, the EKP is firmly applied to the cornea. The prosthesis cannot be moved after it contacts the tissue and must be perfectly centered before application. Pressure is maintained on the EKP, with the eye stationary, for at least 1 minute, and even after removal of the suction holder, the field should be kept dry for at least an additional minute. If fluid comes in contact with the cornea too early, the adhesive will become whitish and powdery, and the bond between the EKP and the cornea will not be firm and long-lasting. Since some patients get a moderate iritis and irritation from removing the epithelium, we dilate the pupil for a few days. The amount of reaction and discomfort varies greatly from patient to patient, and usually disappears within a day or two. In some patients, especially in children whose epithelium is traumatically removed by vigorous scraping, the eye may be inflamed for 2 weeks. Beginning approximately 1 hour after the insertion of the prosthesis, antibiotic drops are used 3 or 4 times until the next morning and then discontinued. Steroids are not generally used.

It is important that a new tube of adhesive be used each day, since the adhesive, on standing, loses its ability to polymerize and form a firm bond.[3, 4]

Results

In all, 30 eyes have been treated with EKP and the prostheses have been in place up to 5 months (Table 13-1). The procedure and approach to different pathologic conditions have varied and the use of the EKP has varied with the specific condition to be treated.

Bullous keratopathy. The epikeratoprosthesis has been applied to 10 patients with bullous keratopathy. All of these patients were aphakic; the bullous keratopathy in most patients was from a Fuchs' endothelial dystrophy which became worse after cataract extraction.

In all patients, the epikeratoprosthesis relieved pain. Two of these patients complained that if they rubbed the eye there was some discomfort, but since they could refrain from this maneuver, the prosthesis was extremely well tolerated. One patient without significant previous symptoms had mild discomfort after the application of the prosthesis. Since vision was 20/20 after keratoplasty in the other eye, the prosthesis was removed.

It was anticipated that the epikeratoprosthesis would provide considerable improvement of vision in patients with bullous keratopathy. Zucker showed that in the rabbit stromal hydration reduced vision relatively little compared to the irregular astigmatism of the epithelium.[5] The removal of this irregular epithelium and its replacement by an optically smooth contact lens might cause dramatic improvement in vision. In addition, some of the distortion and haze in patients with bullous keratopathy comes from a haze above Bowman's membrane. This is easily removed with a knife blade at the time of application of the EKP, and this, too, might improve vision.

In fact, the visual results in patients with bullous keratopathy were variable. Three patients had significant improvement of vision to a level better than 20/200 and could function in ordinary ways which were previously impossible. In other patients, although visual acuity was slightly improved, the change was not significant, and not adequate to permit ordinary activity. Clinically, these patients seem to fall into two different categories. Some patients developed many folds in Descemet's membrane and exhibited relatively slight improvement in visual acuity. Others, even with a thickened stroma in which Descemet's membrane was not folded, appeared to have considerable improvement in vision. Since the irregular epithelial astigmatism was removed and stromal haze did not seem adequate to account for the poor vision, it

Table 13-1. Conditions treated with epikeratoprosthesis

	Number of eyes	Best postoperative visual acuity	Therapeutic result
Bullous keratopathy	10	20/60	9 patients had relief of pain; 3 had significant visual improvement to 20/200 or better
Neuroparalytic keratitis	5	20/30	Recurrent ulceration prevented; visual acuity improved in all cases
Stevens-Johnson disease	6	20/20	4 had relief of pain and improvement of vision; 1 became infected, and 1 spontaneously came off and was not replaced
Keratitis sicca	1	—	Recurrent ulcerations stopped, pain disappeared and vision improved in spite of mature cataract (20/200)
Epidermal dysplasia with abnormal lids, corneal irregularities, and photophobia	1	—	Pain and photophobia decreased; vision improved
Old ulcerating eye burn	1	—	Symptoms relieved; vision improved
Unexplained juvenile corneal epithelial irregularities—vascularization with photophobia	2	20/60	Photophobia and pain disappeared
Corneal epithelial dystrophy—type previously undescribed	1	—	Corneal thickness decreased, but symptoms and photophobia only improved slightly
Monocular aphakia, corneal scar (child)	1	20/25	Asymptomatic, binocular fusion
Normal corneas—blind eyes	2	—	Irritated eye for 7 to 14 days after epithelial debridement; then corneal thickness became normal and symptoms disappeared

seemed, clinically, that the folds in Descemet's membrane contributed a significant irregular astigmatism and interfered with the optics of the eye enough to maintain the reduced visual acuity.

In three patients, the cornea was observed to become thicker, and blood vessels began to grow into the thickened cornea. All of these patients had been treated early in our experience with the epikeratoprosthesis. During the early phase, the importance of keeping the cornea dry and maintaining the dryness and pressure on the EKP for some time after application of prosthesis was not appreciated. The powdery appearing glue apparently did not bond well, and in all of those patients, it could be shown that epithe-lium was growing under the prosthesis, partially elevating the membrane. Experimental work by Green,[6] and recent work in our laboratory indicates that the stroma cannot be left exposed or it becomes cloudy and markedly swollen.[7] When the stroma is protected by a properly sealed prosthesis, this swelling does not occur. It seems likely that the prosthesis did not adequately protect the stroma and was partially elevated. In one of the patients when the prosthesis was removed and reapplied, the stroma immediately dehydrated and the vessels markedly regressed.

In spectacle-wearing patients with good aphakic vision in one eye and bullous keratopathy with aphakia in the other eye, a choice between a plano EKP and an aphakic correction could be made. Both were tried and, in general, patients who wore spectacles preferred a plano EKP.

Neuroparalytic keratitis. Six cases of neuroparalytic keratitis have been treated with an epikeratoprosthesis. In all cases, exposure and sensory deficit had resulted in corneal ulceration and topical medication had been inadequate to protect the cornea. Most of these patients had deficiency of both the fifth and seventh nerve on the involved side. Some were handicapped by hemiplegia and other deficits that prohibited any other type of therapy which would still preserve vision. One had no sensation after an attack of herpes zoster and, despite persistent iridocyclitis, had an EKP to treat recurrent corneal ulceration. In this case, steroid administration was continued after the EKP as before.

In all cases, the cornea was protected uneventfully. In no case was there any decrease in vision under the epikeratoprosthesis, and in those patients in whom the epithelial surface was somewhat roughened, the epikerato-

prosthesis improved vision with the best visual acuity being corrected to 20/30.

Stevens-Johnson disease or essential shrinkage of the conjunctiva. Six patients with Stevens-Johnson's disease, or essential shrinkage of the conjunctiva received EKP's. Three were patients who had not tolerated flush-fitting scleral lenses. Although the EKP's provided good protection, it appears that they were more likely to remain in place for a prolonged time if Bowman's membrane was intact, and were more likely to come off sooner if affixed directly to stroma. Fig. 13-4 shows one patient with early Stevens-Johnson's disease treated with an EKP.

Miscellaneous disorders. A variety of additional conditions were also studied. Keratitis sicca and an old corneal alkali burn with late ulceration responded well to application of the EKP. Four children's eyes with irregular epithelium, vascularization, and photophobia were treated. After scraping the epithelium with a knife and application of the EKP, the eyes were red and sensitive for about 2 weeks. Mydriatics were given, but corticosteroids were not used and the irrita-

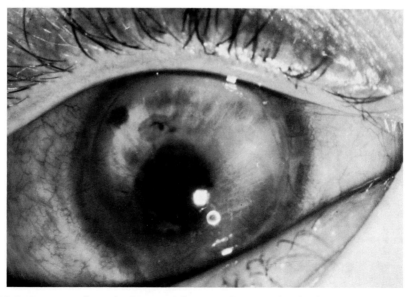

Fig. 13-4. Patient with early Stevens-Johnson's disease who had a previous epithelial defect. The EKP has been in place for 4 weeks. Visual acuity is 20/20.

tion disappeared. This is similar to the reaction seen with corneal scraping alone, and was felt to be caused by the traumatic epithelial removal rather than the EKP or adhesive. One of these children had epidermal dysplasia with clearly abnormal lids. This patient was dramatically improved both in terms of visual acuity and of symptoms. In 2 eyes the etiology of the superficial corneal disease was unexplained, but both had significant improvement of visual acuity and symptoms. One additional child had a bizarre epithelial dystrophy, a thickened cornea and deafness. She had previously been studied at many medical centers and no definite diagnosis of her condition had been made. The EKP caused her cornea to become thinner; however, very slight improvement of her subjective symptoms occurred.

Three normal corneas have tolerated the EKP up to 3 months. The corneal thickness, as measured by the Haag-Streit pachometer, initially slightly increased, returned to normal within 2 or 3 weeks, and has remained normal. One of these was a child with monocular aphakia after a corneal laceration and traumatic cataract who could not tolerate a corneal contact lens. The EKP is being used solely for optical correction and vision is 20/25 despite the laceration scar in the pupillary area. There are no symptoms attributable to the lens.

Complications

Five of the EKP's came off spontaneously. This occurred, for the most part, early in our experience before we realized the importance of maintaining a dry field and using fresh adhesive. No damage to any cornea appears to have resulted from this, and most were easily replaced on an outpatient basis.

Six of the EKP's were intentionally removed. Because of the experimental nature of the technique, if benefits were not significant the eye was dried, the EKP was grasped with a forceps, and the prosthesis was lifted off. One of these patients had the EKP removed to permit penetrating keratoplasty. In three others, the bond was imperfect, epithelium was seen under a margin of the lens, and the unprotected stroma began to swell and vascularize. The lenses were easily removed and replaced.

Three patients had a transient local infiltration under the EKP. In one patient, cared for elsewhere, this appeared to be a significant infection. In the others, the infiltrates disappeared after treatment with topical antibiotics without significant residue. These infiltrates were seen before we realized the necessity for having absolutely sterile lenses and performing the procedure aseptically.

Discussion

In our laboratory we have studied adhesives since 1962. Since 1964, we have investigated the use of various substances, including silicone membranes, for corneal protection. Our experience indicates that silicone, with a soft surface that is easily scratched, is optically poor and is an inferior substance for corneal protection to the hard, optically perfect, easily obtained methacrylate. Although Dohlman and colleagues originally believed that methacrylate would not be a good material to bond to the cornea,[8] our experimental and clinical results have shown it to be suitable[1, 9] and Dohlman and colleagues have had similar results.[10]

Clinical experience indicates that when the epithelium is removed and the stroma exposed, corneal swelling and vascularization occur. When, however, the stromal surface is protected by the EKP, this seems not to occur. Although metabolic benefits to the stroma from the epithelium cannot be ruled out, this experience indicates that the most essential function of the epithelium is protection of the underlying stroma and perhaps the prevention of loss of essential metabolites and electrolytes.[6] Anoxia and problems of lens movement which can damage the epithelium under normal contact lenses appear to be of no consequence with the EKP.

Previous work indicates that cyanoacrylate adhesives can persist more than 14 months.[11]

The bond, however, depends not only on the persistence of the adhesive, but on the persistence of the tissue to which the EKP is bonded. If a lens were bonded to epithelium, the epithelium would come off and the bond would be of no value. Bowman's membrane, especially in its superficial portions, appears to have little or no turnover without an epithelial cover, and seems an ideal site for tissue bonding. It is not clear whether stromal lamellae and keratocytes are so inert and it may be that the bonding to bare stroma will be less permanent. This may be why we observe that in Stevens-Johnson's disease the EKP's provide good protection if used early (Fig. 13-4) (before Bowman's membrane is destroyed), but tend to loosen in the more advanced cases.

The adhesion to the cornea denuded of epithelium may be facilitated by the collar of epithelium around the EKP. In addition, the negative stromal swelling pressure should draw the methacrylate prosthesis against the surface and hold it firm. Although the longest observation of an EKP in man is 5 months there is every reason to believe that the EKP may stay on the cornea considerably longer.

The successful use of the EKP on normal corneas suggests that it will provide an alternative to refractive keratoplasty and intracameral lenses. The EKP seems to offer less risk and can be changed if differing corrections are required.

Any new development with a short period of observation must be accepted cautiously, but the procedure is so simple and so effective in most cases that additional information should soon become available.

Summary

The epikeratoprosthesis is a special methacrylate lens which is bonded to the corneal surface after removal of the epithelium. The bonding agent is octyl cyanoacrylate adhesive. The application can generally be done as a simple outpatient procedure under topical anesthesia, although meticulous attention to detail is necessary for optimal results.

Bullous keratopathy, neuroparalytic keratitis, Stevens-Johnson's disease, keratitis sicca, and other conditions have been successfully treated. The EKP may also be used as an alternative to refractive keratoplasty or intraocular lenses to provide essential optical correction when regular corneal contact lenses cannot be used.

REFERENCES

1. Gasset, A. R., and Kaufman, H. E.: Epikeratoprosthesis; replacement of superficial cornea by methyl methacrylate. Presented to the Association for Research in Ophthalmology, Tampa, Florida, April, 1968, Amer. J. Ophthal. 66:641, 1968.
2. Hood, I., Ellison, E. D., Gasset, A. R., and Kaufman, H. E.: Histological evaluation of corneal epithelium removal. In preparation.
3. Ethicon, Inc. Medical Research Department Review: Methyl 2-cyanoacrylate monomer; a biodegradable plastic tissue adhesive, Feb., 1966.
4. Gasset, A. R., Ellison, E. D., and Kaufman, H. E.: Ocular tolerance to cyanoacrylate monomer tissue adhesive analogues. In preparation.
5. Zucker, B. B.: Hydration and transparency of corneal stroma, Arch. Ophthal. 75:228, 1966.
6. Green, K.: Epithelial ion transport in relation to the corneal hydration. Presented to the Association for Research in Ophthalmology, Tampa, Florida, April, 1968.
7. Gasset, A. R., and Kaufman, H. E.: Comparative study of the effect of the absence of corneal epithelium with and without the protection of the epikeratoprosthesis. In preparation.
8. Dohlman, C. H., Refojo, M. F., Carroll, J. M., and Gasset, A. R.: Artificial corneal epithelium, Arch. Ophthal. 79:360, 1968.
9. Gasset, A. R., and Kaufman, H. E.: Epikeratoprosthesis. Presented at the Corneal Research Meeting, Philadelphia, June, 1968.
10. Dohlman, C. H., Carroll, J. M., and Refojo, M. F.: Artificial corneal epithelium. Presented at the First South African International Ophthalmological Symposium, Johannesburg, September, 1968.
11. Reynolds, R. C., Fassett, D. W., and Astill, B. D.: Absorption of methyl 2-cyanoacrylate-2-^{14}C from full thickness skin incisions in the guinea pig and its fate in vivo, J. Surg. Res. 6:3, 1966.

Chapter 14

Uveitis in children

Moderator:
Robert S. Coles

Panelists:
Herbert E. Kaufman
Rudolf Witmer
Samuel J. Kimura
Dan M. Gordon

The challenge

Herbert E. Kaufman

Robert Oppenheimer once defined the Institute for Advanced Study at Princeton as a place where we go to explain to each other what we don't understand. I think our position in the field of uveitis is very similar to that.

Uveitis in children is not as common a problem as uveitis in adults. Three to 5% of all cases of uveitis occur in children, although, on the average, children make up approximately 20% of the population.

As such statistics are examined one cannot help but wonder whether uveitis is in fact less common in children, or whether its detection is less common. One of the points I would like to make is that the presenting signs and symptoms of uveitis vary greatly according to the age of the child. Therefore, considering children as a group is a fallacy; they tend to be grouped according to age, and there are unique problems that are not seen in adult patients. One of the most fruitful things that we can do is to consider the ways in which uveitis in children differs from uveitis in adults.

For example, in the neonate, primary iritis is rarely seen unless there is severe corneal disease. The typical diagnoses made in the neonate are toxoplasmosis, cytomegalic inclusion disease, and uveitis associated with a systemic disease. These specific syndromes will be discussed in detail by others.

There are two points about this I would like to make. First, with both toxoplasmosis and cytomegalic inclusion disease, it must be understood that the serologic titers in the proved cases may be extremely low, and the height of the titer is of no significance. I have been making this point for the last 8 or 9 years. The neonate is the one group in which a definite diagnosis of these infections, when they present in an eye, can be made by serologic means. Although the mother makes antibodies, they are high molecular weight antibodies (the gamma-M antibody and 19-S antibody), which do not cross the placenta. If antibodies to a specific organism, such as toxoplasmosis or a salivary gland virus of this specific type of immunoglobulin, are found in a neonate, there is very good evidence with a single determination that this is a definite diagnosis.

The other point is that these eye symptoms are associated with systemic disease in the neonate. There are formes frustes of toxoplasmosis in which only the eye or the brain may be involved. I had two patients with ocular toxoplasmosis who had clear signs of encephalitis with cells in the spinal fluid. It is known both from animal studies and from several case reports of acute toxoplasmosis, that the acute disease with proliferative organisms responds well to pyrimethamine (Daraprim) and sulfa. These two children had an almost immediate disappearance of the cells and other signs of inflammation in their cerebrospinal fluid. I am convinced that we saved some brain tissue which otherwise would have been lost, so

143

I think it is important to think of neonatal uveitis as a symptom of a systemic disease.

The worst problem in uveitis in children is chronic cyclitis, and this syndrome is different in children than it is in adults. It is a specific kind of syndrome that causes everyone great concern. There are just a few comments I would like to make about it.

Almost nothing is known about the causes of chronic cyclitis in children. Initially it was thought that if band keratopathy was present, it was related to rheumatoid arthritis. I think now the overwhelming evidence is that this clearly is not the case. Any chronic cyclitis can cause band keratopathy, whether it is related to the rheumatoid arthritis or not, and the band keratopathy per se is of very little diagnostic significance.

A second problem in chronic cyclitis involves steroid therapy. If these children are given steroids and then the dosage is changed (especially if it is reduced), the steroid withdrawal syndrome results with typical arthralgias, pain, and malaise, which in the past has been interpreted as rheumatoid arthritis. There is, I think, good reason to believe that at least many of the children who were previously thought to have rheumatoid arthritis may well not have had it. They may have had only a steroid withdrawal syndrome. Although we find occasional children with rheumatoid arthritis, in most of them we do not really know what is going on. If it is assumed that this disease is a medical disease and it is treated with the same general philosophy as rheumatoid arthritis, I think an enormous amount of good can be done for these children.

Just as in arthritis, it is not known what causes this syndrome. The syndrome cannot be cured in a short period of time, but with proper management these children can be made to see over a prolonged period of time. There are several things about this syndrome I think are of crucial importance. First of all, children, especially the age group from 1 to 10, do not generally have pain, redness, and photophobia from the uveitis. If a young child has pain, the possibility of herpes, lues, or one of a variety of corneal diseases should be considered.

Typically, these children are seen by the ophthalmologist not because of the usual symptoms of uveitis, or even because of blurred vision, but because they have band keratopathy, secondary cataract, glaucoma, or some other complication of juvenile uveitis.

These children are generally brought to the ophthalmologist because of the complications, and almost always the child has had uveitis for several months before he is brought in for treatment.

I think it is necessary to have a totally different philosophy about this type of uveitis than, for example, the typical posterior uveitis which will be well within 6 weeks to 3 months. I think the ophthalmologist should assume that this disease will not stop; this uveitis will remain active for months or years. As it becomes difficult to see through the cornea, it may be thought to be inactive; however, it is better to act as if the uveitis is never inactive. As the lens becomes cloudy it becomes difficult to see cells and flare, and although it appears to be inactive, it is not; in fact, all the secondary complications are occurring. Dilatation in these children needs to be constant and assiduous. These children frequently develop band keratopathy. In my experience EDTA by itself has sometimes worked perfectly well. Frequently it is necessary to chip off Bowman's membrane with the calcium in it. It is often said that if Bowman's membrane is damaged in any way this will produce permanent corneal haze and decrease vision. This has simply not been my experience in any case, and I have chipped the membrane a number of times.

This is a chronic type of iritis that goes on forever. If surgery is done and a small pupil results, it will rapidly and completely occlude. If a hole is ever made in this eye, it is important to make an opening in the iris as large as possible, or the surgery will be worth nothing, at least in my experience.

Again, in this problem of chronic cyclitis, associated arthritis is occasionally found, but an etiologic diagnosis is rarely made. It goes on for months or years, but with intelligent management it can usually be controlled, at least to the point that vision can persist until the disease eventually burns itself out, which, in my experience, is often during the teen-age period.

One of the typical syndromes unique to children is a typical larval granuloma of the macula caused by the *Toxocara canis*. Another syndrome that can occur from larval granulomatosis is a complete detachment of the retina that simulates either a retinoblastoma or a proliferative retinitis with a total retinal detachment. In very young children a complete detachment of the retina usually occurs; in the older ones there is usually a macular granuloma.

Sarcoid uveitis in children may present with the pink nodules (that are diagnostic when they occur) and the big mutton-fat keratitic precipitates. These begin to occur generally from age 7 to 10 years. Paradoxically, in Scandinavia they occur in the very fairest white persons, and in this country they tend to occur most frequently in the darkest Negroes. Exactly why this is so, no one knows.

Typical recurrent posterior chorioretinitis and sarcoid are seen in adults. Pars planitis and acute plastic iritis occur in older children. Older children (from 8 to 15 years of age) complain of pain, redness, and photophobia, whereas this is extremely rare in the younger children. The problem in young children is really the problem of chronic cyclitis, which is a very difficult problem.

Detection

Rudolf Witmer

Incidence, symptoms, and clinical picture

Uveitis in children is not so very rare, particularly if all cases of central chorioretinitis are included. Uveitis should be suspected in every case of amblyopia, especially bilateral amblyopia. Among all uveitis patients, from 6 to 10% are either children below the age of 16 or those with a history of uveitis beginning before that age.

Amblyopia may be the only symptom. Usually the disturbance of central vision is very slowly progressive. The children will, therefore, often come at a late stage, with one eye almost blind and visual acuity below 6/20 in the other eye. An acute onset is rare, but may occur in the so-called articulo-ocular syndrome. The children usually do not complain of any pain. Their eyes may become red and inflamed, usually after some physical effort or mechanical irritation, such as rubbing.

The patterns of uveitis in children will be discussed later by Dr. Kimura. I will, therefore, only mention those features which seem important for the detection of uveitis and possibly for the etiologic diagnosis.

Three main types can be differentiated:

Anterior uveitis. Anterior uveitis may start with an acute onset, or it may be chronic from the very beginning. It leads often to the typical syndrome of band-shaped keratopathy, anterior uveitis with many posterior synechiae, early complicated cataract, and eventually secondary glaucoma. It has been found in combination with Still's disease. Most children do not have any sign of this very rare disease, although many have a history of monoarticular arthritis.

Anterior uveitis may also be combined with keratitis, usually metaherpetic. Circumscribed iris atrophy may be the only sign of this type of iritis.

Chronic cyclitis. Chronic cyclitis is characterized by little or no irritation in the anterior segment. Posterior synechiae are rare, and the lens remains clear for a long time.

The most important alteration is found in the vitreous body where heavy infiltration occurs. Vitreous floaters may be adherent to the posterior capsule of the lens.

Membrane formation over the lower part of the pars plana, perivasculitis of peripheral retinal vessels, or edema of the posterior pole and cyst formation in the macula are typical features. Vision is often very much reduced. The term "pars planitis" not only is monstrous from the ethnologic point of view, but is also wrong morphologically, since most cases of chronic cyclitis are characterized by inflammation of the whole uveal tract. The term "panuveitis" would therefore be more appropriate.

Posterior uveitis. Posterior uveitis can be differentiated into central, juxtapapillary, and disseminated chorioretinitis.

Diagnosis

Biomicroscopy. Examination with slit lamp and contact lens, therefore, is most essential in all these different forms of uveitis. Indentation of the pars plana by scleral depression in combination with the three-mirror Goldmann lens reveals the extreme periphery of the fundus. Cells in the vitreous can be localized, as well as vitreous detachment and retinal tears, which may occur as late complications in cases of uveitis. Fresh infiltration of the retina and choroid is easily seen with the slit beam.

Fluorescent angiography is also very helpful and permits differentiation between quiet scars and active inflammatory infiltration.

The very important question now arises of whether or not the clinical appearance or the localization of the inflammation within the uveal tract will permit an *etiologic diagnosis*. I do not think that this is possible in the strict sense of the word. The differentiation of the clinical picture and its combination with other systemic diseases will only help to clarify the uveitis, but, with the exception of some of the very typical types of central chorioretinitis, it will not reveal the etiology. I would like to discuss this problem on the basis of a survey of over 120 children suffering from uveitis.

The procedure in a case of uveitis in a child is very similar to that in the adult. The *case history* is very important: one should inquire about infectious diseases, allergic conditions, joint diseases, pets, familial incidence, and so on.

Laboratory tests should include sedimentation rate and complete blood picture. Serologic tests in our laboratory include hemagglutination for tuberculosis, dye test for toxoplasmosis, and antistreptolysin-O test. Furthermore, we make agglutination tests for salmonellosis, brucellosis, and leptospirosis, and the usual complement-fixation test for syphilis; in a limited number of patients we have done complement-fixation tests for influenza, adenovirus, mumps, psittacosis virus, and for PPLO, and other tests for the detection of the rheumatoid factor.

The number of patients with *anterior uveitis* is small; this disease concerns more small children. Many of these children had a history of monoarticular arthritis, but very rarely did we find a typical rheumatoid arthritis. An additional survey for the presence of the rheumatoid factor was completely unrewarding. In only one girl could the diagnosis of Still's disease be made. We, therefore, cannot prove the rheumatoid nature of this severe disease, and even if we could prove it in a few cases, we still do not know the etiology of rheumatoid disease. It is interesting that at an early age more girls are found to suffer from so-called rheumatoid uveitis, while in young adults, many more males are affected, often in combination with ankylosing spondylitis. In the adult, rheumatoid arthritis becomes rather common, but its combination with uveitis is very rare. Therefore, we must assume that hormonal factors may be of some importance in this disease.

The group with *chronic cyclitis* and panuveitis is the largest. There are definitely more boys than girls affected. Different factors speak in favor of an infectious etiology. Many of these childern suffer from recurrent bacterial infections of the respiratory tract (sinus, tonsils, pneumonia). Many have had streptococcal infections. An additional survey for the presence of complement-fixing antibodies against mycoplasma pneumoniae (PPLO) gave a higher incidence of positive titers in this group than in others. Many give a history of allergic conditions (asthma, hay fever). There is also a rather high incidence of increased sedimentation rate and lymphocytosis among these children. We can, therefore, assume that different infections may be the

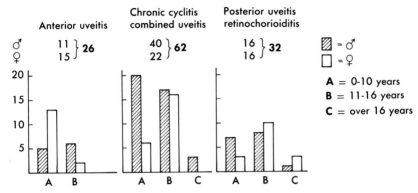

Fig. 14-1. Distribution of age, sex, and localization in 120 cases of uveitis in children.

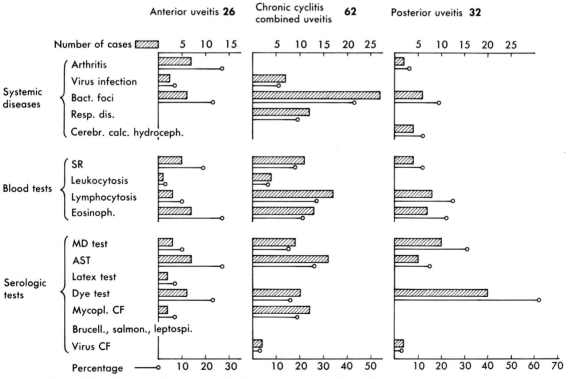

Fig. 14-2. Clinical and laboratory findings associated with uveitis.

cause of this typical entity, that perhaps microbial or viral allergies and even parasites may be responsible for these cases.

The group with *posterior uveitis* is smaller. There is no sex difference. It is not surprising that there is a very high incidence of positive dye tests, and in four of these children cerebral calcifications could be demonstrated, which suggested congenital toxoplasmosis. But there are also other infections to be kept in mind. In two of the children there was strong evidence that the choroidal disease was caused by a tuberculous infection.

Puncture of the anterior chamber is of limited value in these cases, in which there is practically no inflammatory reaction in the anterior segment. Among the 120 children only thirty were subjected to this diagnostic procedure, which in children of the younger age group requires general anesthesia. The method of quantitative serology gave positive results in only 2 cases. About 2 years ago we started to study aqueous humor cytology with the electron microscope. This technique may be very useful in the differentiation between inflammatory and tumor cells.

I would like to mention the value of electron microscopy in the examination of iris biopsies. We were able to demonstrate virus particles in the iris of a patient with metaherpetic iridocyclitis. With children this procedure may eventually be justified.

Conclusion

Uveitis in children is not very different from what is usually seen in adults. The only exception seems to be the anterior uveitis syndrome of a probably rheumatoid nature, but this has still be be proved. Chronic cyclitis corresponds to the clinical picture observed in young adults, and posterior uveitis does not differ from the appearance of chorioretinitis later in life.

The prognosis of uveitis in children is rather poor, but I strongly believe that some cases do heal. Although many have serious visual loss, very remarkable improvements are possible.

Patterns*

Samuel J. Kimura

Uveitis in children has been of particular interest to us and has been the subject of two previous reports.[1, 2] This report brings up to date the analysis of all the cases of uveitis studied in patients 16 years of age or younger.

Approximately 3,900 patients with uveitis have been studied thoroughly in our Uveitis Survey Clinic in the past 18 years. Of these patients 444 were 16 years of age or younger when their initial symptoms and signs of uveitis became manifest. The series is not a random sample of uveitis in the population, for many patients are referred to us from

*This study was supported in part by United States Public Health Program Research Project grant NB 6207. I wish to thank Mrs. Myra Scalarone and Mrs. Peggy Yamada for their help in preparing this paper.

all parts of the world because of the severity of the disease. Our clinical impression, however, is that the figures presented here are probably close to the true incidence of the various types of uveitis seen in our area (California). This impression is gained mainly by comparing our data with those from our private practice files and the outpatient clinic data.

The classification of uveitis that is used in the Uveitis Survey Clinic is the following:

    I. Anterior uveitis
      A. Iridocyclitis
        1. Juvenile rheumatoid arthritis (Still's)
        2. Ankylosing spondylitis
        3. Behçet's syndrome
        4. Sarcoidosis
        5. Trauma
        6. Unknown
      B. Cyclitis
        1. Chronic cyclitis
        2. Cyclitis, possible nematode
        3. Fuchs' syndrome of heterochromic cyclitis

C. Keratouveitis
   1. Herpes simplex
   2. Herpes zoster
D. Lens–induced
E. Syphilis
II. Posterior uveitis
   A. Chorioretinitis
      1. Tuberculous
      2. Unknown
         a. Juxtapapillary chorioretinitis
         b. Disseminated chorioretinitis
   B. Retinochoroiditis
      1. Toxoplasmic
      2. Syphilitic
      3. Toxocara (nematode)
III. Diffuse uveitis
   A. Vogt-Koyanagi-Harada's disease
   B. Sarcoidosis
   C. Sympathetic ophthalmia

This classification is an old one and not an ideal one, but we feel that categorizing uveitis as to the area of maximum disease is helpful in teaching. The diagnosis of uveitis includes so many entities of unknown etiology that an etiologic classification is not possible. The classification proposed by Woods,

Table 14-1. Distribution of types of uveitis

Type	Number of patients
Anterior uveitis	250
Posterior uveitis	178
Diffuse uveitis	16

which separates the different uveitis entities into granulomatous and nongranulomatous[3] has not been too useful for us, for it is not often possible to fit our cases into this classification, particularly in posterior uveitis.

Analysis of cases

Four hundred forty-four patients ages 16 years or younger, out of a series of over 3,900 uveitis cases were studied during the past 18 years. These cases are drawn from our Uveitis Survey files, and many were referred because of the special problem a given case presented.

There is more anterior uveitis in our series than posterior uveitis. Table 14-1 shows the distribution of the 444 cases classified as anterior, posterior, and diffuse uveitis. Fig. 14-3 plots the age at onset of uveitis in children of our series. The 49 cases with onset of disease during the first year of life are of patients with congenital toxoplasmosis.

Anterior uveitis

Of 250 children with anterior uveitis, all except 18 cases had an onset of disease between the ages of 4 and 16. Fig. 14-4 shows that anterior uveitis occurs with almost equal frequency after 3 to 4 years of age. Table

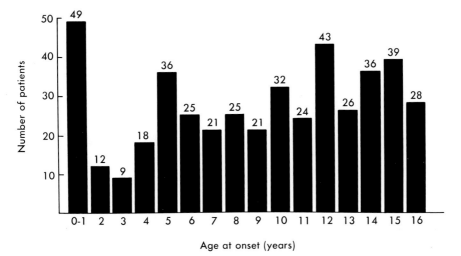

Age at onset (years)

Fig. 14-3. Uveitis in children (444 patients).

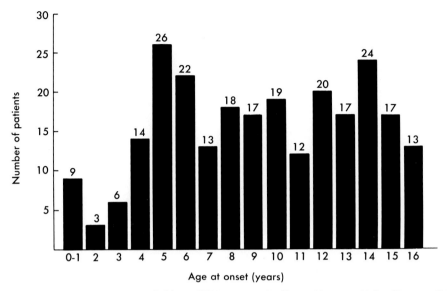

Fig. 14-4. Anterior uveitis in children (250 patients). (From Hogan, M.J., Kimura, S.J., and Spencer, W. H.: Visceral larva migrans and peripheral retinitis, J.A.M.A. **194** [13]: 1345-1347, 1965.)

Table 14-2. Sex distribution of anterior uveitis

Type	Male	Female
Juvenile rheumatoid arthritis	6	37
Iridocyclitis, type unknown	32	52
Cyclitis	55	36

Table 14-3. Distribution of types of anterior uveitis (250 patients)

Type	Number of patients
Juvenile rheumatoid arthritis	43
Iridocyclitis unknown	85
Iridocyclitis associated with spondylitis	2
Iridocyclitis associated with sarcoidosis	2
Chronic cyclitis	82
Cyclitis-nematode	10
Keratouveitis	10
Fuchs' heterochromic cyclitis	9
Behçet's syndrome	1
Other	6

14-2 shows the sex distribution of the three most common types of anterior uveitis. Uveitis associated with juvenile rheumatoid arthritis is much more frequent in female children. Iridocyclitis of unknown etiology or disease association occurs in both sexes but slightly more often in female children. Chronic cyclitis, however, was seen in more males than females.

Table 14-3 lists the types of anterior uveitis that have been studied in our series. Roughly one-third of the iridocyclitis patients have juvenile rheumatoid arthritis, and almost all of the cases are chronic and very low grade. By the time iridocyclitis is recognized there is usually a band keratopathy present. Fig. 14-5 charts the age at onset of the iridocyclitis in patients with an associated juvenile

rheumatoid arthritis. There is 17.2% of the anterior uveitis (low grade chronic iridocyclitis) associated with juvenile rheumatoid arthritis.

Iridocyclitis associated with spondylitis is rare; however, when it occurs, it is in older children. There are 2 cases in this series, and in both the iridocyclitis became chronic after an acute onset. By the Woods' classification, these cases are nongranulomatous.

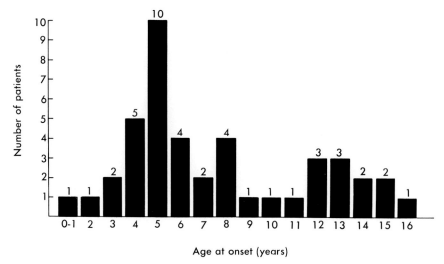

Fig. 14-5. Juvenile rheumatoid arthritis (43 patients.) (From Hogan, M. J., Kimura, S. J., and Spencer, W. H.: Visceral larva migrans and peripheral retinitis, J.A.M.A. **194** [13]: 1345-1347, 1965.)

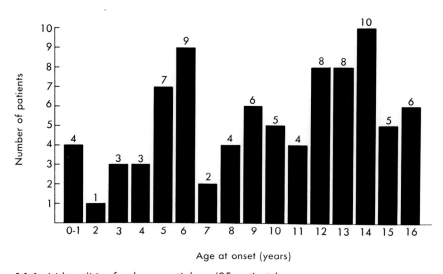

Fig. 14-6. Iridocyclitis of unknown etiology (85 patients).

There are 85 cases of active and chronic iridocyclitis of unknown etiology. Roughly 50% of these cases are chronic iridocyclitis similar to that associated with juvenile rheumatoid arthritis. However, a thorough examination failed to reveal any signs or symptoms of joint disease either past or present. Fig. 14-6 charts the ages at onset of the uveitis in 85 patients with anterior uveitis of unknown cause. There seems to be no age range during which the anterior uveitis appears more frequently.

Chronic cyclitis appears to be an entity which is a very chronic form of anterior uveitis in children. The main feature of this type of uveitis is the vitreous opacities mainly in the anterior and inferior vitreous. The opacities in the vitreous are fine and cellular.

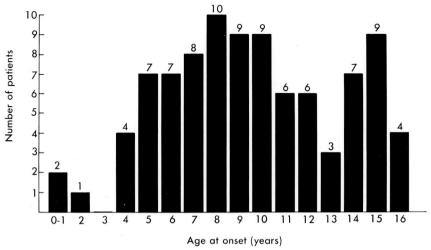

Fig. 14-7. Chronic cyclitis (92 patients).

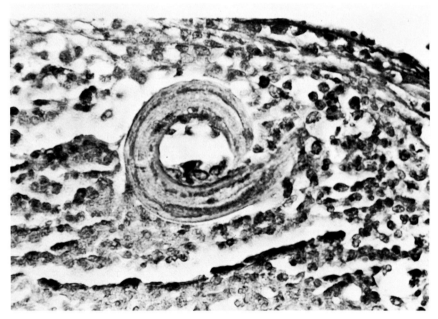

Fig. 14-8. Toxocara microlarva in retinal eosinophilic granuloma (high power).

Frequently there are large "snowball" type of opacities deeper in the vitreous. Fig. 14-7 shows that the age at onset is primarily after the age of 4. Ten of the eighty-two patients had unilateral chronic cyclitis with large amounts of white exudate over the pars plana inferiorly. This exudate appears as a "snowbank," piling up around the equator of the lens inferiorly. These cases are thought to be associated with *Toxocara,* a common nematode larva of puppies and kittens. One of the patients in this series was brought to autopsy, and a microlarva (Fig. 14-8) was found in an eosinophilic granuloma (Fig. 14-9) in the retina.[4]

Fuchs' syndrome of heterochromic cyclitis

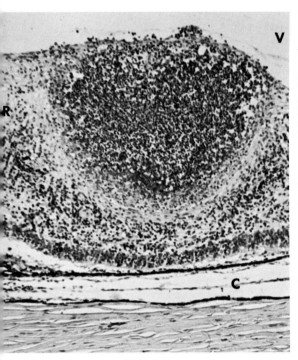

Fig. 14-9. Low power view of eosinophilic granuloma containing nematode larva. V = vitreous, R = retina, C = choroid. (From Hogan, M. J., Kimura, S. J., and Spencer, W. H.: Visceral larva migrans and peripheral retinitis, J.A.M.A. **194** [13]: 1345-1347, 1965.)

Table 14-4. Distribution of types of posterior uveitis (178 patients)

Type	*Number of patients*
Toxoplasmosis	129
Chorioretinitis, etiology unknown	36
Nematodiasis	4
Choroiditis, etiology unknown	9

Table 14-5. Distribution of types of toxoplasmosis (129 patients)

Type	*Number of patients*
Congenital, healed	43
Congenital, recurrent	83
Probably acquired	3

occurs in older children. There are seven patients in this series, and the uveitis is in the lighter colored eye.

There are ten patients with keratouveitis, and all except 1 case are caused by herpesvirus hominis. The remaining case is thought to be caused by *Mycobacterium tuberculosis.* This patient had a granulomatous keratouveitis with iris nodules, mutton-fat type of keratitic precipitates, and active pulmonary tuberculosis. The keratouveitis cleared rapidly on systemic therapy for pulmonary tuberculosis.

Two patients have sarcoidosis of the outer segment, and both are Negro children in the older age group.

There are 6 assorted cases that were caused by lens–induced uveitis, trauma, Reiter's syndrome, Cogan's disease, virus, and syphilis.

Posterior uveitis

There are 178 patients with posterior uveitis in our series of 444 cases of uveitis in children.

Table 14-4 lists the types of posterior uveitis studied in children. Toxoplasmosis produces a clinically recognizable posterior uveitis. Of the 178 cases of posterior uveitis, 129 were caused by toxoplasmosis. Table 14-5 lists the types of toxoplasmosis seen in our series. One-third of the patients show congenital, healed chorioretinal scars. Typically one eye has a healed macular lesion and a peripheral healed lesion in the fellow eye. Few of these children have a monocular squint. Roughly two-thirds of our cases have recurrent retinochoroiditis. The active lesions are usually near a healed chorioretinal lesion forming a satellite lesion which is typical of recurrent toxoplasmic uveitis. Three cases are thought to be acquired toxoplasmosis because of the lack of healed chorioretinal scars, and the lesion is a retinochoroiditis with heavy exudation into the vitreous.

There are thirty-six patients with chorioretinal lesions that are clinically unlike the typical toxoplasmic lesion described above, and the methylene blue dye test titer was negative even in undiluted serum. We are unable to make even a presumptive etiologic diagnosis.

Nine cases of choroiditis are in this series. The lesions are clinically choroidal lesions with little or no exudation into the vitreous. We are not able to determine etiology in these cases.

Four cases are given a presumptive diagnosis of nematodiasis. The posterior fundus lesions are primarily a retinochoroiditis resembling the lesions described as being caused by *Toxocara*.[5]

Diffuse uveitis

Diffuse uveitis is fairly rare in children. Table 14-6 shows the types of uveitis involving both the anterior and posterior segments of the eye in sixteen patients.

Sympathetic ophthalmia is a relatively rare disease, but we have studied 6 cases. Most of these cases were referred to us because of management problems; therefore, the true incidence of this dreaded uveitis appears to be very low. Once the disease de-

velops, there is usually a severe visual loss in spite of treatment with corticosteroids.

Vogt-Koyanagi-Harada's disease occurred in two patients. Both were 15 years of age. This is a serious type of uveitis associated with pleocytosis, ringing in the ears and hearing loss, alopecia, vitiligo, and a granulomatous type of diffuse uveitis.

Behçet's syndrome and sarcoidosis are rare types of uveitis. Only 1 case of each was seen.

There are 6 cases in which a diagnosis or a disease association cannot be made.

Summary

Four hundred forty-four patients 16 years of age or younger with uveitis were studied. There were more cases of anterior uveitis than posterior uveitis (250 to 178). Diffuse uveitis was a relatively rare type of uveitis in children. This series is not a random sample of uveitis in our population, but it is a representative series in discussing patterns of uveitis in children.

REFERENCES

1. Kimura, S. J., Hogan, M. J., and Thygeson, P.: Uveitis in children, Arch. Ophthal. **51:**80, 1954.
2. Kimura, S. J., and Hogan, M. J.: Uveitis in children; analysis of 274 cases, Trans. Amer. Ophthal. Soc. **62:**173, 1964.
3. Woods, A. C.: Endogenous inflammations of the uveal tract, Baltimore, 1961, The Williams & Wilkins Co.
4. Hogan, M. J., Kimura, S. J., and Spencer, W. H.: Visceral larva migrans and peripheral retinitis, J.A.M.A. **194:**1345, 1967.
5. Ashton, N. C.: Larval granulomatosis of the retina due to *Toxocara*, Brit. J. Ophthal. **44:**129, 1960.

Table 14-6. Distribution of types of diffuse uveitis (16 patients)

	Number of patients
Sympathetic ophthalmia	6
Vogt-Koyanagi-Harada disease	2
Behçet's syndrome	1
Sarcoidosis	1
Type unknown	6

Solutions

Dan M. Gordon

The therapy of uveitis has not been altered radically during the past decade, although it has been refined by experience. The solution to the problem of management of uveitis must be divided into its two facets: (1) The

immediate care of the patient who is presently ill, and (2) the long-term attack upon the disease itself with an effort to solve its etiologic implications. Long-term treatment is especially concerned with the specific therapy of uveitis and the prevention of recurrences. This automatically implies solving the problem of etiology. The sick patient would also like to have further attacks prevented, which in most cases is an impossibility in the light of present-day knowledge.

Etiologic attack

Uveitis is a "wastebasket term" which includes every inflammation or apparent inflammation of the iris, ciliary body, or choroid. Many neoplasms, as well as living (blood) and nonliving materials, which enter the globe during trauma or by any route including the bloodstream, may cause an inflammation simulating endogenous uveitis. The multiplicity of causes and lack of knowledge concerning specificity automatically indicates a nonspecific approach to therapy as the initial step. It would simplify matters considerably if the etiology could be readily determined and there were specific therapeutic agents available.

I shall dismiss the etiologic approach with a few words; not because it is unimportant, but because often so very little is known about the actual cause of the disease in a specific patient. Much has been written, but little said, about the etiology. There is no question that some types of childhood uveitis differ from uveitis found in adults. For example, zonular dystrophy is almost exclusively a uveitic complication of the young. An almost similar distinction occurs with uveitis associated with rheumatoid arthritis; the young exhibit a much higher incidence of uveitis than do adults with rheumatoid arthritis.

Many patients require a comprehensive medical examination. One should not overlook the possibility of syphilis as the cause of the disease. Attention to possible rheumatic and genital diseases is also important. I have been impressed by the number of recurrences following the excessive use of alcohol, the influence of psychic trauma, as well as recurrences following certain immunologic inoculations for influenza, upper respiratory tract diseases, and tetanus. When it becomes necessary to immunize a patient who has or has had uveitis, it is wise to use less than the usual minimal dose of the immunizing ma-

terial initially, and to increase the dosage by very small increments. Otherwise, one might precipitate a new attack of uveitis or aggravate one already present.

I do not believe in an extensive course of specific (antitoxoplasmic) therapy in adult uveitis unless the patient is severely afflicted and has failed to respond to conventional forms of therapy. However, I do have one youngster who had a typical toxoplasmic picture with many, many recurrences, and who, following months of treatment with pyrimethamine (Daraprim) and sulfa, has had several recurrence-free years.

Uveitis may be associated with various systemic disorders. These include, among many others, rheumatoid arthritis, Reiter's syndrome, vaccinia, lymphogranuloma venereum, Behçet's disease, generalized cytomegalic inclusion disease, and various viruses, especially herpes simplex and herpes zoster (which is rare in children). The association of uveitis with certain collagen diseases is too well known to require comment. In children with severe vitreous reaction, proliferans, or vitreous bleeding, *Toxocara* and retinoblastoma should be considered. A small inflammatory focus near or around a blood vessel even in the periphery may cause macular edema and visual loss out of all proportion to the size of the lesion.

Therapy of uveitis

The management of uveitis falls into three categories: (1) nonspecific therapy with very generalized measures, (2) corticosteroid therapy, and (3) specific therapy (which is usually unavailable). If one is fairly certain of the etiology, the specific therapy, if available, is that described in most textbooks.

Nonspecific therapy. There are many measures which may be of value in the management of an individual patient. These are directed at improving his general welfare and perhaps removing him from his environment. While few patients require hospitalization during the period of therapy, hospitalization removes the patient from a possibly psychically traumatic environment.

Mydriatics are among the oldest forms of therapy in uveitis, especially in anterior uveitis. All patients should be dilated at the first visit for the purpose of facilitating a complete examination. However, with corticosteroid therapy, it is unnecessary to employ local mydriasis routinely in the treatment of uveitis, unless the patient is actively forming synechiae. Mydriatics would then be employed only during the active stage of adhesion formation. Local heat, in the form of hot packs, is comforting.

The use of antimicrobials is of no value in the treatment of endogenous uveitis. Radiation therapy, light therapy with ultraviolet light, or the Finsen carbon arc have been employed by several workers. Various anti-inflammatory medications, including aspirin, indomethacin, and phenylbutazone, have been utilized in the treatment of uveitis. These are probably more valuable for the comfort they produce than for their anti-inflammatory activity. Foreign proteins injected intramuscularly or intravenously to stimulate resistance to infection and inflammation have been utilized in the past. These have fallen into disuse since the introduction of corticosteroid agents. However, they have been, perhaps, too often overlooked in patients who prove difficult to manage with corticosteroids.

The specific therapy of histoplasmosis with amphotericin B is toxic and is not to be recommended except in dire emergency. The photocoagulation of areas of presumed histoplasmosis away from the macula sounds promising and deserves a trial, if necessary. This also applies to cryotherapy of choroiditis. I have almost the same attitude concerning the so-called specific therapy of toxoplasmosis with pyrimethamine in combination with sulfadiazine as I do toward amphotericin B. However, the former is less toxic and at times does help. The chief function of these regimens should be the prevention of recurrences. I still use the pyrimethamine-sulfadiazine combination in patients who have recurrences of macular choroiditis with a suspected etiology of toxoplasmosis. Success has been questionable, however, except as noted. It may be that our courses of such therapy are too short.

The antimicrobial therapy of tuberculosis is the antimicrobial therapy of the disease itself. I doubt that tuberculosis is an important etiologic factor in the production of uveitis today. The drugs commonly employed are the sulfonamides, para-aminosalicylic acid (PAS), isonicotinic acid hydrazide (INH, isoniazid), and rarely streptomycin. Tuberculosis has been the chief target of uveitis-conscious ophthalmologists in the past. However, human uveal tuberculosis is not common today.

Boeck's sarcoid is found in teen-agers, especially Negroes. There are associated granular, lung, and other organ involvements. Although there is no known cure, the condition often responds to corticosteroids.

Lawton Smith's work on missed cases of syphilis renders this a more important agent than is often realized, especially on a geographic and ethnic basis.

Corticosteroid therapy. Corticosteroid therapy is the backbone of uveitis management today. This statement reflects the thinking of virtually every responsible ophthalmologist. An adequate amount of steroids will control most cases until the pathogenic mechanism exhausts itself. I feel that most failures with steroids are caused by inadequate dosage, especially initially, and undue fear of those usually unimportant side effects which can often be controlled. Children do tend to gain great quantities of weight. I have seen weight gains of 50 or more pounds. This can be somewhat mitigated with the thiazides or other diuretics. The price is worth paying if the patient does well, as the weight can later be lost. This is not to minimize the severe side effects of corticosteroid therapy, but rather to emphasize that one should not be frightened into cessation of therapy merely because the patient is gaining weight. If the patient also has a secondary glaucoma, the carbonic anhydrase inhibitors are the diuretics of choice.

I believe that herpes simplex uveitis is usually missed and that many of the patients with uveitis who exhibit a dendritic keratitis during steroid therapy for uveitis actually are cases of missed herpes simplex uveitis. This is rarely recognized as a problem in children.

The intelligent use of the available corticosteroids makes for greater success in treating children. The physician must be fully aware of the potentialities and the best routes of administration for his specific purposes. The two most important points in the use of corticosteroid therapy are the route by which it is administered and the dosage. In an anterior uveitis (iridocyclitis), frequently applied topical steroids (initially every 15 to 30 minutes, with an increasing interval between applications) will probably control a large percentage of the cases. It is wise to shorten the course of the disease with several days of systemic therapy, or by initially adding a subconjunctival (sub-Tenon's) injection of 0.5 to 1 ml. of 5% cortisone, depo-6 methyl prednisolone, triamcinolone, or other corticosteroid suspension. If there are synechiae present, 2 drops each of 1% atropine and 10% phenylephrine can be added to the subconjunctival injection. Often, this will effectively break up recent dense adhesions. Occasionally, I substitute lid injection for the subconjunctival injection. That is, I inject the topical steroids through the lower lid aiming at the superior cul-de-sac with a 25 gauge, 5/8 inch needle. I find children good subjects for sub-Tenon's injections. The injections can be utilized to eliminate, decrease, or supplement systemic corticosteroids and will be accomplished without the attendant discomfort of the conjunctival route. In binocular cases, I do not hesitate to inject both eyes at the same sitting, although oral medication is often preferable.

One cannot determine the severity of a specific case from the clinical picture. A seemingly severe case may respond overnight to minimal dosage, and a seemingly mild case may prove very difficult to control.

If there are symptoms and signs of an anterior uveitis, I always use topical steroids as frequently as possible. I like drops, and rarely use ointments during the waking hours. If the posterior uveal tract is involved, as denoted by vitreous cells or veils, retinal edema, or an inflammatory focal lesion, then systemic steroids are absolutely mandatory. Topical applications are of no value in posterior inflammations. At times, subconjunctival (sub-Tenon's) steroid administration may be substituted for the systemic therapy. If the patient is hospitalized, then my treatment of choice is the intravenous administration of ACTH, in doses of 20 to 40 units in 1,000 cc. of saline administered slowly, preferably over a period of 12 to 16 hours. The long-acting forms such as Acthar Gel can be used in initial doses of 120 to 160 units intramuscularly daily followed by decreasing doses as the disease responds.

If the patient is treated solely on an ambulatory basis, it is easier to employ oral steroids with or without the subconjunctival injections. If the macula is involved, I immediately give the patient a subconjunctival injection, as well as an initial injection of 160 units of Acthar Gel. These are the patients I would be apt to hospitalize. It is important that the initial dosage of oral steroids be large enough to ensure rapid control of the process. This usually means a minimal initial dose of 8 to 10 tablets of the preferred steroid initially. The dosage may have to be increased to 12 or more tablets in some patients. At this point, after several days of daily medication, the question arises whether to use alternate-day therapy; that is, whether to give 16 tablets at one sitting every other day rather than 8 tablets daily in an effort to minimize the systemic side effects.

I have not been enthusiastic about alternate-day dosage. However, some recent work may point up the reason for that. The various steroids have varying durations of activity. The shorter-acting ones, such as prednisone, prednisolone, and methylprednisolone, are more appropriate for alternate-day dosage. Dexamethasone and betamethasone last longer and are better for daily therapy; triamcinolone and paramethasone fall in between these two groups. Here again one may have to rely on trial and error. Alternate-day therapy has been unsuccessful in severe inflammations, in my experience, but it may be useful in milder cases, or those first controlled by large daily doses.

As indicated above, the geographic site of the lesion determines the urgency and degree of therapy. A lesion in the macula demands immediate intensive therapy and any effort to search for the etiology at the beginning may result in permanent central blindness. When the lesion is away from the macula, and especially in the pars plana or ciliary body, then the loss of vision is undoubtedly due to the resultant central retinal edema and vitreous opacities. Here the urgency of treatment is lessened, although its necessity is probably still present. If the lesions are small, fairly peripheral, and do not cause any special symptoms, one may watch them without any therapy, instituting treatment only if the lesions tend to become larger.

As stated above, treatment consists of starting with good initial doses (8 tablets—6 mg. dexamethasone, 4.8 mg. betamethasone, 40 mg. prednisone) and continuing until improvement in vision or improvement in the clinical picture takes place. At this point, the amount of steroids being given can be gradually decreased. If the youngster responds early in the course of therapy, therapy may be stopped abruptly, but it must be immediately reinstituted if the disease proves to have been only suppressed but not abolished. If an acute uveitis has not shown evidence of response within the first 72 or 96 hours, the dosage should be immediately increased by at least 25 to 50%. If the disease still does not respond after several days, one of two courses is available; a different corticosteroid should be used and/or the diagnosis should be reevaluated. This might also be a good time to add subconjunctivally injected steroids if these have not already been employed. If the anterior uveitis has not responded to topical applications after several days, systemic therapy or subconjunctival injections are indicated.

The patient with chronic or recurrent uveitis presents a problem. Often the recurrences are mild and are treated as are any acute attacks. If the patient is taught to institute therapy at home immediately upon suspicion of a recurrence, the intensity and duration of these attacks will be shortened appreciably. There are, however, some patients who never seem to respond completely to therapy. I have no real answer for these other than giving large initial doses in an effort to subdue the process as rapidly as possible. The disease is then controlled with a minimal amount of systemic and/or (preferably) subconjunctivally injected steroids.

I find that childhood uveitis is either very easy or very difficult to manage. There seem to be few cases occupying the middle group.

The greatest single fault in management is omitting steroids entirely or the use of inadequate doses of steroids for too short a period of time.

Management of complications

Space does not permit a full discussion of the management of systemic side effects. The intelligent use of diuretics will help control many of the annoying problems of overweight. This is not as true, however, in treating children who show a decided predilection for the accumulation and retention of water, and who do not respond to diuretics as do adults.

Synechiae. Synechiae, especially when fresh, often melt away under corticosteroid therapy. Cycloplegics or mydriatics can be employed until the synechiae have been broken. If these are resistant, an injection of 2 minims each of sterile 1% atropine and 10% phenylephrine can be used. These should be obtained from previously unopened bottles or "one shot" applicators.

Myopia. During the active stage of uveitis, the average patient will become temporarily more myopic. Very few patients come out of the attack with a conspicuous increase in myopia. The treatment is obvious. The tendency of uveitic retinal edema to produce myopia often serves to differentiate it from central serous retinopathy, which produces hyperopia.

Secondary glaucoma. Secondary glaucoma is probably the most serious complication of uveitis. This may occur during the active stage, or when the inflammation is inactive. It follows that routine tonometry as well as routine use of the slit lamp and ophthalmoscope are mandatory in the management of active uveitis, and the follow-up of inactive uveitis. When the uveitis is inactive and secondary glaucoma is present, it is usually on the basis of a bombé mechanism; although if steroids are being employed (and they are of no value as a prophylactic mechanism during inactive uveitis), the question of steroid glaucoma should be considered. This can be proved if the glaucoma subsides with discontinuance of the steroids. Early in the course of an active uveitis the intraocular pressure is usually decreased and then returns to normal or above with response to therapy. I have rarely found steroid glaucoma to be an important factor during an active uveitis. Only once have I been forced to operate on a teen-ager for steroid glaucoma, because the patient would have gone blind without steroids, and with steroids would have gone blind with glaucoma. Following filtering surgery, he was easily cured. Medical therapy which can be employed in the management of secondary glaucoma consists of the following:

1. Carbonic anhydrase inhibitors (dichlorphenamide, ethoxzolamine, acetazolamide)
2. Cycloplegics, after tests in the office
3. Miotics (rarely) after tests in the office
4. Levo-epinephrines (these need ample time to take effect)
5. Steroids, if uveitis is active
6. Retrobulbar procaine plus massage
7. Paracentesis, often excellent in breaking up a vicious cycle, but rarely necessary
8. Intravenous urea, acetazolamide (Diamox), mannitol
9. Oral glycerol may break up a vicious cycle

The filtering procedures seemed to be somewhat better than iridectomy. The most common single reason for surgery is a seclusion mechanism. During active uveitis, the angle may become clogged with debris and edema.

The choice of a mydriatic or a miotic depends upon the reaction of the pressure to the particular drug in the office. Usually, dilation is more successful than miosis.

Cataracts. Cataracts occur ultimately in 100% of patients with chronic uveitis whose uveitis is not controlled and in practically 100% of uveitic eyes with years of chronic uveitis even when the uveitis does respond to therapy. Monocular uveitis in young children very often goes undetected for a long period, so that a cataract may be present at the first examination. When surgery is indicated in a patient with active uveitis or a history of uveitis, he should be placed on adequate systemic corticosteroid therapy before, during, and after surgery. In most patients, I find a subconjunctival injection of steroids away from the site of operation at the time of surgery sufficient to prevent recurrences, unless the uveitis is still active. Perhaps there would have been no recurrences in the inactive cases. It is safer, however, to use this prophylactic procedure. In many patients when the cataracts form, the inflammation dies down. This is difficult to explain but it has been seen frequently enough to be significant. The role of the lens and its capsule in perpetuating uveitis must be an important one.

Retinal detachments. Uveitic retinal detachments seem to be related to inadequate steroid therapy. I have never had a patient who exhibited a retinal detachment in an eye with active uveitis while on adequate steroid therapy. I have had several patients with hopeless retinal detachments, who had previously been on minimal or no doses of steroids. The other eye in all of these patients responded to steroid therapy without retinal detachment. Surgery is not as successful in uveitic detachments as it is in other forms of detachment. However, it should be given a trial.

Vitreous membranes. Vitreous membranes can often be lysed if long-term steroid therapy or repeated subconjunctival injections of corticosteroids are employed.

Band-shaped keratitis (zonular dystrophy). Band-shaped keratitis can be managed by the employment of a chelating agent, such as sodium versinate or 2% hydrochloric acid.

Optic neuritis. Optic neuritis may occur as part of the uveitis and responds to the systemic therapy. Children tend to have very engorged veins during posterior uveitis.

Conclusion

Little is known about the specific etiology or the specific therapy of uveitis. Therefore, most therapy is directed toward nonspecific management, more especially with corticosteroid therapy. Too often children are treated with inadequate dosages for insufficient periods of time, or there has been failure to initiate corticosteroid therapy initially when the patient is seen because of undue fear of the side effects of corticosteroid therapy.

A good history and a comprehensive medical examination occasionally will reveal the existence of disease which has not been previously suspected.

Discussion

Moderator:
Robert S. Coles

Dr. Coles: Thank you very much. I am not going to summarize any of the speakers' comments because time is running short. The give and take of the question period is much more important. Dr. Herbert Kaufman has one comment he would like to make on corticosteroids.

Dr. Kaufman: I think a lot of you may remember when the Alan Woods School of Uveitis held sway and the role of the consultant was to do one more test. Then Dr. Gordon, really more than any other single person, I think, was a voice crying in the wilderness, saying we have got to consider this as a disease, treat the disease, and forget the academic part of it. I think he really focused our attention on treatment and on the use of corticosteroids. I think also he has really never received the credit he deserves. As far as corticosteroid treatment is concerned, there are just a few points that come to my mind.

First of all, most biologic responses represent a large dose response. That is, the biologic response is an exponential function of the dose. When you are increasing or decreasing you might as well consider it this way, and, for example, if one is decreasing the doses of steroids, cutting it from 80 to 40 is really very similar to cutting it from 10 to 5. It is an exponential function. This is a convenient and very practical way, I think, to approach this.

Secondly, not all uveitis responds well to steroids. Not uncommonly there are patients who respond initially, who go on with a low grade level of activity and when you stop the steroids you find that it really doesn't make any difference. I think it is worthwhile to periodically stop steroids, or reduce them, or at least be absolutely certain in your own mind that you are accomplishing what you wish to accomplish. One other thing is to consider the possible use of depot steroids in the retrobulbar space. I think Hindrich in our laboratory has good evidence in monkeys that you can get enormous concentrations posteriorly with retrobulbar steroids, and in selective patients for whom systemic steroids really represent a very great hazard. I think this is something we ought to keep in mind. Clinically it seems to work, although that is very hard to tell for sure.

Dr. Coles: Thank you very much, Dr. Kaufman. I would like to open the questioning by differing a little with Dr. Gordon on the use of cycloplegics. I happen to feel that in all forms of cyclitis and iridocyclitis cycloplegics are terribly important, and I have found that if you neglect to use them, especially in children, you really end up with a bound-down pupil despite steroids.

I would like to find out what Dr. Kimura and Dr. Witmer feel about this form of therapy. Do you use cycloplegics or mydriatics? I think it is an important decision to make.

Dr. Kimura: Yes, it has been our policy to gauge it by the flare more than anything else. If there is a good strong flare then we certainly will prescribe mydriatics, and I think Dr. Gordon will agree that it is not a terrible imposition to have patients use a couple of drops of mydriatics.

Dr. Gordon: Actually, this is based on about 14 or 15 years of experience and unless there is fibrin in the anterior chamber or unless the patient seems very sick, I don't use mydriatics routinely. And so far I have not had any real reason to regret doing that.

Dr. Witmer: I think we are more old fashioned and we still use it, but I agree with Dr. Gordon that I think there are cases which do form posterior synechiae, and there are others which don't. In those cases, mainly the anterior uveitis group of so-called rheumatoid arthritis, you can give as much atropine as you want to, and you will always end up with a seclusion and a cyclitic membrane.

Dr. Coles: You mentioned the rheumatoid arthritis group. Dr. Kimura, would you like to clarify a little bit further the concept of rheumatoid arthritis uveitis—whether it really exists, and if it does, what it is?

Dr. Kimura: Originally, we thought that there was a definite association of rheuma-

toid arthritis with uveitis. But we have had to retract on that because with a larger series we have found that rheumatoid arthritis in an adult is really not significantly associated with anterior uveitis. However, in juvenile rheumatoid arthritis, which probably is an entirely different disease, there is a native rheumatoid factor and other things, too, that the rheumatologists will tell you. The ocular lesion that we associate with rheumatoid arthritis is mainly nodular scleritis. It is in spondylitis that from 15 to 25% of the cases will have a very severe iridocyclitis which often becomes chronic. Actually, we prefer not to use the term "rheumatoid arthritis uveitis."

Dr. Coles: The next question is one which plagues us all. In children we get hypotony, I think, almost as frequently as we do secondary glaucoma. These eyes do tend to go into phthisis bulbi more rapidly than in adults. But when you do have a child who has secondary glaucoma, which has been unresponsive to *all* medical therapy, what surgical procedures should be attempted?

Dr. Witmer: Well, I am very fortunate not to have come across a case like that. But I would be very hesitant to do any surgery on it. On the basis of what I showed this morning, I think one should try a filtering procedure.

Dr. Kimura: In the few cases that we have seen recently, we have been doing cyclocryosurgery; not overdoing it (about 8 spots, 4 mm. from the limbus), and we have had fairly good clinical results. We haven't had any of them go into phthisis yet.

Dr. Gordon: I have had the same experience. I have had some experience with iridectomy glueing back down again, so now I prefer to do a filtering operation. Fortunately I have not had to operate upon too many of these, but I had two patients who, on steroids, had an intractable steroid glaucoma, and off steroids, had an intractable uveitis. Both of these had filtering operations, and have done extremely well, and in both cases the uveitis is no longer active.

Dr. Coles: The other complication which follows glaucoma is cataract formation in children. This occurs very early and very rapidly in children. If the eye is relatively quiet, do you do surgery, and if so, what type of surgery would you do? Let us pose the problem of a 5-year-old child with a mature cataract, secondary to uveitis, which is mildly active.

Dr. Gordon: Whenever I operate upon any eye which has or has had uveitis I always do a large sub-Tenon's capsule injection away from the site of the incision. On one occasion some of the steroid got into the anterior chamber and that was the nicest, whitest eye I ever had; perhaps we ought to do that deliberately.

At an early age—under 20 or 25—I would use the conventional methods for young cataracts that have been discussed here today by Dr. Scheie. I have tried, with enzyme, intracapsular extraction, and sometimes I have been lucky, and sometimes I haven't. I think probably for the older group one might be wise to try an intracapsular procedure, and in very young patients do the procedures that Dr. Scheie described.

May I say a word about sub-Tenon's injections. I have tried retrobulbar injections not too successfully. However, in a number of people I started out as though I were doing a retrobulbar, using a 25 gauge, 5/8 inch needle. Having gone through the lower lid, I point up towards the eye, and I think in effect I have given sub-Tenon's injections. Sometimes it seems to have worked very well, and it is not as painful as a subconjunctival injection may be.

Dr. Kimura: I think it depends on the type of uveitis. Fuchs' heterochromic cyclitis, regardless of the flare and cells, gives no trouble. We prefer aspiration and they respond well. However, with cases of juvenile rheumatoid arthritis, it is another problem, and we do the same thing that Dan Gordon does; that is, we do pretreat them, and then treat them postsurgically. I use a lot of Depo-Medrol, and I must give Dr. Coles credit for

that, because about 10 or 12 years ago he convinced me that it was a good way of treating children.

Dr. Witmer: I agree with Sam Kimura.

Dr. Coles: One other comment that I would like to make about Depo-Medrol in sub-Tenon's injections. In the past few years I have been palpating the globe, looking for a tender spot. Sometimes you can find a focal area of inflammation in the anterior uveal tract. Instead of injecting routinely in the upper outer fornix, I now give the injection directly over the tender area, because we know that the steroid goes into the eye directly through the tissues. I think this is a better method.

I would like to ask Dr. Witmer if he would be good enough to tell us some of his results. Dr. Witmer has been doing a great number of aqueous taps in children and in adults with uveitis. Now, I think we would all be interested in learning just a little bit more about the results, because this is such a desperate situation and we frequently feel that we want to do something more. Paracentesis is something that offers this opportunity, along with iris biopsy, on occasion.

Dr. Witmer: I must admit that in children this has very limited value. Among the 120 children I have studied, only 30 were submitted to this diagnostic procedure, which in children of this young age group usually required general anesthesia.

The method of quantitative serology gave positive results in only 2 of these 30 cases, which is a very low percentage. But in these 2, toxoplasmosis could be confirmed by this method. About 2 years ago we started to perform aqueous humor cytology with the electron microscope and this technique may be quite useful in the differentiation between inflammatory and tumor cells.

You mentioned that we could also do iris biopsies. We have not done this in children. We have done it in about 4 adult cases and only 1 was positive, but it does show that iris biopsies may be helpful in making an etiologic diagnosis.

OPHTHALMIC PLASTIC SURGERY

Presiding Chairman: **Byron Smith**

Chapter 15

Radiation therapy of lid tumors

M. A. Bedford

There have been lucid and well-reasoned pleas advocating the use of surgery or radiotherapy for the treatment of lid tumors.[1, 2] Each specialty can produce a list of the most damning complications and recurrences caused by the other specialties' treatment.[3, 4, 5] This paper arises from the assessment of cases seen at the tumor clinic of Moorfields Eye Hospital and the general clinic of St. Bartholomew's Hospital, London. It is unique in that it is, in effect, a plea for radiotherapy by an eye surgeon.

At first visit each case is considered on its own merits and under two main headings: the site of the tumor and its nature. The tumor is measured accurately; its site and proximity to the lid margins, the canaliculae, the pliability of the skin and tarsal plates, and the age and debility of the patient are all considered. A biopsy is done in all cases before any treatment is planned, whether surgical or by radiotherapy.

After treatment each case is then reviewed in a similar fashion and a note made of any side effects. It has become apparent in the last year that the number of cases being referred for radiotherapy is increasing, as the side effects after treatment are only minimal. Surgery is now restricted to a simple excision, perhaps combined with a Wolfe graft in selected cases. The more complicated surgical procedures are usually reserved for recurrences of previous radiation treatment, which are uncommon. The dangers of irradiation cataract, glaucoma, symblepharon, and so on are nonexistent, as the eye is virtually completely protected by a lead contact lens during treatment. With conventional x-ray therapy using 140 kv machines the eye receives less than 1% of the total radiation dose.

The lid, of course, receives a full thickness dose of radiation and does show changes. On the skin, epilation and telangiectasia are to be expected; on the conjunctival aspect telangiectasia may also appear but is of no significance. However, on this aspect of the lid, changes may occur that can be troublesome to a minor degree. These changes are formation of keratin plaques.[6, 7] These are formed as the smooth, moist conjunctiva is converted to a dry, crumbling, flaky area, which may be large or, more commonly, small. Its size is really of no consequence; what is more important is the site. If this is in the center of the lid, particularly the upper one, Bengal rose staining may be seen on the cornea and the eye may be so irritable that occasionally a conjunctival graft may be needed. This is the only significant side effect that has occurred after radiation of a lid tumor.

Two other minor complications may be seen. Epiphora may occur from radiation stricture of the lower canaliculus, but in no case have the symptoms been severe enough to need surgery. Sometimes with a lesion of the outer aspects of the upper lid, the lacrimal gland secretion may be reduced. This appears to be rarely significant, but in an extreme case may lead to all the signs and symptoms of a dry eye. One other interesting fact has emerged. If a recurrence after radiotherapy does occur, further surgery does not appear to be made difficult. Tissue planes can still be dissected easily and rapidly.

The number of cases referred for radiotherapy in the tumor clinic of Moorfields Eye Hospital has increased rapidly in the last few years as it has become apparent that the side effects are minimal from the treatment of most cases. From 1961 to 1966, for every patient treated by radiotherapy, approximately two were treated surgically. (Out of a total of 196 patients 124 were treated surgically and 72 were treated by radiotherapy.) The recurrence rate for surgery was 14%; for radiotherapy the rate was 8%. From March 1967 to March 1968, for every patient in the general clinic who was treated by radiotherapy, two were treated by surgery. In the tumor clinic, for every nine patients treated by radiotherapy, one was treated by surgery.

The current indications for radiotherapy are: (1) all tumors involving the lid margin for more than a few millimeters, and (2) all tumors adjacent to the lacrimal puncta or canaliculae. Surgery is reserved for all cases of recurrence from radiotherapy, all tumors in the center of the upper lid, and those tumors with at least 2 or 3 mm. of normal tissue on all sides not encroaching on the lid margin, the lashes, or the canaliculae.

My thanks are due Dr. Lederman and Mr. Williams, the radiotherapists to Moorfields Eye Hospital and St. Bartholomew's Hospital, London, for their skilled treatment of the cases that I have referred to them.

REFERENCES

1. Stallard, H. B. In Boniuk, M., editor: Ocular and adnexial tumors, St. Louis, 1964, The C. V. Mosby Co., p. 109.
2. Lederman, M. In Boniuk, M., editor: Ocular and adnexial tumors, St. Louis, 1964, The C. V. Mosby Co., p. 104.
3. Jones, I. S., and Reese, A. B.: Focal scleral necrosis; a late sequel of irradiation, Arch. Ophthal. **49:**633, 1953.
4. Blodi, F. C.: The late effects of x-radiation on the cornea, Trans. Amer. Ophthal. Soc. **56:**413, 1958.
5. Stallard, H. B.: Treatment of malignant neoplasms of the eyelids—surgery or irradiation? Brit. J. Ophthal. **43:**159, 1959.
6. Lederman, M.: Radiotherapy of non-malignant diseases of the eye, Brit. J. Ophthal. **41:**1, 1957.
7. Bedford, M. A.: The corneal and conjunctival complications following radiotherapy, Proc. Roy. Soc. Med. **59:**529, 1966.
8. Duke-Elder, S.: Textbook of ophthalmology, vol. 6, St. Louis, 1954, The C. V. Mosby Co., pp. 654-658.
9. Reese, A. B.: Tumors of the eye, ed. 2, New York, 1963, Paul B. Hoeber.

Chapter 16

Complications of periocular radiation therapy

Herbert L. Gould

The fact that cancerous tissue is susceptible to alteration of its biologic behavior by ionizing radiation in a far more sensitive manner than the normal tissue that surrounds it establishes a gratifying therapeutic opportunity. However, a radiotherapeutic impasse can occur if contiguous normal tissue fails to have a greater ability to recover from the effects of ionizing radiation than the diseased tissue.

Periorbital neoplasms usually involve eyelids and arise from skin epithelium or skin appendages. Generally, they are radiosensitive, but only moderately so. Therefore, the radiotherapeutic ratio between cancericidal effectiveness and damage to normal tissue is small.

This paper concerns those ocular complications that follow radiation therapy that has been directed toward the eye.

General considerations

Most radiotherapists consider radiation therapy preferable to surgery, since not only is the disease well controlled, but satisfactory cosmetic and functional results can be obtained with a minimum of hospitalization and incapacitation of the patient.[1] On the other hand, ophthalmic plastic surgeons, having developed their skills in tissue reconstruction, strongly favor excision.

No method is infallible, however, and recurrences of tumor may occur following either surgery or radiation. Merriman states that many surgical recurrences are treated by radiation,[2] while Dollfus and Shulz state that, as a rule, radiation is used initially followed by surgery, if necessary.[1, 3] Mustardé, Hughes, Bodian, Reeh, and Smith strongly feel that the surgical approach should be primary.[3]

Stallard emphasizes complications from irradiation for lid carcinoma and advocates surgical excision. He points out that an important pathologic feature of basal cell carcinoma which favors surgical treatment is its slow penetration, since its infiltration is delayed by fascia.[4]

Iliff, in discussing orbital tumors, emphasized that the choice between surgical excision and irradiation depends on the extent, location, and sensitivity of the tumor.[5] While benign tumors are most amenable to surgical excision and malignant ones may require sacrifice of the globe and orbital contents, poorly delineated lymphomas respond dramatically to irradiation. In some instances, a combination of surgery and irradiation gives the best results.

Principles of ophthalmic radiotherapy

Two methods of delivering radiation to carcinomatous lesions of the eyelid and canthi are currently in vogue—x-ray and radium needle implants.

Low voltage or superficial x-rays (60 to 100 kv.), which have limited powers of penetration, are used for superficial lesions of the lids and canthi. High voltage (deep) x-ray therapy (200 to 250 kv.) is used in the treatment of malignant disease and is applicable for intraocular or orbital tumors.

Radon seeds or radium needles are gamma-ray sources used as surface applicators and interstitially placed needles. Generally, these are used in epibulbar melanosis, although there are still reports of radiotherapists using radium for lid tumors.[6-8]

Shielding of the globe is essential, and a variety of devices are available, both direct and indirect. In direct shielding a lead shield is placed over the eye. When this is not applicable, indirect shielding is used in which an absorbing material is interposed in the beam of radiation to absorb that part of the beam which would otherwise reach the eye.

The direct method of protection can be used for voltages up to 250 kv. and for tumors of the lids, epibulbar region, and orbit. The lead shields are 1 or 2 mm. thick with a plastic or paraffin coating. There is no figure that can be given as a cancericidal dose for lid neoplasms. However, a single dose of 2,250 R will sterilize most cancers, although as little as 1,600 R may be adequate in certain cases.

Effect of radiation of ocular tissue

Skin. The skin of the eyelids generally reddens and is residually hyperpigmented at a dose of 200 to 300 R; 800 to 1,000 R will produce desquamation of epithelium; 1,500 to 3,000 R will cause ulceration, resulting in atrophy and scarring. Single doses in excess of 3,600 R will lead to necrosis.

Eyelashes. Transient epilation will occur with single doses of approximately 300 R. Permanent loss of eyelashes occurs with 1,200 R.

Cornea. While an erythema dose will produce a superficial keratitis, a cancericidal dose of x-rays usually results in severe ulceration and scarring. In some instances, a relative neurotrophic keratitis is residual.

Lens. The principal clinical effect of ionizing radiation on the lens is production of cataract. In 1953, Schulz and Stetson stated that the human lens could tolerate 800 R without production of cataract.[9] In 1958, Merriam and Focht demonstrated cataract formation with as little as 200 R and concluded that a dose of 700 R had approximately a 50% chance of producing a cataract.[10] Generally, in the treatment of lid cancer with x-rays combined with proper shielding, cataracts were rare. However, with radon seeds, the incidence was significantly higher.

Uveal tract. Excessive doses of irradiation may produce an iritis with secondary glaucoma.

Nasolacrimal system. Metaplasia of the

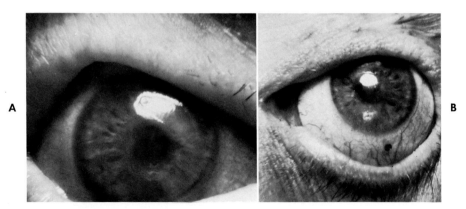

Fig. 16-1. A, Thirty-five-year-old woman who underwent irradiation of right upper lid for basal cell carcinoma. Three years later she had lid deformity, corneal anesthesia, and corneal ulcer. **B,** After she was fitted with a flush-fitting lens she has had a quiet eye, clear cornea, and 20/70 vision for 3 years.

columnar epithelium of the nasolacrimal duct and sac following therapeutic irradiation is not uncommon when treating canthal tumors. In spite of frequent postradiation probings, epiphora finally occurs as a result of lacrimal duct stenosis.

Lacrimal glands. Transient changes in secretory activity of lacrimal glands follow doses of 300 to 600 R. Cancericidal doses result in permanent loss of secretory activity. This may lead to extreme xerosis and loss of the eye.

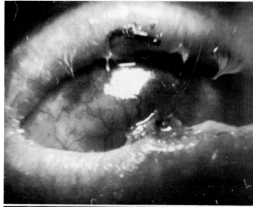

A

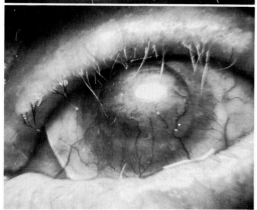

B

Fig. 16-2. A, Sixty-eight-year-old male who had undergone irradiation treatment to the left eye for tumor 20 years prior to coming to the clinic. A tarsorrhaphy was performed, but the right eye became blind. The left eye was opened and was found to be xerotic and hypoesthetic. The cornea was ulcerated. **B,** A scleral lens was fitted (all day wear). The eye became quiet and the cornea healed. Visual acuity is 20/100.

Case reports

Case 1. M. C., a 35-year-old white secretary was referred to the scleral lens clinic for recurrent corneal ulcerations in February 1965. Three years previously she had undergone radium irradiation at a university center for a basal cell midline carcinoma of the right upper lid. The following radiation complications were seen: (1) deformity of the upper lid with vertical cicatrix and leukoplakia, (2) chronic conjunctivitis, (3) xerosis, (4) extensive superior corneal ulceration, (5) corneal anesthesia, and (6) radiation cataract. She was treated with a flush-fitting scleral lens with clearing of the corneal ulcer, reduction of conjunctival infection, restoration of a moist milieu, and a visual acuity of 20/70 (Fig. 16-1).

Case 2. H. K., a 68-year-old retired white jeweler who had extensive x-radiation to the left eye for a retrobulbar lymphoma in 1945. He developed (1) keratitis and recurrent corneal ulceration, (2) lid deformity, (3) epilation, (4) radiation cataract, and (5) xerosis. A cataract extraction was performed, but the cornea developed an indolent ulcer and a lamellar keratoplasty was performed in 1959. The donor tissue was rejected and a permanent tarsorrhaphy was performed. Unhappily, the right eye developed optic atrophy following cataract surgery. In June 1965 a flush-fitting scleral lens (with optical correction) was fitted after opening the tarsorrhaphy. Despite corneal vascularization he has maintained useful vision (20/100) and a moist eye for 3 years (Fig. 16-2).

Case 3. H. B., a 72-year-old white woman with squamous cell carcinoma of the left brow, treated intermittently with radiation over the past 10 years. In spite of multiple treatment with surface irradiation, the tumor has recurred with: (1) cicatrix of the left upper lid, (2) corneal ulcer, (3) exposure keratitis, (4) symblepharon, (5) conjunctivitis, (6) keratinization, (7) glaucoma, and (8) radiation cataract. She was fitted with a flush-fitting scleral lens in June 1966. Since that time, the left upper lid has melted away, but the eye has been well-preserved with useful vision and comfort (Fig. 16-3).

Case 4. L. S., a 26-year-old white soldier treated with extensive, deep x-ray for right ethmoidal carcinoma in 1965 while on active duty in the army. He developed: (1) keratitis with ulceration, (2) epilation, (3) xerosis, (4) radiation cataract, and (5) conjunctivitis-keratinization, progressing over a 3-year period. Six months prior to his initial visit, he had useful vision in the right eye; however, there was gradual loss of vision from the development of a deep corneal ulcer. He was fitted with a scleral lens with resolution of the ulcer but opacification and vascularization of the cornea (Fig. 16-4).

Case 5. M. C., a 16-year-old school girl with vernal conjunctivitis treated with high dosages of beta-radiation, left eye, in an attempt to destroy

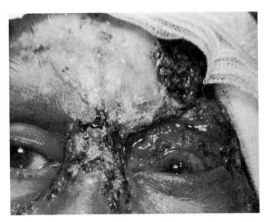

Fig. 16-3. Seventy-two-year-old woman with exposure keratopathy. She had worn a scleral lens constantly for 3 years. The upper lid was lost after extensive radiation for carcinoma, but eye maintains useful vision.

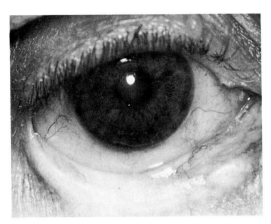

Fig. 16-5. A 59-year-old woman who had been treated with radiation for basal cell carcinoma of left lower lid. She developed chronic conjunctivitis, leukoplakia, lacrimal stenosis, lid deformity, epilation, glaucoma, and cataract.

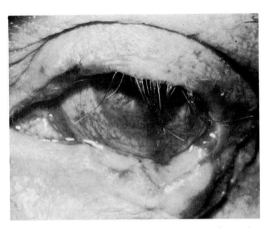

Fig. 16-4. Deep irradiation treatment for ethmoidal carcinoma which had been treated with a scleral lens. The patient had corneal ulcer, epilation xerosis, leukoplakia with lid deformity, cataract, and chronic conjunctivitis prior to therapy.

the papules of the tarsal mucosa. She developed: (1) tarsal conjunctival keratinization and (2) a secondary corneal ulcer. She was fitted with an optical scleral lens with dramatic increase in comfort, and normal vision.

Case 6. I. B., a 59-year-old saleslady seen as a private patient following the death of her ophthalmologist. In March 1965 a basal cell carcinoma in the left mid-eyelid was referred for radiotherapy. Her corrected vision in the left eye at

this time was 20/25. From March 3 through April 5 a total of 5,250 R was delivered to the involved area with low-voltage therapy (100 kv., 1 mm. Al filtration, T.S.D. 15 cm., H.V.L. 1.8 mm. Al). She had a lower lid erythema lasting 1 month and a recurrence was suspected. A biopsy showed only focal hyperplasia. The lower lid remained inflamed and irritable over the next 4 months. She returned in June 1966 with a history of chronic conjunctivitis in the left eye. Her best vision was 20/60, and intraocular tension was 36. She was placed on pilocarpine with control. In May 1967 glaucoma was controlled but the best vision was 20/200 in the left eye. and a diagnosis was made of a posterior cortical radiation cataract. She is awaiting cataract surgery. This patient had the following postirradiation complications: (1) chronic conjunctivitis, (2) leukoplakia at the tarsal conjunctival site of irradiation, (3) lacrimal stenosis, (4) lid deformity, (5) epilation, (6) glaucoma, and (7) radiation cataract (Fig. 16-5).

Discussion

For a quarter of a century, the majority of authors of standard surgical textbooks have written in favor of radiation for the treatment of eyelid carcinoma. There is, however, a notable lack of consideration for some of the serious ocular complications that sometimes follow radiation.[4]

While radiation may be the therapy of choice for surgically inaccessible tumors and lymphomas, lid cancer offers the reconstructive surgeon a significantly competitive therapeutic opportunity.

Over the years, reports on the use of radiation in the treatment of lid and canthal carcinoma have appeared in the literature. However, only recently has statistical attention been paid to post-treatment complications. The highlights of these reports will be reviewed in the following.

In 1953, Shulz and Stetson reported on the treatment of 400 patients with eyelid carcinoma (simultaneously reporting only 67 cases of ocular lymphomas). All patients were treated with x-ray alone. The following complications were reported: radiation necrosis, 6 cases (3%); stenosis of tear ducts, 11 cases; tearing, 6 cases; conjunctivitis and keratitis, 10 cases; and cataract, 1 case. There was a notably low total complication rate of 8.5%. There were 46 recurrences; secondary surgical attack was successful in 7 cases.[9]

In 1962 Fayos and Wildermuth reported on 111 cases of eyelid carcinoma treated with x-ray. The overall complication rate was 29%, including conjunctivitis, 12 cases; conjunctival ulcer, 1 case; epiphora (stenosed lacrimal duct), 13 cases; ectropion, 1 case; entropion, 2 cases; and late skin necrosis, 3 cases. There were 7 recurrences of tumor of which 3 were further controlled by surgery.[11] In 1962, McKenna and MacDonald reported on 157 cases treated with superficial x-ray and reported a complication rate of 3% with 1 case of glaucoma, 2 cases of telangiectasis, and 1 case of entropion. It must be emphasized that low radiation dosages were used in this series.[12]

In 1964, Cobb and colleagues found a 30% rate of complications in 119 patients treated by x-ray alone. In addition to 36 complications, there were 8 recurrences. The complications included cataract, 1 case; scarring and atrophy of lids, 9 cases; telangiectasis, 4 cases; ectropion, 2 cases; nasolacrimal occlusion and epiphora, 12 cases; and conjunctival telangiectasia, 2 cases.[13]

In 1962, Domonkos advanced the Philips contact x-ray as the treatment of choice for lid and canthal carcinoma and reported on 104 patients treated with this method. He had a complication rate of 5%, the only complication being lacrimal duct stenosis.[14]

Those investigators who recommended the routine use of radium in the treatment of eyelid carcinoma report few, if any, complications after treatment. Pipkin noted only tear duct stenosis in 3 out of 928 cases.[6]

McAuley found the following complications in eighteen patients treated with radon seeds: lens changes, 1 case; pain, 3 cases; epiphora, 1 case; scarring, 4 cases; and late radiation reaction, 3 cases. In spite of a 66% complication rate, he advocates radium therapy as the treatment of choice.[7]

In 1966 Levitt and colleagues reported on 63 cases treated during the period 1946 to 1962.[15] Radium needle implantation or x-irradiation was used. A complication rate of 47% was noted in 29 cases including 15 cases of conjunctivitis, 4 cases of cataract, 3 cases of keratitis, 2 cases of corneal ulcer, and 1 case each of conjunctival scar, iritis, leukoma, glaucoma, and symblepharon. Skin atrophy occurred in 21 cases, cicatrix in 20, telangiectasis in 11, skin necrosis in 4, and cartilage necrosis in 1. The significant finding in this study was the high incidence of postirradiation complications following radium implantation as compared with x-ray. They conclude that routine radium implantation is contraindicated for eyelid and canthal lesions. This conclusion is in complete disagreement with other authors[6-8] and sharply emphasizes the controversy surrounding this mode of therapy.

Recently, another manifestation of x-ray complication was reported—conjunctival leukoplakia at the site of treatment.[16] This was seen in Cases 1 and 6. This was asymptomatic and required no treatment.

Summary

A review of radiation techniques and principles has been presented with emphasis on the response of ocular tissue to irradiation. Therapeutic attitudes have been discussed in respect to surgery versus radiation or in consort. Recent radiographical literature has been surveyed as to the incidence of complications and new cases have been presented. It is to be emphasized that both surgery and radiation offer valuable therapeutic approaches to the management of ocular tumors and both carry with them the possibility of complications.

REFERENCES

1. Shulz, M. D., and Wang, C.: Radiotherapy of lesions of the lids, Int. Ophthal. Clin. **4**(1): 239, 1964.
2. Merriman, G.: Radiation therapy of lid lesions. In Smith, B., and Converse, J. M., editors: Proceedings of the Second International Symposium on Plastic and Reconstructive Surgery of the Eye and Adnexa, St. Louis, 1967, The C. V. Mosby Co., pp. 62-64.
3. Hughes, W. L., moderator: Panel discussion on tumors of the eyelids. In Smith, B., and Converse, J. M., editors: Proceedings of the Second International Symposium on Plastic and Reconstructive Surgery of the Eye and Adnexa, St. Louis, 1967, The C. V. Mosby Co., pp. 101-104.
4. Stallard, H. B.: Treatment of lid tumors, Highlights Ophthal. **6**:120, 1964.
5. Iliff, C.: Primary orbital tumors; therapy. In Smith, B., and Converse, J. M., editors: Proceedings of the Second International Symposium on Plastic and Reconstructive Surgery of the Eye and Adnexa, St. Louis, 1967, The C. V. Mosby Co., pp. 116-120.
6. Pipkin, J. L.: Comment on Domonkos paper, Arch. Derm. **91**:370, 1965.
7. McAuley, F. D.: Implantation irradiation of epitheliomata of the eyelids and adjacent areas, Brit. J. Ophthal. **47**:257, 1963.
8. Breed, J. E.: Radium therapy in cancer of the eyelid, Illinois Med. J. **125**:237, 1964.
9. Shulz, M. D., and Stetson, C. G.: Radiation therapy of malignant lesions about the eye, Radiology **61**:786, 1953.
10. Merriman, G. R., and Focht, E. F.: Radiation dose to lens in treatment of tumors of the eye and adjacent structures, Radiology **71**: 357, 1958.
11. Fayos, S. V., and Wildermuth, O.: Carcinoma of the skin of the eyelids, Arch. Ophthal. **67**: 298, 1962.
12. McKenna, R. J., and MacDonald, I.: Carcinoma of the eyelid treated by irradiation, Calif. Med. **96**:184, 1962.
13. Cobb, G. M., Thompson, G. A., and Allt, W. E.: Treatment of basal cell carcinoma of eyelids by radiotherapy, Canad. Med. J. **91**:743, 1964.
14. Domonkos, A. N.: Treatment of eyelid carcinoma, Arch. Derm. **91**:364, 1965.
15. Levitt, S. H., Bogardus, C. R., and Brandt, E. N.: Complications and late changes following radiation therapy for carcinoma of the eyelid and canthi, Radiology **87**:340, 1966.
16. Kopf, A. W., Allyn, B., Andrade, R., and Strichland, M.: Leukoplakia of conjunctiva; complication of x-ray therapy for carcinoma of eyelid, Arch. Derm. **94**:552, 1966.

Chapter 17

Late repair of chemical, thermal, and radiation burns

Richard R. Tenzel

Healing by severe cicatrization is common to all chemical, thermal, and radiation burns. Whether or not the patient develops entropion, ectropion, symblepharon, or corneal edema depends upon which layer or layers received the most severe injury. If the skin surface is primarily involved, ectropion will result; if the injury is mainly to the conjunctiva, entropion will ensue. Severe injury to the cornea may result in opacification or pseudopterygium with symblepharon formation.

Ectropion usually develops from thermal or radiation burns and occurs only rarely after chemical injury. The treatment is *not* small grafts to the lids with tarsorrhaphies in an attempt to control contractures; rather, the lids should be deeply undermined even to bringing the involved lid over its fellow lid and utilizing a large, adequate skin graft. A bolus should be used to place the graft firmly against its recipient bed to prevent hematoma formation beneath the graft. In re-formation of the entire upper lid, I try to place one graft from the lid margin to where I want the lid fold, and then to place the rest of the graft (or another graft) from the lid fold upward (Fig. 17-1).

Entropion is a frequent occurrence, especially after chemical injuries. An excellent technique of repair is anterior marginal rotation or transverse blepharotomy. An incision is made 3 to 4 mm. below the lid margin through the skin and muscle. The lid is everted. The same distance is measured from the lid margin, and a second incision is made through the tarsus. These two incisions should then be joined and continued the length of the lid. The control of the depth of the incision, both on the anterior and the posterior surfaces of the lid, is essential to maintain a good vascular supply to the lid margin. A double-armed horizontal mattress suture is brought from the lower cut tarsal edge to the upper cut skin edge and is tied tight enough to rotate the lid into slight ectropion (Fig. 17-2). The sutures are left from 5 to 10 days depending upon the amount of marginal rotation desired. A complication of this procedure is loss of the central one-third of the lid. If this occurs in the upper lid, it usually has to be repaired as one would repair a full-thickness loss of the lid. When it occurs in the lower lid, it may heal without requiring another procedure.

Another excellent operation for entropion of the upper lid is the modified Cuenod-Nataf procedure, which utilizes lash recession with tarsal fracture and skin excision to obtain the result desired (Fig. 17-3). It is important not to tie these lid sutures too tightly, and to make certain that the lashes are recessed a full 2 mm. from the lid margin. Touch-up cutting into the gray line incision is frequently necessary.

If trichiasis is mild, electrolysis should be used to remove the lashes. I prefer the Pro-Electro epilator for this purpose. One point should be stressed here: the patient must hold the machine in order to complete the

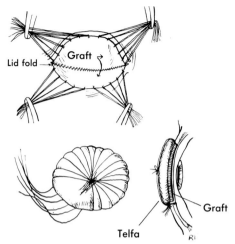

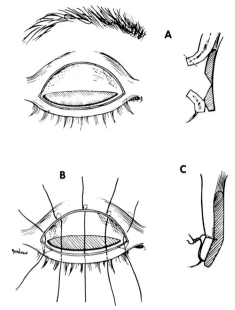

Fig. 17-1. With the upper lid below the lower lid, a large graft is cut in two and placed in the defect as two grafts, with the junction points being the lid fold that is to be formed. (From Tenzel, R. R.: Cul-de-sac reconstruction, Arch. Ophthal. **76**:580, 1966.) The lower drawings show the Telfa bolus being tied into place. (From Tenzel, R. R.: Repair of entropion of upper lid, Arch. Ophthal. **77**:675, 1967.)

Fig. 17-3. A, The incision of skin to the tarsus: a 2 mm. groove in the gray line; a wedge excision of the tarsus, and excision of the redundant skin in the upper lid. **B,** Placement of sutures with additional triangular areas of skin excised in each end of the original incision. The three central sutures go through the gray line incision, take a bite in the levator, and come out through the upper skin incision. The medial and lateral sutures go through the gray line incision and then out through the upper skin incision. **C,** The sutures are tied with the lash margin recession and tarsal fracturing.

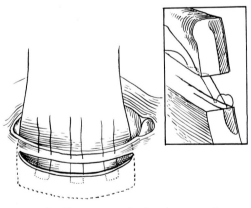

Fig. 17-2. Placement of the horizontal mattress suture joining the lower cut edge of the tarsus to the upper cut edge of the skin.

circuit. The lash should almost fall out and should not have to be pulled out after electrolysis. If trichiasis is more severe on the upper lid, modified Cuenod-Nataf procedure should be used. On the lower lid, I prefer splitting the anterior and posterior lamellae,

excising the lashes, and suturing the skin to the inferior tarsal margin (Fig. 17-4).

Symblepharons that extend on the cornea require more than a simple excision. The procedure that works best in my experience is excising the symblepharon and transposing a 5 mm. wide bipedicle conjunctival flap from 180 degrees across the cornea. One should leave at least 1 mm. of conjunctiva next to the limbus in taking the graft to facilitate closing the donor site. If another graft is needed deep in the cul-de-sac, then a split-thickness mucous membrane or free conjunctival graft can be used (Fig. 17-5).

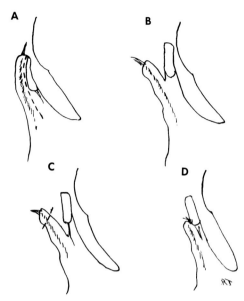

Fig. 17-4. A and **B,** Division of the lid into the anterior and posterior lamellae. **C,** Excision of the lashes. **D,** Suturing of the lid to the inferior tarsal margin.

If molded scleral shells are used at all, they should be confined to the first 48 hours postoperatively. Longer use will lead to extensive corneal vascularization.

Mucous membrane keratinization is especially troublesome after x-ray therapy to the lids in the treatment of malignant disease. The therapy is replacement of the keratinized mucous membrane with a free conjunctival graft from the other eye or a split-thickness mucous membrane graft from the lip. If a patient has had symblepharon repair with a tendency toward corneal vascularization, a keratinized mucous membrane on the inner surface of the lid will aggravate the vessels present and give further vascularization. The technique that I have successfully used for treatment of this vascularization is to put a 0.2 mm. shim in the Castroviejo keratome. A suture is placed on the inner and outer corners of the lid. The lid is everted, and

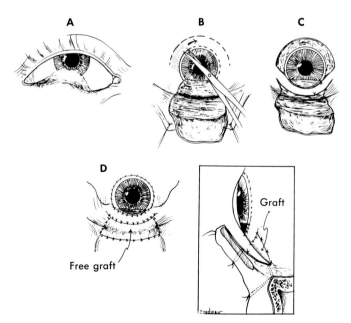

Fig. 17-5. A, Symblepharon present with pseudopterygium on cornea. **B,** Excision of pseudopterygium from the cornea with dissection of inferior cul-de-sac. A bridge flap is taken 180 degrees from the defect after a 360 degree peritomy is made 1 mm. from the limbus. **C,** The bi-pedicle flap sutured into position. **D,** Closure of the donor site, use of the previously dissected symblepharon to line the lid, and a free graft in the remaining defect. Inset shows proper placement of sutures to anchor the graft into the inferior cul-de-sac.

the keratome is used to shave off the keratinized surface. A mucous membrane graft from the lip, taken with the keratome, is used to cover the defect in the lid. By tying the knots on the skin surface, further abrasion of the cornea is prevented when the graft is sutured to the lid.

In treating severely contracted sockets after chemical injury, the only technique I have found to be successful is to place a split-thickness skin graft within the socket. I personally utilize the same technique used in placing the graft on the skin with a bolus dressing of Telfa.

Any treatment for these injuries should be aimed at removal of all irritation from the cornea and repair of the contracted surfaces. The procedure that will give the fewest complications and the best cosmetic result is the one that should be used.

REFERENCES

1. Besnainou, R.: L'entropion-trichiasis trachomateux et sa cure chirurgicale, Rev. Int. Trachome **33**:3, 1956.
2. Converse, J. M., and Smith, B.: Repair of severe burn ectropion of the eyelids, Plast. Reconstr. Surg. **23**:21, 1959.
3. Cutler, N. L., and Beard, C.: A method for partial and total upper lid reconstruction, Amer. J. Ophthal. **39**:1, 1955.
4. Tenzel, R.: Chemical Burns of the Eye and Eyelids. In Smith, B., and Converse, J. M., editors: Proceedings of the Second International Symposium on Plastic and Reconstructive Surgery of the Eye and Adnexa, St. Louis, 1967, The C. V. Mosby Co.
5. Tenzel, R.: Cul-de-sac reconstruction, Arch. Ophthal. **76**:580, 1966.
6. Tenzel, R.: Repair of entropion of the upper lid, Arch. Ophthal. **77**:675, 1967.
7. Wies, S. A.: Spastic entropion, Trans. Amer. Acad. Ophthal. **59**:503, 1955.

Chapter 18

Oculorotary muscle imbalance associated with orbital fractures

Margaret Fealy Obear

Oculorotary muscle imbalance is the most common complication following orbital fractures. Immediate diplopia after a blow to the orbit indicates an orbital fracture until proved otherwise. All too often, lid edema, unconsciousness, or other severe injuries obscure the patient's vision and the doctor's observation, resulting in the diagnosis being delayed weeks or even months after the initial injury. Prolonged muscle imbalance and diplopia in undiagnosed fractures lead to secondary deviations and ocular suppression.

Muscle imbalance of immediate onset can usually be completely cured with early orbital exploration and reduction of the fracture of the floor of the orbit (Fig. 18-1). Late imbalance with secondary deviation and suppression, on the other hand, requires primary reduction of the orbital fracture and usually secondary ocular muscle surgery. Therefore, the early ocular muscle imbalance is quite different from the late imbalance, even though the injury-fracture etiology may be the same.

The mechanism of ocular muscular imbalance in orbital fractures may be direct, indirect, or secondary. The direct intraorbital injury to the ocular muscles occurs at the time of impact when the muscle or its fascial sheath may be caught in the fracture, torn by a loose bone fragment, or hemorrhagic from the severe contusion. The degree of injury varies with the severity of the contusion force.

Indirect imbalance is the result of trauma to the third, fourth, or sixth cranial nerves, to their branches to the ocular muscles, or to their intracranial connections. Facial fractures are often associated with cranial fractures or concussions in severe automobile accidents or military injuries. Obviously, the repair of the orbital fracture will not eliminate the ocular imbalance in nerve or cranial injuries.

Secondary muscle imbalance may be caused by latent or marginal ocular balance prior to the injury which is made obvious by the separation of fusion due to the orbito-ocular injury. Occasionally, secondary ocular imbalance results from the actual surgical reduction of the orbital floor fracture; it may be temporary (if caused only by edema) or permanent. In these instances the ophthalmologist has created a greater problem than he has cured by reducing the orbital fracture.

The initial examination of an orbital injury includes vision, an external examination, a careful intraocular examination, ocular tension, an exophthalmometer measurement, a prism muscle measurement in all six cardinal fields (distance and near), and a subjective diplopia record. The actual tests used are not as important as the information obtained. The uninjured eye is usually the fixing eye. Severe diplopia is usual in adults unless previous amblyopia or intraocular injury exists. These patients have a great desire for fusion.

Vertical imbalance is the rule with a reverse hypertropia, which is almost pathog-

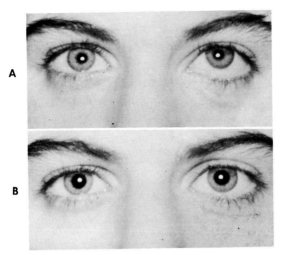

Fig. 18-1. A, The preoperative appearance of a patient with a fracture of the floor of the orbit is characterized by hypertropia and increased scleral show on the affected side. **B,** The postoperative correction of the muscle imbalance by reduction of the floor fracture.

nomonic of a fracture of the floor of the orbit. Horizontal deviations are secondary to the vertical imbalance, with exotropia being the most common. Esotropia is rare and, if it occurs, probably indicates a stab wound near the medial rectus or a previous esotropia-phoria.

The primary treatment of extraocular muscle imbalance associated with fracture of the floor of the orbit is reduction of the orbital fracture with implant of a prosthetic strut. Early imbalance is often cured by this procedure alone. It is preferable to wait 3 to 4 months after the reduction of the fracture before performing surgery to correct any persistent ocular deviation. Monthly muscle measurements will indicate any change in the imbalance. When the muscle picture is stable over two examinations, surgery can be advised. We aim to repair all the vertical and horizontal imbalance in one operation, but frequently numerous surgeries are necessary. Two to 3 months should be allowed between operations for adequate recuperation. We operate on both the injured and the non-

injured eyes and do not hesitate to operate on paretic or fibrotic muscles. It is often necessary to sacrifice fusion in the upward position of gaze for fusion in the more functional primary and downward positions of gaze. The subjective diplopia tests indicate progress toward fusion. But the best test of all is when the patient removes his black patch to resume binocular vision. Even in instances of the loss of central vision, peripheral fusion may be restored by ocular muscle surgery. Traumatic and paretic muscle imbalances are grossly incomitant; therefore, prisms incorported in the glasses are generally unsuccessful.

In order to better illustrate some of the aforementioned points, a recent case will be presented. The patient is a 24-year-old man injured in an automobile accident 3 years prior to being referred to me. He was hit in the face by a wooden post which projected through the windshield. The immediate repair was incomplete because of the severity of the facial tissue avulsion. One year later he had a 5 mm. left inferior rectus resection and a 4 mm. left superior rectus recession without improvement. The patient had no history of previous ocular imbalance. The visual acuity was right eye, 20/20, and left eye, 20/30. He had worn a patch on his left eye for the past 4 years and was incapacitated for his work as an automobile mechanic; he collected state and automotive industry insurance.

My examination revealed gross ocular muscle imbalance with diplopia in all fields of gaze. The patient also had a hypertelorism, a lacrimal obstruction, lid lacerations, and trichiasis with corneal erosion and multiple facial scars embedded with dirt (Fig. 18-2). It was obvious at the first examination that several operations would be necessary to restore the patient to a functional existence. The muscle measurement in primary position was 10 prism diopters of exotropia and 15 prism diopters of left hypertropia, increasing in the downward fields.

Primary surgery was the reduction of the

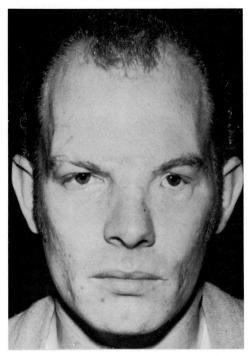

Fig. 18-2. A typical preoperative appearance of a traumatic naso-orbital injury with hypertelorism, muscle imbalance, and lid deformity.

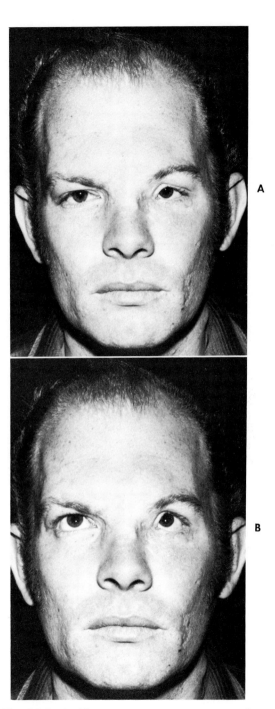

Fig. 18-3. A, The postoperative correction of the muscle imbalance, hypertelorism, and reduction of the lid deformity are noticeable. **B,** Upward gaze postoperatively shows the range of fusion which enabled the patient to resume work as an auto mechanic.

fracture of the floor of the left orbit with a Supramid plate and revision of the left upper lid notch and trichiasis and dermabrasion. One month later, the patient had a medial canthoplasty and binasal wiring, a canaliculoplasty and dacryocystorhinostomy. Two months following, a 10 mm. right lateral rectus recession, a 10 mm. left lateral rectus recession, and a 5 mm. resection of the left medial rectus were performed. There was a significant amount of scar tissue in the medial canthal area extending back towards the posterior ethmoids.

Following this surgery, the patient had binocular single vision to the left and above. One month later his measurements were 25 prisms of exophoria, 10 prisms of left hypertropia down, and 5 prisms of right hypertropia up.

The last operation, performed 3 months after the first muscle surgery, was a 5 mm.

Patient—24-year-old white male

Occupation—Auto mechanic

    March 1964—Auto accident; hit by wooden post
           Midfacial injuries; immediate repair incomplete

    August 1965—5 mm. LIR recession, 4 mm. LSR resection
           No improvement

    July 1967—Referred
           Fracture, floor left orbit and nose, multiple facial scars
           Diplopia all fields
           30 to 40 prisms XT, 15 to 20 prisms LHT up and down
           (incomitant)

    August 1967—Surgery
           Reduction of fracture floor of orbit
           Excision of lid notch and trichiasis
           Dermabrasion

    September 1967—Surgery
           Medial canthoplasty—transnasal wiring
           Canaliculoplasty and DCR

    November 1967—Surgery
           10 mm. RLR recession
           10 mm. LLR recession and elevation
           5 mm. LMR resection and elevation (marked scarring)

    January 1968—15-20 prisms XT (incr. to rt.) 5 RHT up, 10 LHT down
           B.S.V. to left and up

    February 1968—Surgery
           5 mm. RMR resection
           2-3 mm. LIR resection
           Tarsal graft L.L.L.
           Overgraft L. medial canthus

    March 1968—15 prisms X prim., 10 XT to right
           5 prisms RHT up
           B.S.V. primary 30 degrees horiz. range
               45 degrees vertical range

right medial rectus resection and 2 mm. left inferior rectus resection. A tarsal graft was performed to the left lower lid to elevate the lid, and an excision of some scar tissue on the left lower lid. Following this surgery, the patient had binocular single vision in the primary position of gaze with a range of 15 degrees medial and lateral rotation, and binocular single vision inferiorly. He is now able to resume his previous work as an auto mechanic without the patch except when working under the car which necessitates superior field of vision (Fig. 18-3).

In summary, extraocular muscle imbalance is a common complication of orbital fractures. Immediate imbalance can often be cured by the reduction of the orbital floor fracture. Late ocular imbalance usually requires muscle surgery. Repeat muscle measurement records are emphasized to best follow the progress of recovery of muscle function and surgical improvement.

REFERENCES

1. Converse, J. M., Smith, B., Obear, M. F., and Wood-Smith, D.: Orbital blowout fractures; a ten-year survey, Plast. Reconstr. Surg. **39:**20, 1967.
2. Obear, M. F.: Complications of fractures of the floor of the orbit. In Smith, B., and Converse, J. M., editors: Second International Symposium of Plastic and Reconstructive Surgery of the Eye and Adnexa, St. Louis, 1967, The C. V. Mosby Co.
3. Obear, M. F.: Post-traumatic ocular muscle imbalance and enophthalmos; diagnosis and treatment. Presented at The Second International Corneo-Plastic Conference, London, 1968. (In press.)

Chapter 19

Upper lid reconstruction

History

Wendell L. Hughes

Reference to facial mutilation and repair goes back in history for many, many centuries; it goes back to the Chinese period, in which there are very few scattered references before 5000 B.C., and to the Indian period after 5000 B.C. in which there are scattered references to various plastic procedures.

The eye was an ancient Egyptian symbol which was worshiped as something very valuable. The conventional symbol of the eye, "the ouidjat eye," was used as a symbol for the 1937 International Congress of Ophthalmology in Cairo. The Egyptians divided the eye into 64 parts. The most valuable part was the medial canthus, and was given the value of 32. The pupil was the next and had a value of 16. The upper lid and brow area was given a value of 8, the lateral canthus had a value of 4, the lower lid a value of 2, and the lacrimal apparatus had a value of 1. These figures come to a total of 63. There was one part left for that peculiar sense of sight which was not understood. Sight was thought to emanate from the eye to the object—the proof being that if an obstruction was put in front of the eye the object could not be seen.

In a collection of writings from the sixth century B.C. there are references to sliding flaps. Around the time of Christ, Celsus wrote a summary of some of the plastic procedures that were used, for the most part, to reconstruct the nose. There were two main types of sliding flaps that Celsus recorded—one to cover a rectangular area, the straight sliding flap, and another to repair a triangular defect, the circular sliding flap. In the early

Buddhist period (250 B.C. to 750 A.D.) these procedures were done by the Brahmans or the priests; when the Hindus took over, it was relegated to a lower caste, because the priests would not contaminate themselves by contact with diseased flesh. Later, in the Mohammedan era, this was relegated to a still lower caste.

There was very little progress until the mid-fifteenth century. The Greeks and Arabs had added very little to the progress of medicine in general, and plastic surgery in particular.' When flaps were used for repair of lids around the eyes, there were gross scars and contractures. This led to the development in about 1400 of the so-called Italian method, a technique that was brought from India by some physicians who had joined the Crusades and had learned the technique from some of the Indian medical men. This method consisted of putting the arm to the head with the inside of the upper arm adjacent to the area to be repaired. The skin flap was raised from the inner arm and was brought over the area to be repaired. The arm was left in this position for 8 days. The pedicle was then cut, and the arm freed after the piece of skin from the arm had healed onto the area of the face to be repaired.

This method was used by several families in Italy—notably the Branca, Bojano, Pavone, Floraventi, and Montigore families—between 1400 and 1500, and was practiced as a secret art. Finally Gaspar Tagliacozzi, about 1500, popularized this technique and wrote extensively about it. He was particularly concerned with repair of noses. A statue of Tagliacozzi with a nose in his hand was erected in the square of Bologna to his memory. This method was further improved by Paul Berger in 1895, who developed a harness to hold the arm up to make the procedure somewhat less uncomfortable for the patient.

The first record of this method being definitely used for blepharoplasty was by Jules Sichel in 1834.

In the latter part of the eighteenth century and in the early nineteenth century, there was a great deal of animal experimentation and a resurgence of medical curiosity. Several investigators (Dzondi, Zeis, Fricke, and Deiffenbach) did a great deal to advance the modern concept of plastic surgery. Deiffenbach has been called the father of modern plastic surgery, and many of his procedures were performed on animals. He transplanted hair, feathers, and teeth, in addition to transplanting areas of skin from one part of the body to another. Even then there was curiosity about free transplantation of skin. Most of Deiffenbach's skin transplant procedures were failures because of lack of understanding about infection; many were lost through suppuration.

The double Celsus flap modification by Herman Knapp utilized the sliding of two flaps from opposite sides toward each other for lid reconstruction. Deiffenbach originally utilized a type of transposition flap from the temporal site for reconstruction of a lower lid. Later, after the work of Reverdin showed that tissues could be transplanted from one place to another, Budinger added a graft of ear cartilage to the inside of the flap (the so-called Deiffenbach-Budinger type of reconstruction).

In Spain, D'Argumosa did very much the same as Deiffenbach. Hysern y Molleras was another Spaniard who designed various flaps based at the temple, which were planned to replace the greater portions of the upper and lower lids. In the 1830's many of these grafts were failures; infection almost invariably occurred and there was no proper anesthesia.

Von Walther in 1826 was the first to use lid adhesions to prevent the contractures that were present in so many of these cases. Mirault, in 1842, and Keiker, at about the same time, also utilized them.

Reverdin, when an intern in Hôpital Necker, demonstrated conclusively for the first time that tissues could actually be transplanted from one part of the body to another using pinch grafts.[1] Reverdin started a whole new era in plastic surgery. He was able to transplant skin to areas that had been burned and to stimulate healing in these areas. Ollier transplanted split skin in 1872, and Thiersch in 1875 used very large skin grafts. Gradenigo in 1870 postulated that the best repair of lid tissues could be done by lid tissues themselves. This was emphasized by D'Antreue Tartois and Wheeler during the first world war. Esser used blood vessels in the transplantation of a biologic flap, and he also transplanted parts of the lid margin from one lid to another for correction of coloboma of the lower lid.

There have been many methods developed that are in use today for reconstruction of part of or an entire upper or lower lid. The Cutler-Beard procedure for the reconstruction of an entire upper lid and other methods will be demonstrated by other members of the panel.

REFERENCE

1. Reverdin, J. L.: Greffe epidermique—expérience faite dans le service de M. le Docteur Guyon à l'hôpital Necker. Reprinted from Bull. Imp. Soc. Chir. Paris **10**:511, 1869; Plast. Reconstr. Surg. **41**(1):79, 1968.

Modern techniques

Byron Smith

In the preceding section terminology was mentioned that was used in some of the earlier writings regarding sliding, advancement, rotation, and transposition. The terminology was somewhat different than it is today. The flap referred to as a circular sliding flap, for example, is usually called a rotational flap by plastic surgeons today. Transposition means taking up a flap and putting it in another place without disturbing its base. These flaps may be lined or unlined.

In addition to the flaps, which carry circulation, free grafts may be used, and they may consist of skin, mucous membrane, cartilage, or other tissues. In the past few years plastic surgeons have come to use a great deal of foreign material instead of actual tissues.

In the closure of lid tumors there are many methods of closing the defect across the margin. The overlapping or halving technique, as it was described years ago, is still used by some people. However, I think most surgeons now do an end-to-end anastomosis after block excision of tumors, just as they repair through-and-through lacerations of the lids. At the Manhattan Eye, Ear, and Throat Hospital, the end-to-end anastomosis is frequently done under the microscope using very fine sutures that are buried in the pretarsal fascia. If this technique is carried out with fine sutures, fine instruments, and fine needles, there is no need to use any type of overlapping method or figure-eights. It is simply a matter of common sense and accurate suturing.

After looking in an anatomy book one day I decided that perhaps some of the tumors of the orbit could be approached by a transmarginal incision, and I tried it out. In this procedure a transmarginal incision is made with a razor blade and extended with a Mayo scissors up to the cul-de-sac, in order to expose the tumor and resect it. The closure is direct. There is no overlapping and no notch postoperatively.

Another type of lid tumor is known as a "phantom tumor" because the encapsulated tumor of the anterior orbital region often bobs around in the orbital fat. The tumors are frequently operated upon and missed, because they slide back into the orbit when the surgeon goes after them. To keep these from going back something should be put behind them: either the surgeon's finger, a contact lens or lid plate, an Ehrhardt clamp, or a pack in the cul-de-sac. They may then be removed through a horizontal incision in the lid.

A common phantom tumor is an encapsulated hemangioma. I recall one case in which I removed an upper lid tumor and carried it to the laboratory myself, where it was diagnosed as an encapsulated hemangioma. A week later I was surprised to note its return in the lower lid of the same eye. It was summarily removed again, taken to the laboratory, and diagnosed again as an "encapsulated hemangioma." I think what happened was a diversion of circulation into a second, small hemangioma in the lower lid as result of cutting into and excising the co-existing one in the upper lid.

Tarsoconjunctival grafts used to be taken by splitting the lid margin of the graft side. Some complications arose from this procedure, such as scalloping of the lid margin, entropion, and trichiasis, with their attendant difficulties. If one chooses to utilize the upper lid for a tarsoconjunctival graft, the incision should be made about 2 mm. above the lid margin and not at the margin. There should be no splitting of the lid margin. I think that anytime a lid margin is split, whether for ectotropion or for a tumor, it leads to trouble. I, therefore, like to preserve the lid margin and do an end-to-end anastomosis.

In repairs of defects of the lower lids, we interdigitate the graft flap from the upper lid into the vertical sides of the lower lid defect, and advance a skin flap over it from below. This carries circulation, and after it has healed for a month, a lash graft is taken from the brow for appearance, and for stability of the new lid margin. The bridge is subsequently opened. Some people have criticized this procedure because it denies the patient vision in the eye during the 4 to 6 weeks interval. However, in my opinion, this is a small price to pay for the excellent results that may be achieved by this operation.

In defects of the upper lids, the same type of procedure described for repairing lower lid defects may be used. The principles and procedure are the same. There is no lid-splitting or free skin grafts from the opposite upper lid, or from any other lid, since lid-splitting or free grafts result in trichiasis, entropion, and general tissue shortage. The incision, parallel to the lid margin, should be placed 2 to 3 mm. below the lid margin, leaving the margin with its arterial supply intact, as well as the integrity of the lid margin itself. The advancement flaps are no trouble—I have measured these flaps and they sometimes double in length in the time that they are left uncut, which should be approximately 4 weeks.

The operating microscope is useful in sewing up the lid margins and for microresection of small lid tumors. Lashes will grow back after careful resection of superficial lesions; the reason for this is that the roots of the lashes are not disturbed by slicing across superficially.

Chapter 20

The use of major flaps versus other methods of lid reconstruction

Moderator:
Byron Smith

Panelists:
John Marquis Converse
Alston Callahan
Sidney A. Fox
Peter Ballen

Reconstruction of the lower lid by means of flaps

John Marquis Converse

The present trend in lid reconstruction, under the leadership of Dr. Wendell Hughes, is to employ local tissue. The most popular type of flap is the tarsoconjunctival flap, but there are occasional indications for the use of flaps taken from the temporal area or from the cheek area adjacent to the lid. As you know, Mr. Mustardé has been one of the advocates of this latter method. The following is a case in which there was a definite indication for the use of a temporal flap.

The patient, a 72-year-old male, originally came to me for the excision of a basal cell carcinoma situated at the level of the infraorbital margin (Fig. 20-1). The patient had received radiation previously and had had two previous excisions. After I excised the lesion, I realized the extent of the tumor. I had no other surgical alternative than to perform an exenteration of the orbit. Mohs' chemosurgery technique was employed and saved the patient's eye (Fig. 20-2).

The technique consists in the application

of a sclerotic, which fixes the malignant tissue. A careful histologic verification is then done on the extent of the propagation of the tumor. This technique permits following extensions into normal tissue even at a distance.

After the cure and verification that the patient had no more tumor, the problem of reconstruction of the lid was considered. A temporal flap was used in this case.

After the lid had healed, there was ectropion. There was also a bony defect in the infraorbital margin and a portion of the anterior floor of the orbit as a result of the destruction of the tissue by the chemical paste.

The remaining portion of the lid was raised and it became obvious that bone would be exposed. This is a primary indication for the

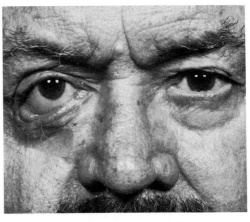

Fig. 20-1. Patient with lower lid basal cell carcinoma at the level of the infraorbital margin.

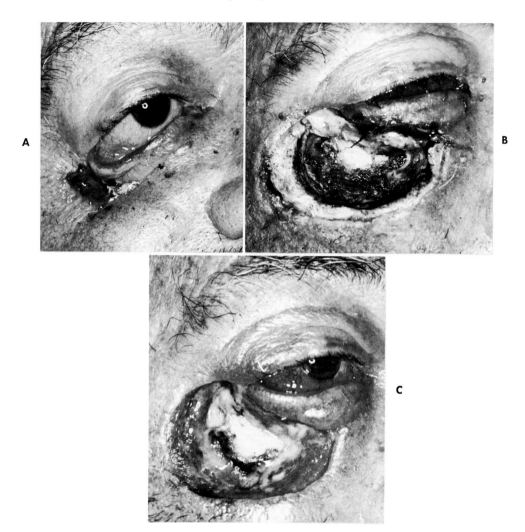

Fig. 20-2. Progressive results through use of Mohs' chemosurgery technique from initial treatment, **A,** to final extent, **C.**

use of a flap, since it is usually not possible to obtain satisfactory survival of a free skin graft over bare bone.

After the lid was repositioned, a defect occurred in the lower portion of the lid and the upper portion of the cheek area with bone exposed. A classical temporal flap was outlined, the lid was shortened in its horizontal dimension, and the temporal flap was transposed. Later, the reconstruction procedure in this patient was completed by the addition

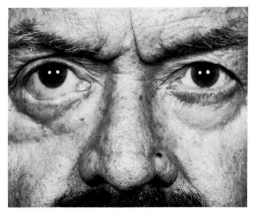

Fig. 20-3. Postoperative appearance of patient after reconstruction by temporal flap.

of a free graft taken from the upper eyelid. The graft was inserted into the area situated immediately above the flap and this was also accompanied by a further shortening of the horizontal dimension of the lower eyelid (Fig. 20-3).

I would like to add one point, which I think is rarely made. In reconstructive plastic surgery there is a great difference in the procedure to be employed and the procedure that will give the best result according to the age of the patient. There is a difference between the young patient and the elderly pa-tient. A young patient has tight tissues and does not have the generous supply of addi-tional tissue that the older person has. This is perhaps one of the few compensations of old age! Flaps can be widely employed in older patients because the tissue is available.

The lower lid can readily accept a flap, because it is a less mobile structure than the upper eyelid. The upper eyelid, on the con-trary, does not do well with a flap because the flap interferes with the normal mobility of the eyelid.

Mustardé transfer of lower lid for loss of upper lid*

Alston Callahan

Mustardé has pointed out that the normal lid elasticity is adequate for the lateral three-fourths of the lower lid to be stretched out to form most or all of the upper lid. In this way the medial fourth of the lower lid with its important lacrymal drainage structures can be left undisturbed in the formation of a new upper lid. The lower lid is replaced by the connective flap of skin and muscle from the zygomatic area of cheek. The flap is lined by a mucosal graft from the buccal mucosa or nasal septum.

The film "The Reconstruction of the Lower Lid by the Mustardé Technic" shows an 8-year-old girl who had an epidermoid carcinoma throughout most of the extent of her left upper lid. The lateral three-fourths of the upper lid is excised, and a normal zone of 1 cm. surrounding the tumor is re-moved with it. After the removal of the upper lid, the lower lid is cut so that the lateral two-thirds will be transferred up and rotated up and laterally, so that the base of the lower lid is sutured to the stump of the former upper lid. The sutures extend from the tarsus of the lower lid to the levator edge. The cheek flap is undermined and as it is rotated medially to permit the rotation of the lower lid into the upper lid defect, buccal mucosa is sutured to the undersur-face of the new lower lid.

After 3 weeks, the pedicle extending from the lateral end of the lower lid is divided and both lids are shaped as normally as pos-sible. A scar developed in the new lower lid from the repeated surgery, and this was excised, with a retroauricular skin graft being placed in the proper position.

Examination 2 years after the operation shows that the lower lid has been transferred, functions normally, and appears not too un-like the fellow lid.

---

*Dr. Callahan's presentation utilized three screens and consisted of the simultaneous projection of two motion pictures, "The Reconstruction of the Lower Lid by the Mustardé Technic" and "The Reconstruction of the Upper Lid," with explana-tory slides. The following is a summary of his remarks accompanying the Mustardé technique film.

Lid repairs

Sidney A. Fox

I will discuss techniques of lid repair other than the large rotated flaps. The procedures have been roughly divided into the older procedures that have been in use for approximately 15 years, and the ones of more recent date.

The simplest of the older techniques are the advancement pedicles, horizontal or vertical, which may be used with or without a halving closure. Another favorite technique is the Hughes technique in which a tarso-conjunctival flap is drawn from the upper lid and a skin flap from the lower. The trouble with vertical flaps is the tendency for the repaired lid to ride above or below the limbus, thus exposing too much sclera. This can be avoided to some extent by using free skin grafts instead of advancement flaps. Horizontal temporal advancement flaps give a much better cosmetic result, especially if the lesion is close to the lateral canthus. In these cases the lower lid is not pulled down below the limbus.

Among the newer techniques, the inter-marginal splinting or figure-eight suture has proved extremely useful.[1] It can be used in losses of up to half a lid especially in older individuals. The repair sometimes has to be helped along by a canthotomy and cantholysis at the lateral canthus. This technique gives the best cosmetic results. It is equally useful in traumatic colobomata, congenital colobomata, and tumor resections.

Collar-button resection is a recent technique that is useful when a neoplasm involves more skin muscle than tarsoconjunctiva. The loss of less tarsoconjunctiva simplifies closure and enhances the final appearance of the repair.[2]

The most recent technique is the use of full-thickness grafts which can be transplanted from homolateral or contralateral lids to close defects greater than half a lid.

REFERENCES

1. Minsky, H.: Surgical repair of recent lid lacerations; intermarginal splinting suture, Surg. Gynec. Obstet. **75**:449, 1942.
2. Fox, S. A.: Lid halving with variations, Arch. Ophthal. **65**:672, 1961.

Selected measures to correct various lid lesions

Peter H. Ballen

The ideal procedure to correct lid lesions is one which is the least damaging, is neat, and can be done in the shortest amount of time and competently by the greatest number of individuals. Sheehan stated in 1927, "It is probable that with many, the first thought about plastic surgery is that it is concerned mainly with aesthetic improvement. That has to be unlearned. The first concern is for functional restoration, the superior importance of which no surgeon will think of challenging."[1]

Fig. 20-4 shows a cutaneous horn at the junction of the lateral and middle one-third of the lower lid. A basal cell carcinoma that involved one-third of the lid border was found at the base of the horn. This can be repaired by direct excision and suturing, possibly with release of the lateral canthal ligament. Fig. 20-5 demonstrates the end result after excision and direct suturing.

The principle that the upper lid should not be invaded to provide tissue for the lower lid is based on the possibility that there will be a shortage of tarsoconjunctiva with resultant possible entropion of the upper lid or an excessive pull of the levator on the inner layer of the upper lid. The principle was established some time ago and remains

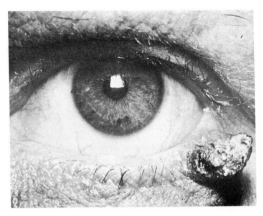

Fig. 20-4. Cutaneous horn.

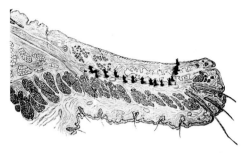

Fig. 20-6. Dotted line indicates incision beginning 1 mm. above lid border to avoid disturbing lid margin.

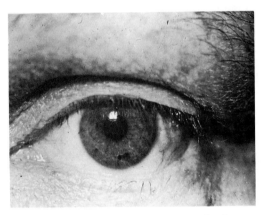

Fig. 20-5. Result following excision of edge-to-edge repair.

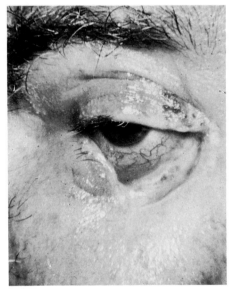

Fig. 20-7. Necrosis of lower lid following attempted reconstruction with large flap.

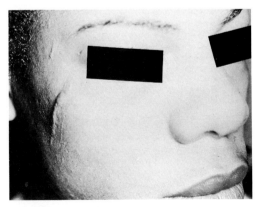

Fig. 20-8. Keloid formation.

true. When the tarsoconjunctiva with its attached levator is placed in the defect in the lower lid, it must show no signs of retraction. The section of the segment chosen to replace the loss of tarsoconjunctiva in the lower lid must be adequate, with lysis of any of the check ligaments and adhesions that may cause complications. If this flap occupies the space required without any sign of retraction, it will not cause any deformity in the upper lid. If one attempts to stretch the tarsoconjunctival layer from the upper lid or pull it down with tension sutures without an adequate dissection into the superior cul-de-sac, then trouble will be encountered. Tarsoconjunctiva from the upper lid, therefore, may be used with appropriate precautions. This procedure can be easily taught and performed, since the modification of using the tarsoconjunctiva with incisions beginning approximately 1 mm. above the upper inner lid border in order not to disturb the lash root has been widely accepted (Fig. 20-6).

Assuming that lid retraction from stretching the tarsoconjunctiva from the upper lid does occur, it does not seem to me to be dismaying and might easily be corrected. Fig. 20-7 shows a major failure which occurred in the moving of a large flap in the lower lid. This is a major loss that will require a major surgical procedure, whereas a shortage of a small amount of tarsoconjunctiva in the upper lid or even a somewhat low-riding lower lid is not as serious.

Another complication not described by the advocates of major flaps of the cheek for the restoration of lid is keloid formation. The author who advocates this method has the advantage of working with individuals who heal well. It would be interesting to hear from Dr. Callahan on this matter, because the population he deals with is subject to such keloid formation. In our experience, as soon as the field of surgery is extended beyond the upper and lower lids into the malar area and the preauricular area in Negroes, there are likely to be unsightly scars. Therefore it is our policy to stay away from these areas (Fig. 20-8).

Fig. 20-9 shows a traumatic defect in the left upper lid which occupies two-thirds of the upper lid in the horizontal and approximately 4 mm. in the vertical dimension. The defect is repaired by the Cutler-Beard procedure.[2] The anterior and posterior layers in the wound edges are split above to provide a tarsoconjunctival layer and a skin orbicularis layer. The width of the defect is measured and outlined on the lower lid with a methylene blue marking stick.

A through-and-through incision is made to the plate beneath with a No. 15 blade and is finished with scissors. The vertical

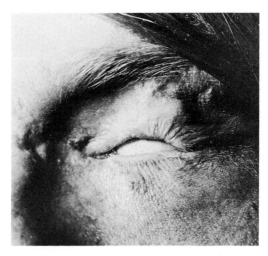

Fig. 20-9. Traumatic defect of upper lid.

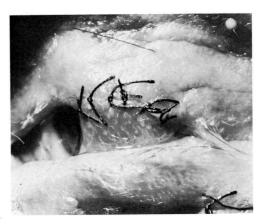

Fig. 20-10. Five days after Cutler-Beard procedure was performed to repair the traumatic lid defect in the patient seen in Fig 20-9.

portions of the flap are completed with scissors. The incision is made 2 to 3 mm. below the lower lid margin to avoid the marginal arterial arcade. This allows from 2 to 3 mm. of tarsoconjunctiva to be transplanted in the upper lid. This procedure is done under a local block anesthesia and does not require major hypotensive anesthesia or infiltration. The posterior layer of the inferior tarsoconjunctiva from the lower lid is sutured with a No. 6-0 nylon running suture.

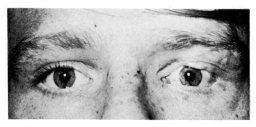

Fig. 20-11. Results 6 months after Cutler-Beard procedure for traumatic lid defect. Left lower lid shows no shortage of tissue.

It is first carried through the skin to tarsoconjunctiva, and then out through the skin and looped around itself to lock it. Three weeks following surgery, the pull-out suture is removed. The skin orbicularis section is sutured with a No. 6-0 silk suture. The wound in the lower lid is not sutured. A moderate pressure bandage is applied after the application of a layer of Telfa and some ointment (Fig. 20-10). The skin sutures are removed 3 to 5 days following surgery, and the pull-out sutures are removed a week to 10 days following surgery. The flap elongates two to three times its original length during the course of the next 2 months, which gives adequate tissue in the lower lid so that there will be no entropion or ectropion. The flap is then severed and the thickened tissue is excised from between the tarsoconjunctival layer and the skin. Posterior and anterior layers are sutured with silk (as well as the anterior layer) back into the lower lid after the wound is freshened.

This simple procedure provides an adequate result (Fig. 20-11). It can be done rapidly and taught easily. It is also tailored to the capabilities of the surgeon and to the peculiar legal atmosphere in which we exist.

REFERENCES

1. Sheehan, J. E.: Plastic surgery of the orbit, New York, 1927, The Macmillan Company.
2. Cutler, N. L., and Beard, C.: Method for partial and total upper lid reconstruction, Am. J. of Ophth. 39:1-7, 1955.

Discussion

Moderator:
Byron Smith

Dr. Smith: Here is a question for the panel members' opinion. At what age would you operate on a congenital coloboma of the upper lid?

Dr. Hughes: I think that depends entirely on whether the eye is in danger of damage. If the eye is in danger due to corneal exposure, which is quite rare, then it should be done within the first few days. It is, however, preferable to wait until the youngster is 1½ to 2 years of age. At that age you have something a little larger to work with and it is easier to obtain a better result. Usually nature provides protection even though a portion of the upper lid is missing.

Dr. Ballen: I think that the coloboma should be operated on when it is presented to the surgeon for repair no matter what the age of the patient.

Dr. Callahan: Well, I don't believe that time makes so much difference. I think that tissues, even at a very early age, will hold the sutures. On the other hand, I have seen cases in which the child has gone on to adulthood with a disturbing coloboma, and reached the age of being inducted into the army without corneal damage occurring. I would schedule it at some convenient time and neither wait nor delay it. I think it is perfectly all right to either proceed on an infant or delay until the child is older.

Dr. Smith: I might say that the earliest one that I have done is 2 weeks of age. The mother was rather upset about it. It was a gruesome-looking thing, and it was my decision to do it at that time. I will say that it worked out perfectly well. What is your opinion about it, Dr. Fox?

Dr. Fox: If the cornea is not involved and

in no danger, I see no point in hastening an operation the first week or two of a baby's life. I think we can afford to wait until the child is a year or two old. If the patient is an adult, he should be operated on as soon as possible. Sometime ago I operated on a girl 16 years old with a large coloboma of the upper lid because the parents were not interested in the operation before then.

Mr. Bedford: I think in Moorfields in London we tend, if the cornea is not in danger, to leave it as long as possible; usually until about the age of 4, because people usually start to school at that age.

Dr. Smith: I have another question for Mr. Bedford. What is the complication rate at 5-year and at 10-year follow-up in radiated lid tumors?

Mr. Bedford: This, in fact, depends a great deal on the radiotherapist one is working with, and I don't feel it is up to me to comment on radiotherapists and their doses. But there is no doubt that the incidence of keratin plaques is much higher if you have a radiotherapist who uses 5,000 R, over a period of only 3 weeks. One of the radiotherapists we work with only uses 3,500 R, and he gets no conjunctival complications whatsoever, but I have a clinical impression that probably his recurrence rate is a little bit greater. We only follow basal cell carcinomas for 5 years and squamous cell carcinomas for 10 years. I think that probably at least 60 to 70% of them get keratin plaques following 5,000 R. However, if it is off center and is not rubbing the cornea, there seems to be no irritation or complications at all.

Dr. Smith: Do you have any surgical treatment for hyperkeratinization of conjunctiva in the lid? Do you have any means of treating it surgically to alleviate the irritation if it is present?

Mr. Bedford: Yes. A free conjunctival graft to the center of the upper lid is done, but I would emphasize that I have seen over 300 cases and there has been only one that has needed a conjunctival graft.

Dr. Smith: I think we will give the next question to Dr. Hughes, because he has always been very interested in prisms, refraction, and muscles as well as fractures and plastic surgery. Discuss glasses for noncommitant diplopias in orbital fractures.

Dr. Hughes: When Dr. Obear was showing her pictures she had some cases in which there was diplopia in one portion of the field and the rest of the field had binocular single vision. For several years I have used a partially frosted lens on one side to eliminate binocular vision in the field in which there is marked diplopia, allowing the patient to see binocularly in the rest of the field. One can experiment with this very easily in the office with Scotch mending tape which has a ground glass appearance. You can put it across one lens to fog the field in which there is diplopia, leaving the rest of the lens clear. The patient is able to carry on very comfortably, and as the diplopia field decreases, as it often does in these cases, one can cut off a little piece of this mending tape and gradually eliminate it all as the diplopia disappears. This is a very useful little trick that is acceptable to many patients to eliminate their diplopia and yet allow them binocular vision in certain parts of their field.

Dr. Smith: I have another question for Mr. Bedford about his experience with and the advisability of using strontium 90 radiation in the treatment of neoplastic diseases of the lids.

Mr. Bedford: Actually we have some experience with this. I am afraid there is rather a schism—yet another schism—between America and England about the treatment of cancerous melanosis, and certainly at our unit we never exenterate them as a primary procedure. What we do is flatten the lesion with a biopsy and give strontium 90 as a definitive treatment. We find it a very curious disease as it waxes and wanes, and it blows up sometimes during menopause. Certainly the treatment we prefer at the moment is strontium 90. Because, as you know, it has only a small penetration, perhaps 3 mm. in the usual doses at which it is used, it isn't cataractogenic. If it is used for over 9,000 R, certainly you can get into trouble with cataract, and secondary glaucoma also. On the other hand, one has to observe that it really is a small price to pay for a disease in which the only other really logical treatment is exenteration. And, of course, we use strontium 90 also for grafts, but this is another problem.

Dr. Smith: I thank you very much. I have one more question. I would like to get the opinion of the panel on brow transplantation in the absence of the eyebrow. What has been your experience, or what is your advice in replacement of the eyebrow? We will start with Dr. Hughes.

Dr. Hughes: I think the transplantation of the eyebrow is always a difficult thing in which to get good cosmetic result. If it is part of one eyebrow that is missing, very often one can take a piece of the opposite brow. That of course gives the best match, if you can take part of the other eyebrow without creating a defect there.

For total loss of the eyebrows the beauticians do a pretty good job—with pencil lining and various other modalities with which some of the female members of the audience may be more familiar than I. They do a pretty good job in imitating the brow, and I think

probably the best replacement of a brow that I have seen is by the beautician.

Dr. Ballen: If it is possible to split one brow 50-50 I think that this is the method that I would prefer, taking half a brow, thinning it out and then using eyeliner and eyebrow shadow to thicken it up some. I think the presence of irregularities of the lashes or the appearance of the slight projection of the lashes is always desirable if you can get some eyebrow hairs from the opposite side.

Dr. Callahan: When one eyebrow is lost and the other one is normal I would prefer to use a free skin graft from the temple area. When the patient got older he might have some hair left and not be troubled by alopecia of the graft that you transplant.

Dr. Fox: These don't happen very often, fortunately. A simple graft sometimes works and sometimes doesn't; earlier in my career I had one case where the growth was so profuse that the man had to cut his brow every once in a while to match the other one. On the other hand, to balance that, I have had a couple of complete failures from the occipital region. So I think I am inclined to go along with Dr. Hughes and leave it to the beautician.

NEW TECHNIQUES IN OPHTHALMOLOGY

Presiding Chairman: **Goodwin M. Breinin**

Chapter 21

Expandable orbital implants

David B. Soll

The cosmetic and psychologic problems associated with enucleation surgery and the care of the anophthalmic socket are well known. Initially patients are usually grateful for the removal of a diseased or painful eye. However, after several months or years have elapsed most of these people are disturbed, consciously or unconsciously, by their cosmetic blemish. Even the very best cosmetic result cannot duplicate the appearance of a normal eye.

It is generally agreed that the greatest problems associated with prosthetic eyes are deepening of the superior lid sulcus, poor motility, displacement of the implant in the orbit, loss of lid tone or upper lid ptosis, and an enophthalmic-appearing socket.[1] A new type of implant has been developed which promises to provide more satisfactory solutions to many of these problems.

Standard implants

Cosmetic results are superior when intraorbital implants are used in conjunction with enucleation surgery.[2] There are many different types of implants available. At the present time buried implants are the most frequently used type. These can be classified in two general groups. The first consists of a Mules' type sphere, which is implanted within Tenon's capsule. There are no muscle attachments directly to the implant. The second group consists of various types of implants in which the extraocular muscles are either sutured to the implant or passed through tunnels within the implant.[4-9]

Integrated or semiburied implants initially give excellent motility and a very satisfactory cosmetic appearance. Their continued use, however, has not proved desirable, because a high percentage of the patients in whom this type of implant has been inserted eventually extrude the implant and develop secondary infections and contracted sockets.[10, 11]

Tunneled implants are still used and, when inserted properly, do give satisfactory cosmetic results. Their insertion, however, requires the stripping of Tenon's capsule from the muscles, and this upsets some of the normal anatomic relationships. They do occasionally tilt.[1, 10]

Eviscerations with intrascleral implants usually give the best long-term cosmetic results; but this procedure cannot always be done.[1]

Stone states that 65% of spherical implants become displaced with subsequent malposition of the extraocular muscles.[1] The insertion of a secondary or delayed implant after slippage or extrusion of an implant is a very tedious and often unrewarding procedure.

Expandable implant*

Evolution and present construction. All of the implants in use today are characterized by the fact that after insertion very little can be done to improve the function or appearance of the socket. During the past few years a new type of enucleation implant has been devised that solves many of the problems

---

*All expandable implants have been made under the direction of Dr. Ethel G. Mullison by the Dow Corning Center for Aid to Medical Research, Midland, Michigan.

formerly associated with enucleation surgery and implants.

The original implant consisted of four Dacron strips, 8 mm. wide, which emerged from under a 4 mm. cap of silicone rubber. The posterior portion of the implant was a solid silicone sphere. At the time of surgery each strip was cut to a length of 4 mm. and the extraocular muscles were sutured onto the strips, but not over the anterior surface of the sphere. Tenon's capsule was then closed over the implant, after which the conjunctiva was closed. This type of implant proved very satisfactory as far as motility was concerned. The four rectus muscles maintained a relatively physiologic position, approximating their position on the normal globe. The implant could not slip out of the muscle cone since the four rectus muscles were solidly attached to the Dacron strips.

The muscles were sutured to the side of this implant rather than imbricated over the anterior surface, because, as previous investigators have shown, imbrication of muscles over a sphere can cause the muscles to exert pressure on the sphere and the extrusion of the sphere between the muscles so that the implanted sphere eventually migrates outside the muscle cone.[1]

This initial implant did give better motility than the original Mules' type sphere, and, with the decreased possibility of slippage of the implant, assurance of better long-term motility and fewer orbital disturbances was given.

Development. The second phase in the development of the implant was the incorporation of a Dacron felt over the anterior surface of the silicone cap. This additional material allowed for the invasion of fibrous tissue between the edges of the four rectus muscle stumps and again allowed for better security of the implant within the muscle cone.

As technical improvements in the manufacturing process of silicones occurred, it became possible to construct an expandable ball type implant which consists of a Dacron mesh under which are incorporated the four Dacron strips. Under this is a self-sealing silicone plate. The posterior aspect of the implant consists of a silicone balloon filled with silicone gel. The entire spheric diameter of the implant is 16 mm. However, this implant is expandable. Sterile saline or antibiotic solution can be injected into the implant by inserting a 30 gauge needle through the anterior surface so that the needle point goes through the Dacron felt, the Dacron mesh, the self-sealing silicone plate, and is inserted into the center of the silicone gel. Thus the implant can be enlarged to an equivalent size up to or even beyond the volume of a 25 mm. sphere (Fig. 21-1).

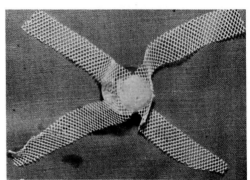

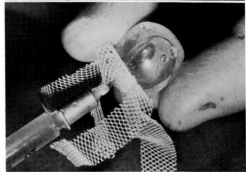

Fig. 21-1. **A,** Anterior view of the implant. Each Dacron strip is cut to a 4 mm. to 5 mm. length at the time of surgery. **B,** The implant is expanded with air for photographic representation. Sterile saline or an antibiotic solution is usually used. The needle passes through the anterior Dacron portion, then through a self-sealing silicone plate, and into the center of the silicone gel.

The present implant is constructed with a seam located at the equator so that when the implant is injected expansion will occur perpendicular to the seam. The medial and lateral Dacron strips are inserted in line with the seam. This property allows for vertical expansion of the implant and filling in of a superior lid sulcus when necessary.

Surgical technique. An enucleation is performed in the usual manner. My preference is a conjunctival perimetry using a Bard-Parker blade as close to the limbus as possible. The four rectus muscles are identified and severed from their insertions. A No. 4-0 chromic catgut suture is inserted through the tendon of each rectus muscle and locked at either end. The inferior oblique and superior oblique muscles are severed as close to the sclera as possible. All adhesions between muscle sclera and Tenon's capsule are then severed. A No. 4-0 black silk traction suture is inserted through the medial and lateral rectus muscle stumps. The globe is then elevated by using both of the No. 4-0 black silk traction sutures. By this maneuver the optic nerve can easily be palpated and even inspected using an Arruga speculum. The optic nerve is severed with a snare or is crushed with a hemostat and cut with a scissors. Only a very small rent in the posterior part of Tenon's capsule should be obtained using this technique.

The implant is then inserted with the seam of the implant in a horizontal position. The Dacron strips are cut to an exposed length of 4 mm. The four rectus muscles are then sutured to the Dacron strips so that the muscles overlay the strips. One or two additional No. 4-0 chromic sutures can be used to secure each rectus muscle to a Dacron strip (Fig. 21-2).

At the conclusion of this phase the Dacron felt should be centrally located in the socket and facing anteriorly. After this maneuver Tenon's capsule is closed over the implant using a purse-string suture of No. 4-0 chromic catgut. The conjunctiva is then closed by using interrupted No. 6-0 chromic catgut sutures. A conformer is inserted into the socket and a pressure bandage applied for

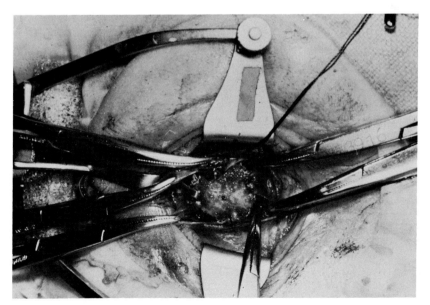

Fig. 21-2. The extraocular muscles have been sutured to the Dacron strips. Hemostats are on Tenon's capsule which is now closed over the surface of the implant. The Dacron felt and self-sealing plate are facing anteriorly.

a period of 4 days. The patient may be fitted with a prosthetic eye any time from 4 to 6 weeks following surgery.

Function. The most significant difference between the solid silicone implant and the new expandable type implant is found in the greatly increased versatility of postoperative management. If at any time during the patient's postoperative course there appears to be a deepening of the superior lid sulcus,

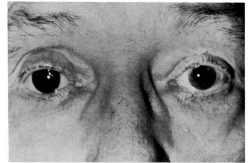

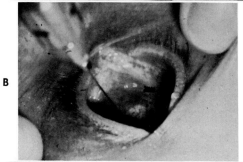

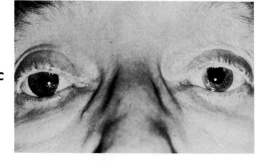

Fig. 21-3. A, Patient with anophthalmic right socket containing an expandable implant. Patient has a deep superior sulcus. **B,** A No. 30 gauge needle is passed into the center of the implant and 1.5 ml. of sterile saline is injected. **C,** Postinjection appearance.

enophthalmos, or any reason to fill the orbital volume, this can easily be done.

The patient's lids are scrubbed with pHiso-Hex. Several drops of topical anesthesia are inserted into the cul-de-sac of the anophthalmic socket. A 30 gauge needle is inserted through the apex of the socket so that it traverses the conjunctiva, Tenon's capsule, the Dacron felt, the Dacron mesh, and the self-sealing silicone plate, and pierces the center of the silicone gel, which is within the walls of the silicone balloon (Fig. 21-3).

After the needle is placed, which is a painless procedure easily done in the office (Fig. 21-3, *B*), sterile normal saline or an antibiotic solution is injected into the center of the implant. As much as 2.5 ml. of additional saline can be easily injected into a 16 mm. silicone balloon implant without exerting undue pressure upon the walls of the implant. Immediately following the withdrawal of the needle it is difficult to find the point of penetration.

Self-sealing property of the implant. Infection has not been a problem so far and it would seem unlikely that the insertion of a sterile 30 gauge needle through a Dacron mesh surface would cause any difficulty. To confirm this, an expandable implant which had been previously inflated and deflated several times in demonstration was selected for study. Each of the previous perforations had been performed with a 30 gauge needle. It was felt that this implant with its previous multiple punctures would make an excellent test object because of the many opportunities for leakage. At the time of this study the implant contained 2.5 ml. of saline in addition to its original volume, and was considered to be in an expanded state.

After being autoclaved, the implant was punctured with a 30 gauge needle and inflated with an additional 0.5 ml. of a specially prepared suspension of live coagulase positive staphylococci. Each milliliter of this suspension contained approximately 2×10^9 organisms. After contamination of the interior of the implant in this manner, the entire implant was immersed in a solution of 70% alcohol to sterilize the exterior. After removal from the alcohol solution, the implant was washed with 500 ml. of sterile saline and placed in a flask of freshly prepared thioglycolate broth and then the material was placed in an incubator. There was no growth after 8 weeks. It, therefore, seems that the self-sealing properties of the implant preclude any extrusion of its internal contents.

Experience with implant

The noninflatable type of implant has been used in six patients since 1966. There were no complications in 5 cases. In the sixth case, a small dehiscence of Tenon's capsule occurred 5 days after the enucleation surgery. This healed uneventfully after the defect was sutured closed.

The expandable implant has been used in eight patients since February 1967. Six of these have been uncomplicated. The postoperative motility was good in all of these patients. A deep superior lid sulcus developed in one patient and was corrected by injecting the implant as an office procedure. In two patients the implant extruded. One patient is a 49-year-old woman with a traumatically ruptured globe and marked tissue edema and protrusion of the globe between the lids prior to enucleation. The implant was inserted under tension and the sutures did not hold. It was possible to insert a silicone sphere in this patient's socket 3 weeks after the injury when all of the orbital edema had subsided. The patient retained the silicone sphere. The other extrusion occurred in a 2-year-old girl whose eye was enucleated because of a retinoblastoma. Tissue healing was poor in this patient and no attempt at insertion of a secondary implant was made.

Discussion and future projections

The concept of an expandable implant offers many possibilities in ophthalmic surgery. For initial trials it was felt that a ball type implant would be most desirable. Technically it is possible to construct this type

of implant in varied shapes and, therefore, use them for different purposes. It is possible that after more experience is gained a shape other than a ball will be chosen.

An expandable implant is also available for use in evisceration surgery. The scleral opening is made smaller than usual and, after the contents of the globe are removed, a deflated sphere is inserted into the scleral shell and expanded to the desired volume. This type of implant has only been used once, but with excellent success.

Until the present time I have used subperiosteal Teflon implants, wired to the orbital floor, for filling of the orbital volume in patients with anophthalmic enophthalmos associated with deepening of the superior lid sulcus. In general this has worked well. Now, however, an expandable subperiosteal implant has been developed; if the desired result is not initially obtained, more implant volume can be obtained by injecting fluid into the silicone gel of the implant.

Expandable conformers are also projected for use in socket reconstruction and expansion of congenitally anophthalmic sockets.

Summary and conclusions

The concept of expandable implants in ophthalmic surgery is a new one that has not yet been fully developed. Initial trials have been rewardingly successful, and it is hoped that its potential can be utilized and developed.

REFERENCES

1. Stone, W., Jr.: Complications of evisceration and enucleation. In Fasanella, R. M., editor: *Complications in eye surgery*, ed. 2, Philadelphia, 1965, W. B. Saunders Co.
2. Hughes, W.: Classification and mechanics involved, Trans. Amer. Acad. Ophthal. Otolaryn. **56:**25, 1952.
3. Mules, P. H.: Evisceration of the globe with artificial vitreous, Trans. Ophthal. Soc. U. K. **5:**200, 1885.
4. Allen, J. H., and Allen, L.: A buried muscle cone implant. I. Development of a tunneled hemispherical type, Arch. Ophthal. **43:**879, 1950.
5. Allen, L., Ferguson, E. C., and Bradley, A. E.: A quasi-integrated buried muscle cone

implant with good motility and advantages for prosthetic fitting, Trans. Amer. Acad. Ophthal. Otolaryn. **64:**272, 1960.

6. Cutler, N. L.: A basket type implant for use after enucleation, Arch. Ophthal. **35:**71, 1946.

7. Cutler, N. L.: A universal type integrated implant, Amer. J. Ophthal. **32:**253, 1949.

8. Milauskas, A. T.: A new orbital implant of fused acrylic plastic, Amer. J. Ophthal. **61:** 1443, 1966.

9. Troutman, R. C.: A magnetic implant, Arch. Ophthal. **43:**1123, 1959.

10. Cutler, N. L.: Principles underlying the surgical technique, Trans. Amer. Acad. Ophthal. Otolaryn. **56:**29, 1952.

11. Troutman, R. C.: Enucleation; recent trends, Arch. Ophthal. **62**(1):161, 1959.

Chapter 22

Nystagmus surgery

Abraham Schlossman

Fifteen years ago nystagmus surgery was introduced by Alfred Kestenbaum of New York and by J. Ringland Anderson of Melbourne. Although at first received with a great deal of skepticism, enough time has now elapsed and surgeons have had enough experience with these operations to prove that they are extremely effective, as well as dramatic in their results. When I visited the Filatov Institute in Odessa I was intrigued to find that the Russians also have a vast experience with this form of surgery.

Surgery is ideally suited for patients with jerk nystagmus who have a position of the head which improves their visual acuity. Such individuals usually have a head turn. Central visual acuity diminishes greatly when these patients hold their head straight. I have examined patients whose vision was as poor as 20/100 or 20/80 while they maintained their head in the so-called primary position, but who improved to 20/40 or 20/30 when they turned their head in the favored position. Conversely, when their head was turned to the opposite direction, acuity diminished to 20/200 or less. Although uniocular acuity usually follows a similar pattern, I use binocular vision as one of the chief criteria.

Such cases are relatively infrequent; nevertheless they can be greatly benefited by surgery. The results are often so dramatic that as soon as the bandages are removed, the patient actually prefers to hold his head quite straight, both to the amazement of his family and to the extreme satisfaction of the ophthalmic surgeon. Patients who have nystagmus with strabismus have individual problems which can only be corrected by strategically planning surgery in a manner which will combat both conditions simultaneously. Since there are no real precedents for these combined operations, each one represents a challenge.

Generally, this type of jerk nystagmus increases in amplitude when the patient looks in the direction of the quick phase, and decreases when he looks in the direction of the slow phase. When surgery moves the position of the eyes sufficiently toward the direction of maximal nystagmus (quick phase), the patient is able to attain maximal visual acuity in the primary position because the amplitude of nystagmus is diminished in this position, and he is relieved of an unsightly and uncomfortable head turn.

Anderson recommended bilateral recessions in order to rotate the eyes toward the side with greatest nystagmus. Kestenbaum advocated recessions or resections of all four horizontal muscles in order to achieve a similar result.

It is difficult to specify how much recession or resection should be performed. If the patient does not have heterotropia, surgery must be planned to alleviate the head turn without creating strabismus. Consequently, the amount of resection that can be performed is limited by the maximal medial rectus recession, which is 5 mm. Generally, surgery is balanced by performing 1 mm. more recession or resection of a lateral rectus than of a medial rectus muscle. A moderate head turn can be improved by bilateral recessions, while a significant alteration of the position of the head calls for resection of the remaining horizontal muscles as well, thus involving all four horizontal recti.

If the patient needs to turn his head to

the left to attain maximal vision, his eyes are shifted to the right (the position of least nystagmus). Surgical correction requires rotation of his eyes to the left (greatest nystagmus) in order to decrease nystagmus in the primary position; recession of the left medial rectus and of the right lateral rectus should be performed. In the presence of a marked head turn, the left lateral rectus and right medial rectus should be resected additionally. On the other hand, patients who must turn their heads to the right for maximal visual acuity should have their eyes rotated to that side. Consequently if only two muscles are to be operated upon, the right medial rectus and left lateral rectus should be recessed. If a greater effect is desired, the right lateral rectus and left medial rectus can also be resected. Since there are no specific rules for surgical correction of strabismus associated with nystagmus surgery, the ophthalmic surgeon divides the procedures on the different muscles by balancing those that benefit the strabismus against those that help combat the nystagmus.

I can give several broad generalizations to illustrate the planning of these combined operations for nystagmus and strabismus. When the patient has esotropia or exotropia, which has already moved one eye in the direction necessary to improve vision in nystagmus, it will be necesary to perform the recession-resection on the fellow eye in order to benefit both the heterotropia and the nystagmus. Thus, if the patient has a right esotropia and it is necessary to rotate his eyes to the left, the surgery should be performed on the left eye. On the other hand, if the patient has a right esotropia and it is also necessary to rotate his eyes to the right because of the nystagmus, it will be necessary to recess the right medial rectus and to resect the right lateral rectus for the correction of strabismus. Since this operation will have to be combined with a calculated amount of recession of the left lateral rectus and perhaps even with resection of the left medial rectus, it is important that the surgery on the right

eye aim at overcorrecting the heterotropia, because the nystagmus surgery on the left eye will neutralize the strabismus surgery to a certain extent. Because of these unorthodox approaches in planning, the ophthalmic surgeon should have a good idea of how much result he can expect from a given amount of recession or resection.

I think it is best to record vision according to the position of the eyes rather than according to the turn of the head. This helps in planning surgery, because it is actually the position of the eyes which the surgeon wishes to alter. Since these combinations of muscle surgery are so infrequently performed, I chart the detailed procedures on a sheet of paper and attach it to the wall in the operating room so that I will be prevented from making a mistake. The following four examples illustrate four different approaches:

Case 1. B. Y., age 8, had a moderate head turn to the left, but no strabismus. When his eyes were rotated to the left (head turned to the right, greatest nystagmus), binocular vision was 20/70. When his eyes were rotated to the right (head turned to the left, least nystagmus), vision improved to 20/25. The turn was moderate and vision in the primary position was 20/60. Surgery was planned to rotate the eyes toward the left (greatest nystagmus), enabling the patient to achieve minimal nystagmus in the primary position. A 5 mm. recession of the left medial rectus and 6 mm. recession of the right lateral rectus resulted in sufficient correction so that the patient attained 20/25 vision in the primary position and held his head straight.

Case 2. P. S., age 7, had to turn her head to the left in an extreme position to gain maximal visual acuity. Her binocular vision was 20/200 when her eyes were rotated to the left (head turned toward right, maximal nystagmus). When the child's eyes were rotated to the right (head turned toward the left, least nystagmus), vision was 20/50–1. This was an extreme case and required maximal surgery to rotate the eyes to the left. Consequently, the following surgery was performed: 5 mm. recession of the left medial rectus, 6 mm. resection of the left lateral rectus, 5 mm. resection of the right medial rectus, and 6 mm. recession of the right lateral rectus. After surgery the patient's vision improved to 20/50–1 in the primary position. (It had been 20/100 prior to surgery.) There was no preoperative or postoperative strabismus, and the patient maintained her head in a straight position.

Case 3. S. L., age 6, preferred to turn his head

moderately toward the right. Additionally, he had about 25Δ esotropia for distance and near. In the primary position his binocular vision was 20/100. When his eyes were rotated to the right (head turned to left, maximal nystagmus), his vision was 20/200. When his eyes were rotated to the left (head turned to right, least nystagmus), vision improved to 20/50. A 4 mm. recession of the right medial rectus and a 6 mm. resection of the right lateral rectus were planned for the correction of esotropia. In order to rotate the left eye further toward the right (nystagmus surgery to accompany recession of the right medial rectus and resection of the right lateral rectus), the left lateral rectus was recessed 6 mm. After surgery the child's head turn had disappeared, and he was able to attain binocular acuity of 20/50 in the primary position. His esotropia was reduced from 25Δ to 12Δ, also with significant cosmetic improvement.

Case 4. K. B., age 14, had right esotropia since birth. At age 4, bimedial recessions (5 mm. each) had been performed. Although immediately after surgery 20Δ of esotropia remained, by the time I examined the patient (ten years later) she had about 4Δ of exotropia for distance and 10Δ to 14Δ of exotropia for near. When she turned her eyes to the right (head turned to the left), she had maximal nystagmus and her vision decreased to 20/200 or less. In the primary position her vision was a poor 20/70. However, when her eyes were rotated to the left (head turned to the right), her vision improved to 20/30 and, of course, this was her preferred position. In this case it was necessary to move both eyes toward the right and at the same time to attempt to improve the girl's exotropia which was quite noticeable because of her

extreme head turn. As a result of the operations performed at age 4, the recession of the right medial rectus favored moving the eyes towards the right, while the recession of the left medial rectus was antagonistic to the nystagmus correction. By advancing the left medial rectus to its original insertion, I would perform nystagmus surgery and at the same time help to improve the exotropia. I felt that a resection of 3 mm. would further correct the exotropia. Recession of the left lateral rectus (7 mm.) was necessary to complete the nystagmus surgery. While it aided the exotropia, its effect was neutralized by resection of the right lateral rectus (also 7 mm.). Thus all the surgical procedures favored correction of the marked head turn. Only the resection and advancement of the medial rectus had been planned to correct additionally the exotropia, which incidentally was greater for near than for distance. I was gratified that after surgery the patient's vision was 20/30 in both eyes with her head held straight, and the resultant esotropia of 8Δ for distance and near gave her a much better cosmetic appearance than her former exotropia.

Nystagmus surgery aims to eliminate a head turn and to enable the patient to attain maximal visual acuity when he holds his head straight. In order to achieve this result, the eyes should be rotated towards the position of greatest nystagmus. If the patient also has heterotropia, combined surgery should be planned in order to attain the best results in correcting each of these disorders.

Chapter 23

Ultrasonics

Diagnostic and therapeutic ultrasonics

Edward W. Purnell

For the past ten years ophthalmologists have been exploring the possible uses of ultrasound in their specialty, both for diagnostic and therapeutic purposes. The practicability of diagnostic ultrasound has been demonstrated; the usefulness of therapeutic ultrasound has not yet been established.

Diagnostic ultrasound

Ultrasonograms may be obtained by either the time-amplitude or scanned-intensity-modulated methods (Fig. 23-1). The comparative advantages and disadvantages of these two methods have been the subject of many discussions in the opththalmic literature. Continued experience shows there are limitations to both methods.[1] While it is difficult to predict just what type of apparatus will evolve for clinical use in the future, those of us who have both the time-amplitude and the intensity-modulated equipment available prefer the intensity-modulated scanner for diagnosis whenever the patient's age and physical condition permit its use. In my opinion, this method of examination is essential for adequate evaluation of retrobulbar disease.

Patients are referred for ultrasonic examination because of intraocular or retrobulbar disease. In our institution referrals for examination of retrobulbar problems constitute 70% of the total number of patients referred. The majority of patients examined for intraocular disease are referred because of suspected intraocular tumor. In approximately one-half of these cases the diagnosis could be made by conventional means without ultrasonography. In the remaining cases the optical methods of diagnosis are not helpful, and ultrasonic examination is essential (Fig. 23-2). Sufficient data have been accumulated on the acoustical characteristics of malignant melanoma to make the diagnosis of this tumor by ultrasound reliable.[2] Intraocular

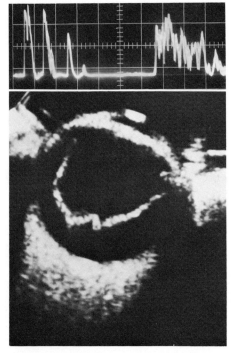

Fig. 23-1. Types of ocular ultrasonograms. Above, the time-amplitude sonogram. Peaks from left to right are from cornea, anterior lens surface, posterior lens surface, artifact, posterior ocular coats, and retrobulbar fat lobules. Below, an intensity-modulated sonogram of an eye containing a retinal detachment, horizontal cross-section. The anterior segment is uppermost; the detachment is represented by a W-shaped echo pattern within the vitreous body. The crescent-shaped echo pattern below represents the posterior pole of the eye and retrobulbar fat. The side walls of the eye are not represented because of their unfavorable orientation to the sound beam.

foreign bodies are not common in the Cleveland area, but among those cases which do occur, ultrasound is occasionally needed to accomplish localization. The examination is helpful in a variety of other intraocular conditions. Retinal detachments may be recognized in the presence of massive vitreous hemorrhage; the extent of proliferative diabetic retinopathy can be evaluated prior to removal of an opaque cataract. The thickness of the lens may be established in cases of traumatic cataracts, thus avoiding the com-

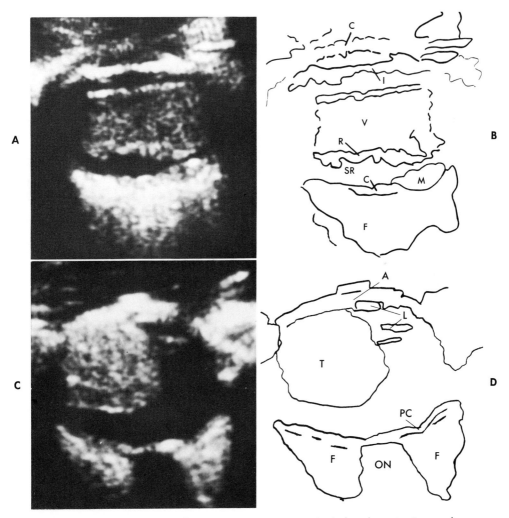

Fig. 23-2. A, Ultrasonogram of an eye containing a retinal detachment, vitreous hemorrhage, and small melanoma. **B,** Explanatory diagram. *C* (above), corneal echo; *I,* iris; *V,* vitreous compartment containing hemorrhage; *R,* retina; *SR,* subretinal space; *C* (below), choroidal pattern; *M,* melanoma. The vitreous hemorrhage is limited anteriorly by the anterior vitreous hyaloid face, and posteriorly by the retina. **C,** Ultrasonogram of an eye containing a large anterior choroidal melanoma. **D,** Explanatory diagram. *A,* anterior segment; *L,* lens surface; *T,* tumor; *PC,* posterior ocular coats; *F,* retrobulbar fat; *ON,* passage of optic nerve. The anterior chamber has been collapsed by the tumor.

plications that follow a standard surgical approach to removing a lens that is nearly completely absorbed.

The most rewarding application of diagnostic ultrasound, however, is to problems of monocular proptosis.[3] Diagnosis depends upon careful analysis of serial cross-sections and comparative views of the uninvolved normal orbit. Diagnosis of orbital disease requires a familiarity with the large variety of ultrasonic retrobulbar patterns seen in normal scans and often depends upon a knowledge of the alterations in the retrobulbar display seen with the examined eye in different positions of gaze. Scans made with the eye in extreme positions of gaze will frequently cause the shifting fat pattern to delineate a retrobulbar lesion, which might otherwise be overlooked.

An analysis of 100 consecutive cases of monocular proptosis is presented in Table 23-1. On the basis of the ultrasonic findings the lesions were reported as either mass lesions (43%) or infiltrating lesions (57%). A further attempt was made to predict the nature of the mass lesions as either invasive or noninvasive. If no mass lesion was observed, the ultrasonic pattern was classified as infiltrative. An attempt was made to identify these lesions as pseudotumor or endocrine-related on the basis of the ultra-

Table 23-1. Analysis of 100 cases of monocular exophthalmos examined by ultrasound

Type of lesion	Percent
Mass lesions	
Noninvasive (hemangioma, lymphangioma, neurilemmoma, xanthogranuloma, lacrimal gland tumor, unknown)	33
Invasive (carcinoma, sarcoma, melanoma)	10
Infiltrating lesions	
Endocrine	25
Pseudotumor	20
Congestive (sphenoid ridge tumors, leprosy, A-V fistula, ophthalmic artery occlusion, sinus disease)	12

sonogram alone. This subclassification agreed with the clinical diagnosis in approximately 80% of the cases. The subclassification of "congestive" was made when the ultrasonic pattern fitted neither the pseudotumor nor the endocrine groups. In only one case was a mass lesion missed.

From the ultrasonic pattern it is often possible to predict the pathologic diagnosis (Fig. 23-3). Lymphangiomas and hemangiomas usually reflect echoes from their interior portions. Carcinomas and other fairly solid lesions are usually seen as echo-free areas within a distorted retrobulbar fat pattern. Granulomatous pseudotumor produces a localized cystic type of ultrasonic pattern, while small cell pseudotumor produces irregular densities throughout the retrobulbar area.

Endocrine exophthalmopathy presents a fairly characteristic ultrasonic appearance. The diagnosis can be made with certainty if there is evidence of enlargement of one or more extraocular muscles, combined with a denser than usual echo pattern from the retrobulbar fat lobules. The extraocular muscles themselves are usually not visualized ultrasonically. Their tone and size can be inferred from the shape of the retrobulbar fat pattern, which is composed mainly of echoes from lobules of the intramuscular or central portions of the fat pad. In more advanced cases echoes are obtained from within the muscle bellies; they are presumably caused by the abnormal material within these muscles.

In addition to indicating the type of lesion, ultrasonic examination will often indicate the proper surgical approach for biopsy or removal of the lesion.

Ultrasound has a unique role in many areas of basic eye research. Both the intensity-modulated and time-amplitude methods can be used to measure intraocular distances with a reliable degree of accuracy. These measurements are valuable in the study of refractive anomalies, especially myopia. Instrumentation is available for measuring small changes

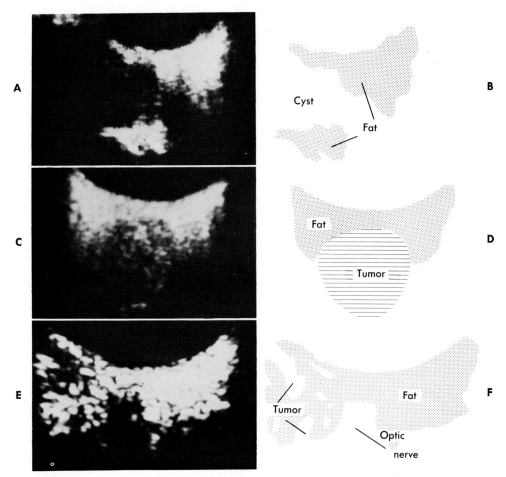

Fig. 23-3. A, Ultrasonogram of the retrobulbar fat pattern in a case of monocular proptosis due to lacrimal gland cyst. **B,** Explanatory diagram. Fat has been forced into the
apex of the orbit by the cystic mass lesion. **C,** Ultrasonogram of the retrobular fat pattern
in a case of monocular proptosis due to hemangioma. **D,** Explanatory diagram. **E,** Ultrasonogram of the retrobulbar fat pattern in a case of monocular proptosis due to giant cell
pseudotumor. **F,** Explanatory diagram. To the left of the optic nerve passage the fat has
been pushed aside by the infiltrating granulomatous material.

in the position of reflecting surfaces within
the eye.[4] It is possible to measure by ultrasound the change in eye length that occurs
with each heartbeat, and to measure the
thickness changes in the lens that occur during accommodation.

Therapeutic ultrasound

High energy ultrasonic devices are under
investigation for possible therapeutic use.[5-7]
The ultrasonic power of these devices is several thousand times greater than that employed in diagnostic examinations. While
there is no known injurious effect from ultrasound at power levels used in diagnosis, the
transducers used in therapeutic research are
capable of producing severe and permanent
injury to the globe. Two characteristics of the
sound beam are of specific interest—the thermal effect at the focal point and the sonic
radiation pressure along the axis of the beam.
Injury caused by the thermal effect has po-

tential use for tumor destruction, for creating chorioretinal lesions, and for ciliary body destruction in certain forms of glaucoma. Radiation pressure has potential use in treating retinal detachment.

After several years of extensive animal and clinical experimentation, we are still unable to evaluate the future therapeutic usefulness of ultrasound. There are too many poorly understood problems concerning the monitoring and reliability of the ultrasonic input to allow us to speculate confidently about its future. Excellent results in isolated clinical trials, however, point out the enormous potential of this form of therapy. The major problems at present are technical and are related to directional control of the sound beam, control of the amount of energy that actually enters the eye, and avoidance of undesirable side effects along the path of the beam.

The equipment developed for ocular therapeutic ultrasound is shown in Fig. 23-4. A variety of interchangeable transducers is available for supplying ultrasonic energy at frequencies ranging from 800 kilocycles to 15 megacycles. Various beam shapes may be produced, from highly convergent to parallel.

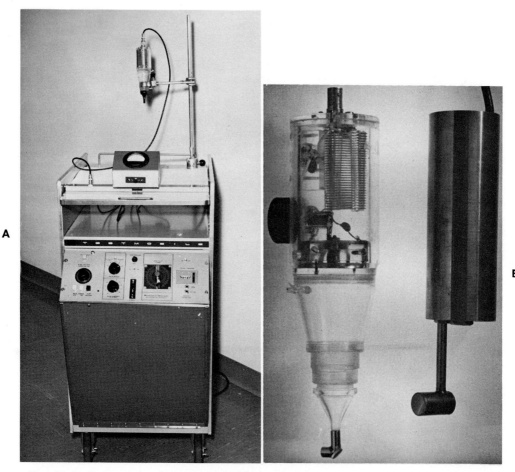

Fig. 23-4. A, Apparatus for production and application of high energy ultrasound to the eye. The transducer, shown in storage position, is held by hand during exposure. **B,** Two ocular transducers. The transducer at left produces a focused beam, which is bent 90 degrees near the tip. The transducer at right produces a broad, parallel sonic beam.

The transducer may be operated continuously or in the form of repetitive pulses with a wide choice of duty cycles. The ultrasonic power is adjustable, up to a maximum of 300 watts/cm.² at the focal point of a convergent beam.

Useful application of therapeutic ultrasound in the treatment of ocular disease depends upon the ability to apply appropriate energy to the intraocular target site without producing cataract. This is best accomplished by avoiding the lens entirely when applying the sound beam. In situations in which the sound beam must pass through the lens, the sonic energy density and duty cycle must be adjusted to avoid cataract production. These two parameters have been evaluated, and the cataract–producing doses for various exposure programs have been determined for each transducer and each frequency used clinically.[8] The energy density of the portion of the sound beam passing through the lens is kept as low as possible. This is particularly important when using convergent (focused) beams, since the exposure time required for cataract production increases as the square of the lens–focal point distance. Pulsing the sound increases the total amount of sound that may be passed through the lens without cataract production.

Chorioretinal lesions may be produced by ultrasound. Injury varies, depending upon the total power employed, from transitory retinal edema to localized perforation of the globe. With focused beams the area of injury may be kept to within approximately 5 degrees of retinal surfaces. The sharp delineation of the area of injury is striking. Even with the more destructive dosage programs leading to perforation of the globe, there is no microscopic evidence of injury beyond 1.4 mm. of a 2 mm. perforation.

The thermal energy of focused ultrasound may be used for cyclodiathermy. Data obtained in animal studies correlate ultrasonic exposure programs with resultant changes in intraocular pressure.[9] Experience with ultrasonic cyclodiathermy in glaucoma patients has been limited. In severely diseased eyes the pressure reduction following ultrasonic therapy is definite but often transitory, and returns to pretreatment levels within several weeks or months. Results are comparable to the results obtained using the conventional methods of cyclodiathermy, which are safer and more convenient.

The greatest potential use of ultrasound is in retinal detachment therapy. Areas of a detached retina may be retro-displaced by the radiation pressure of a sound beam, the total power of which is a fraction of that known to cause cataract or chorioretinal injury. Patients may be treated under topical anesthesia with little or no discomfort. From the small series of detachment patients treated by ultrasound thus far, a number of observations can be made. Movement of the retina and vitreous debris is readily observed and is always in the direction of the beam propagation. When the sound is pulsed, vitreous opacities move a certain distance and remain in the new location for the duration of the pulse. During the "off" interval, vitreous material returns to approximately its original position. The linear amount of movement and the rate of movement are directly proportional to the energy used. Movement of the retina is variable; movement of the retina in the path of the sound beam is in the direction of propagation, and counter movement or billowing is seen in other areas. Response to the sound beam is an indication of retinal motility.

Radiation pressure may be used to alter persistent vitreous traction on the retina. Traction at the site of small retinal tears has been observed to disappear following exposures of pulsed ultrasound. During a 12 hour period following brief exposures, there is frequently a marked flattening of the retina. This has been observed in cases in which there was little or no settling from gravitational forces prior to therapy. The mechanism of this effect is not known. In 2 cases there was complete settling of the detachment.

With one exception, all attempts to "unfold" the overhanging retina on the posterior side of giant retinal tears have failed to yield the desired result of placing the retina in a more favorable presurgical position. The reason for this failure is not entirely clear; however, data obtained from experiments in animals with detachments suggest the problem may be solved by utilizing broader beams, lower frequency, and relatively greater sonic pressure. In one case responding favorably to presurgical treatment with ultrasound, the giant tear was associated with a totally dislocated lens. Sufficient presurgical unfolding was accomplished by ultrasonically moving the lens from its inferior position back to the pupillary area.

As yet we have little clinical experience with the treatment of retinal detachment by divergent or parallel beams of wide diameter, or with the retro-displacement of detached retinas using low power beams for protracted periods of time. Most of our experience to date has been obtained using sharply convergent beams, with radiation pressure limited to a small area of detachment. Use of several beams, entering from different points around the globe, has been considered as a means of stripping the retina free of adhesions. The method must await further refinement in transducers.

REFERENCES

1. Purnell, E. W.: Ultrasound in ophthalmological diagnosis; diagnostic ultrasound. In Preceedings of the First International Conference, University of Pittsburgh, 1965, New York, 1966, Plenum Press, pp. 249-258.
2. Baum, G.: Ultrasonic characteristics of malignant melanoma, Arch. Ophthal. **78:**12, 1967.
3. Purnell, E. W.: Ultrasonic interpretation of orbital diseases. Presented at the International Conference on Ultrasonics in Ophthalmology, Philadelphia, 1968. (In press.)
4. Sokollu, A.: Ultrasound in ophthalmic research. In Proceedings of the First International Conference, University of Pittsburgh, 1965, New York, 1966, Plenum Press, pp. 174-183.
5. Purnell, E. W., Sokollu, A., and Holasek, E.: The production of focal chorioretinitis by ultrasound; a preliminary report, Amer. J. Ophthal. **58:**953, 1964.
6. Purnell, E. W., Sokollu, A., Torchia, R., and Taner, N.: Focal chorioretinitis produced by ultrasound, Invest. Ophthal. **3:**657, 1964.
7. Purnell, E. W.: Therapeutic use of ultrasound. In Goldberg, R., and Sarin, L., editors: Ultrasonics in ophthalmology, diagnostic and therapeutic applications, Philadelphia, 1967, W. B. Saunders Co., pp. 102-123.
8. Torchia, R., Purnell, E. W., and Sokollu, A.: Cataract production by ultrasound, Amer. J. Ophthal. **64:**305, 1967.
9. Rosenberg, R. S., and Purnell, E. W.: Effects of ultrasonic radiation to the ciliary body, Amer. J. Ophthal. **63:**403, 1967.

Foreign body localization

Nathaniel R. Bronson II

The successful extraction of an intraocular foreign body with minimal damage to the eye requires an accurate localization of the object. Occasionally the foreign body can be seen with one of the optical instruments, but all too often the view is obscured by hemorrhage or a cataract.

In the past reliance has been placed on x-ray and metal locators, and these continue to be of great value. With x-ray it is possible to tell the size, shape, and attitude of the foreign body, and to obtain some idea of the consistency and location; the accuracy of

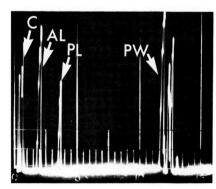

Fig. 23-5. Normal ultrasonogram through the primary axis showing echoes returned from the cornea *(C)*, the anterior lens capsule *(AL)*, the posterior lens capsule *(PL)*, and the posterior wall *(PW)*.

x-ray localization varies with the experience of the radiologist and the ability of the patient to cooperate. The metal locators, such as the Berman or the Roper-Hall instruments, can often be helpful in determining the location of the foreign body if it is near the surface. They will also give some idea as to the magnetic characteristics of the object. Neither, however, give information as to the position of the foreign body relative to the other structure of the eye, nor is it possible to determine the amount of damage the eye has already sustained. Moreover, it is not feasible to repeat x-ray localization in the operating room.

Ultrasonography provides the ideal complement to the older techniques, since localization relative to the structures of the eye is simple and safe and can be repeated in the operating room. In addition, it is possible to determine if there is hemorrhage, retinal detachment, or encapsulation of the object.

Ultrasound functions by sending a beam of sound through tissues. Any structures or object in its path will return some sound which is shown as an upward spike or echo on a cathode ray tube. In the normal eye with the sensor or transducer placed over the center of the cornea, echoes are returned from the anterior and posterior lens capsules, the posterior wall, and the orbital fat (Fig. 23-5). As the lens distorts the sound beam, most examinations are carried out over the sclera.

As compared to the echoes from tissue, foreign bodies return a much larger amount

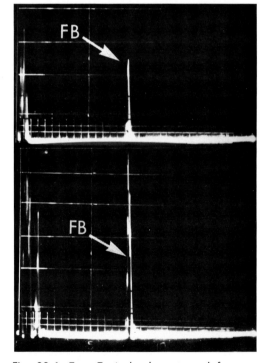

Fig. 23-6. Top: Typical echo returned from an intraocular foreign body *(FB)* (50 db.). Bottom: At higher sensitivity (70 db.) no tissue echoes are seen surrounding it; the foreign body is free in the vitreous.

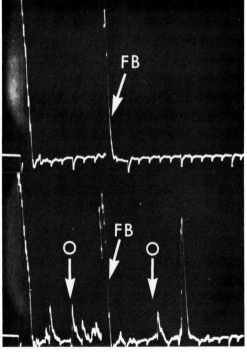

Fig. 23-7. Top: At low sensitivity (50 db.) only the strong foreign body echo *(FB)* is seen. Bottom: With high sensitivity (75 db.) intense vitreous reaction and organization *(O)* can be seen to be present. A cataract prevented optical visualization of this damage.

of sound and the echoes are therefore stronger. Fig. 23-6 (top) shows a typical echo from an intraocular foreign body. The foreign body is 16 mm. away from the sclera, and by increasing the sensitivity tissue echoes would become apparent. In this case (Fig. 23-6, bottom) the area between the foreign body and the sclera is clear and it would be safe to draw the foreign body to the pars plana without risk of traction bands which

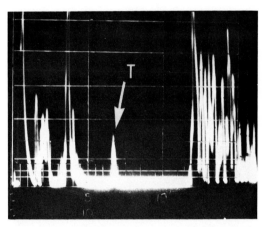

Fig. 23-8. A vitreous traction band is shown *(T)* at a sensitivity of 70 db. This could be traced with the ultrasonic beam back to the foreign body. The reaction in front of the band was a dense secondary membrane.

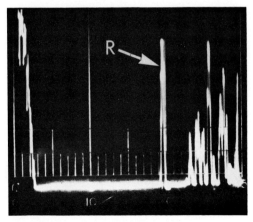

Fig. 23-9. A retinal detachment *(R)* of 3 mm. elevation is seen at 60 db. sensitivity.

might detach the retina. The ultrasonic picture is completely different when there is any change in the vitreous. Fig. 23-7 (bottom) at a high sensitivity (75 db.) shows the extensive changes that have taken place. Low voltage echoes represent hemorrhages or loosely organized vitreous changes. Traction bands appear as stronger echoes (70 db.) and their paths can often be traced through the eye with the ultrasonic beam (Fig. 23-8). A detachment of the retina (Fig. 23-9) shows as a fairly strong echo (60 db.) equal in height to the posterior wall response, while total disorganization of the eye shows multiple strong echoes throughout the vitreous.

A foreign body in the vitreous is usually easy to demonstrate, since it returns a stronger echo than any obtained from the retina or tissue organization. An intrascleral foreign body is more difficult to pinpoint,

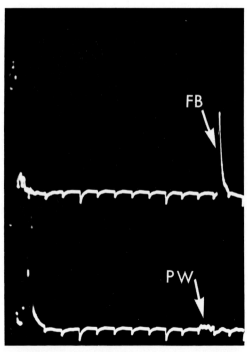

Fig. 23-10. Localization of an intrascleral foreign body by height of the echo at a very low sensitivity (50 db.). The foreign body echo *(FB)* is significantly higher (top) than any obtainable from the posterior wall (bottom).

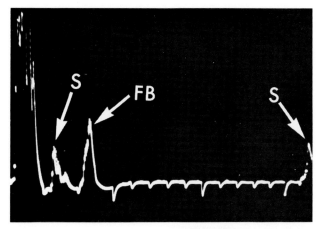

Fig. 23-11. Preoperative ultrasonic localization of foreign body *(FB)* relative to the sclera *(S)*. The transducer was placed over the inferior rectus near the equator and can be seen to be lying 3.5 mm. from the external scleral surface at this point.

and it is helpful to have an approximate idea of the location, such as can be obtained by x-ray or one of the metal locators. To prove a foreign body is intrascleral it is necessary to show that the echo returned is far stronger than any obtained from the posterior wall. Fig. 23-10 shows such a picture.

The value of ultrasound in foreign body management and preoperative estimation of ocular damage is shown in the following cases.

Case 1. The patient was referred as having a nonmagnetic intraocular foreign body. Ultrasound showed the foreign body to be lying near the site (Fig. 23-11) where extraction had been attempted, and a strong magnetic type of response was obtained from a metal locator. It was difficult to understand why magnet extraction had failed. Repeated ultrasonic examination at the time of surgery showed that when the eye was turned upward the foreign body dropped back 14 mm., out of the field of force of the magnet. A site closer to the foreign body was chosen and the object was readily extracted with a magnet.

Case 2. A 5-year-old child who had an intraocular foreign body and such extensive edema that it was impossible to open the lids was referred to us. With the ultrasonic transducer placed on the lid, the foreign body echo was found near the posterior wall. At a high sensitivity extensive vitreous reaction and organization was found, and the eye appeared far too damaged to be retained (Fig. 23-12). With this knowledge the child was anesthetized. Foreign body extraction equipment was available, but the parents understood that

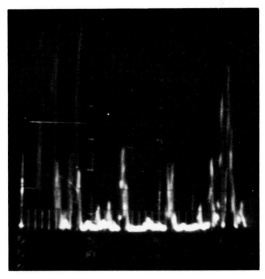

Fig. 23-12. The entire vitreous is filled with intense organization and reactions. The transducer was placed on the lids in this case to allow estimation of the damage before examination under anesthesia.

enucleation would more likely be necessary. When the lids were opened (Fig. 23-13) the case was found to be hopeless as had been suspected by ultrasound, and the eye was removed.

We have had several similar experiences in which ultrasound has given us this important information.

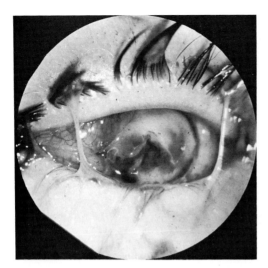

Fig. 23-13. External photograph of the severely damaged eye found under anesthesia.

Ultrasound does not eliminate the need for the use of other techniques. It does complement x-ray and the metal locators by giving an exact localization of a foreign body relative to the sclera. It also shows the amount of tissue damage that has been done by the foreign body and associated injury which allows far better planning of the surgical approach. As localization by ultrasound is easy and safe, it can be done both preoperatively and during surgery to find a shifting foreign body.

Myopia*

Brian J. Curtin

The Myopia Clinic of the Manhattan Eye, Ear and Throat Hospital was initiated with the object of offering to the myopia patient a comprehensive service which would include diagnosis, detection of complications, and treatment.

The diagnosis of the individual myopic eye as physiologic or pathologic represents a clinical problem of considerable magnitude. The axial length of the eye is the major determinant of refraction, but the effect of the other components of refraction, corneal curvature, lens refraction, and, to a limited extent, anterior chamber depth, are such that a 26 mm. eye can be rendered hyperopic and a 22 mm. globe can be made myopic by appropriate combinations of these factors. The degree of refractive myopia is, therefore, a poor basis for diagnosis except at the extremes of the myopia spectrum.

*This study was supported in part by Grant N 3408 of the United States Public Health Service.

Because of this problem in diagnosis, the measurement of axial length must be considered an indispensable tool in the field of myopia management and research. Until the advent of ultrasonography, however, the techniques used for the determination of axial diameter, principally those utilizing x-ray or optical methods, were highly sophisticated and demanded an unusual degree of patient cooperation.[1, 2] In the case of x-ray, a certain amount of risk was also present. Ultrasonography presented to the ophthalmologist an accurate, safe, and objective method of ocular biometry. In 1964, ultrasonic gear was installed in the Myopia Clinic, and since that time axial length mensuration has been an essential part of the myopia survey. The Myopia Clinic patient also undergoes a refraction, ophthalmoscopy by both direct and indirect methods, tonometry, ocular rigidity determination, slit lamp examination, and keratometry. Gonioscopy, fundus biomicroscopy and photography, as well as other special studies, are added as indicated. These data are recorded on a Royal McBee card and a detailed fundus drawing is made on its reverse side (Fig. 23-14).

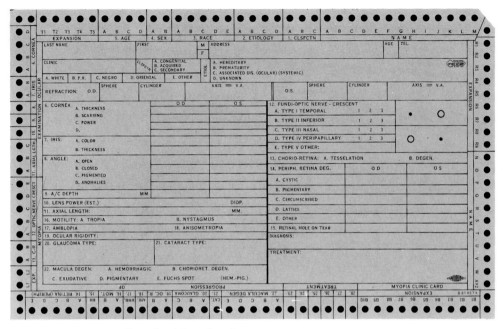

Fig. 23-14. Myopia Clinic Card, Royal McBee type.

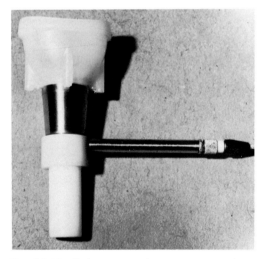

Fig. 23-15. Eight megacycle eye cup transducer with transparent core.

The primary research target of the clinic was the establishment of criteria for the diagnosis of pathologic myopia. The posterior fundus changes of this disease are dramatic in their appearance as well as their extent. They are, furthermore, the present basis for diagnosis in myopia. A correlation of fundus changes with axial length in myopia appeared to be a study which could offer an entirely new basis for diagnosis.

The ultrasonic gear used in this study has evolved gradually over the past 4 years. Originally an 8 MC focused transducer was touched to the cornea. The variability of readings due to corneal flattening and frequent off-axis alignments necessitated the substitution of an eye cup transducer (Fig. 23-15). In this device an 8 MC focused transducer is cored axially and the core is filled with methylmethacrylate. The delay tube and eye cup are filled with saline and the patient fixes a light held below the transducer through the transparent core. A modification of the Coleman-Carlin transducer assembly[3] was also used with a 10 MC transducer and collimator (Fig. 23-16). Neither of these methods provided the rapidity and ease of measurement needed in our clinic operation, so these methods were eventually supplanted by the use of a 10 MC focused transducer with a 36 mm. delay column

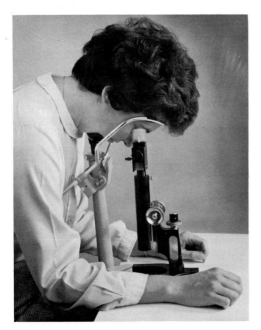

Fig. 23-16. Modified Coleman-Carlin transducer assembly.

sealed with a thin plastic film of 12 μ thickness (Fig. 23-17). These films can be discarded after each examination. The column is filled with distilled water and the patient fixes the tip of an optic fiber, which is inserted into the center of the transducer face. With optimum alignment, the patient sees a bright white spot in the center of a dull gray circle. This transducer can be hand held or used with a micromanipulator (Fig. 23-18).

The ultrasonoscope itself consists of a modified Hoffrel 101 A unit with 5 to 15 megacycle echo receivers. This is used in conjunction with a Hoffrel 705 digital adapter and a Monsanto 1000 H 20 MHZ precision electronic digital counter (Fig. 23-19). The 101 A ultrasonoscope generates the driving impulse for the transducer and receives echo information from it. This is amplified and displayed on a cathode ray tube. It also supplies all the timing signals for the system. This unit generates 450 pulses per second, each with a duration of from 0.3 to 0.5 micro-

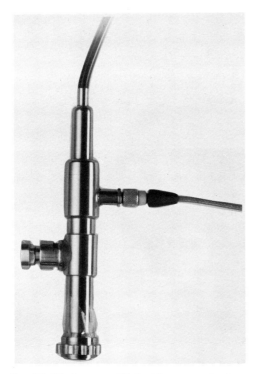

Fig. 23-17. Sprague Clinic 10 megacycle transducer.

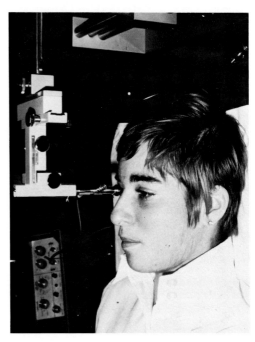

Fig. 23-18. Sprague Clinic transducer with micromanipulator.

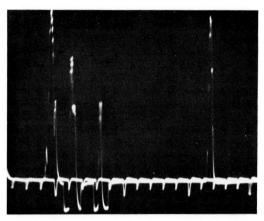

Fig. 23-21. Position 2. Axial A mode display, gates set for lens thickness measurement.

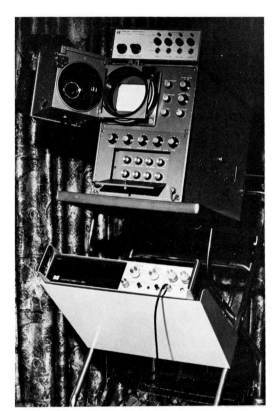

Fig. 23-19. Hoffrel 101A ultrasonoscope with 705 digital adapter (top) and Monsanto 1000 H digital counter (below).

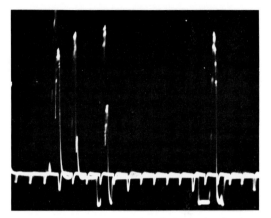

Fig. 23-22. Position 3. Axial A mode display, gates set for vitreous segment measurement.

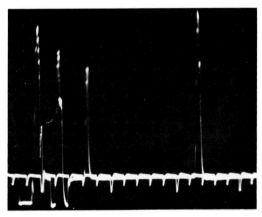

Fig. 23-20. Position 1. Axial A mode display, gates set for anterior cornea to anterior lens surface measurement.

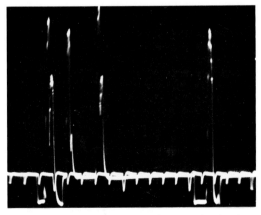

Fig. 23-23. Position 4. Axial A mode display, gates set for anterior cornea to anterior retina composite measurement.

second. It operates at 300 to 350 volts, which translates to a power output from 0.0001 to 0.001 watt. The 705 adapter generates sweep and gain triggers as well as two gate display wave forms. This produces an output of a gated precision crystal controlled oscillator. The oscillator frequency is automatically selected for the sound velocity of the tissue examined. The duration of the oscillator gate is determined by the time interval between gate selected start–stop echos. The impulse is then passed into the Monsanto counter, which displays the gated measurement directly in millimeters. The gate systems used are:

Position 1—anterior cornea to anterior surface of lens (Fig. 23-20)

Position 2—anterior lens surface to posterior lens surface (Fig. 23-21)

Position 3—posterior lens surface to anterior retinal surface (Fig. 23-22)

Position 4—anterior corneal surface to anterior retinal surface (Fig. 23-23)

The gate position switch also automatically selects the proper quartz crystal for the oscillator so that relative sound velocities are accurately compensated for in the final millimeter readout.

The velocities used are:

Position 1—1,532 meters per second

Position 2—1,640 meters per second

Position 3—1,536 meters per second

Position 4—1,536 meters per second

In this study position 4 was used. The exact reproducibility of axial length measurements is currently under study, but there appears to be a level of accuracy of about 0.2 mm. on either side of the averaged readings.

In this study over 1,400 eyes have been examined. It was found that neither conus nor peripheral retinal changes could be considered pathognomonic of pathologic myopia in view of their ample representation among normal eyes with low myopia and even hyperopia. Those fundus changes considered unique to pathologic myopia were the Fuchs' spot, lacquer cracks, and circumscribed

chorioretinal atrophy. This atrophy occurred most frequently in contiguity with conus and was never seen in the absence of this fundus change. These myopic degenerative changes of the posterior fundus have been described in more detail elsewhere.[4]

During the progress of this survey two factors were immediately apparent—the greater axial length of the male eye and the marked effect of age upon the incidence of degenerative changes of the posterior fundus. A difference of approximately 0.5 mm. in minimal ocular length between male and female eyes was detected, and the same difference was noted in median readings up to age 20. This disparity is of special interest inasmuch as the median axial length for degenerative posterior pole lesions in the female eye was 29 mm. compared to that of 30 mm. in the male. A similar disparity in size between male and female eyes has been reported in several other studies.[5-7] Age was a factor of great importance in the appearance of posterior pole degeneration. In eyes of 27 mm. length there was an increase in incidence of these degenerative changes from 15% to 55% between the age groups 30 to 45 years and 46 to 90 years, respectively. Eyes of 29 mm. length showed an increase of from 33% to 76%, respectively, in these same age groups.

Because of this effect of age, a plot was made of 330 eyes of patients 45-years-old and above (Fig. 23-24). The dramatic effect of axial length upon the incidence of posterior pole degeneration is obvious. What is equally obvious, however, is that there is no sharp delineation of axial length at which such changes will and will not occur. From these data it appears that eyes with an axial length below 25 mm. are physiologically myopic, and eyes with axial lengths of 31 mm. or more are pathologically myopic. Between these figures the axial length determination alone cannot give the clinician more than a probability of the disease.

There can be little doubt as to the importance of the association of axial elongation

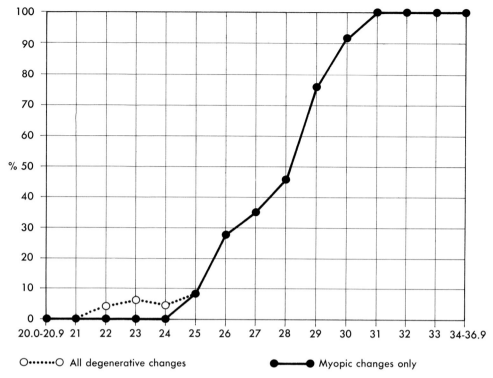

O········O All degenerative changes   ●———● Myopic changes only

Fig. 23-24. Incidence of posterior pole degeneration at each axial length (330 adult eyes; patients from age 45 to 90 years).

with pathologic myopia and, as a consequence, little doubt as to the importance of axial length determinations in cases of myopia. It does appear, however, that other, more subtle changes can be better correlated with axial length for the diagnosis of the myopias than the gross damage of degenerative fundus changes. The electrophysiologic changes of the electroretinogram and especially the electro-oculogram would seem most suitable in this regard, and it is in this direction that our subsequent efforts are to be made.

REFERENCES

1. Stenstrom, S.: Variations and correlations of the optical components of the eye. In Sorsby, A., editor: Modern trends in ophthalmology, Vol. 2, New York, 1947, Paul B. Hoeber, pp. 87-102.
2. Sorsby, A., Benjamin, B., Davey, J. B., Sheridan, M., and Tanner, J. M.: Emmetropia and its aberrations; a study in the correlation of the optical components of the eye, Medical Research Council Special Report, Series No. 293, London, 1957, Her Majesty's Stationery Office.
3. Coleman, D. J., and Carlin, B.: A new system for visual axis measurements in the human eye, Arch. Ophthal. **77**:124, 1967.
4. Curtin, B. J.: Physiopathology and therapy of the myopias, Trans. Amer. Acad. Ophthal. Otolaryng. **70**:331, 1966.
5. Sorsby, A., Benjamin, B., and Sheridan, M.: Refraction and its components during the growth of the eye from age of three, Medical Research Council Special Report, Series No. 301, London, 1961, Her Majesty's Stationery Office.
6. Jansson, F.: Measurement of intraocular distances by ultrasound and comparison between optical and ultrasonic determination of the depth of the anterior chamber, Acta Ophthal. **41**:25, 1963.
7. Gernet, H.: Über Achsenlange und Brechkraft emmetroper, lebender Augen, Graefe Arch. Ophthal. **166**:424, 1964.

Chapter 24

Cryosurgery

Moderator:
Charles D. Kelman

Panelists:
Tadeusz Krwawicz
Andrew de Roetth, Jr.
Donald M. Shafer
John G. Bellows
R. David Sudarsky

Cataract

Tadeusz Krwawicz

Cryoextraction of cataract continues to be the most interesting application of low temperature in ocular surgery. This is a natural consequence of the fact that cataract extraction constitutes a vital problem for every ophthalmic surgeon, and that significant advances in the operative treatment of cataract are eagerly looked for. Everyone who performs such operations is familiar with the often considerable difficulties that accompany them. A need for stabilization was felt, regarding the method of grasping the lens capsule to alleviate the risk of damaging the capsule. This stabilization can now be obtained with the use of low temperature. The advantages offered by the cryogenic method of cataract extraction have been noticed in a comparatively short time, and it is now possible to speak of progress in the art of restoring sight to people affected with cataract.

Cryoextraction of cataract has freed the operator from the distressing uncertainty resulting from the question of which will break first: the delicate zonule fibers or the sometimes even more delicate and vulnerable capsule of the cataractous lens. A successful out-come of the operation has become possible for a great number of specialists, even to those with less experience, and this has, in turn, contributed to a speedy development of cryosurgery of cataract. The almost complete absence of capsular complications has gained this method a large number of adherents.

The first reports, dating from 1960, on the possibility of applying low temperature in ophthalmology gave rise, especially in the United States, to experimental and clinical investigations on further prospects offered by this method, and development of new instruments for application of cold to ocular tissues.[1]

The number of excellent, up-to-date modifications of the cryosurgery apparatus now available is so great that it is hardly possible to gain practical knowledge of all of them. The merit of some cryoextraction units is that the temperature of the working part can be controlled. Kelman's thermoelectrically cooled instruments,[2-4] Bellow's cryoextractors and liquid nitrogen cryosurgical unit,[5-7] and Sudarsky's Freon-cooled probe[8] are very well known and popular in the United States.

Some more complicated appliances fail to gain wider popularity and give way to simpler instruments. All may be useful in the hands of operators who employ them habitually, because the basic idea is always the same; but even the most ingenious technical achievement cannot replace the delicacy of the operator's hand. The basic idea is that the refrigerated instrument—either the original simple cryoextractor or one of its more elaborate modifications—grasps not only the capsule of the opaque lens, but also the congealed subcapsular masses.

The cryogenic method of cataract extraction eliminates the risk of complications that result from damaging the capsule or from leaving behind its fragments; it can be said that such accidents now belong to the past.

Cryoextraction has a wide range of indications and practically no contraindications; it is used for all types of cataract, including complicated cataract.

The problem of transmission of low temperature to other parts of the eye, resulting in possible damage to the surrounding tissues, has been studied. It has been found that during cryoextraction of cataract, the fall of the temperature of the ocular tissues is not greater than when the traditional operative methods are used.

I would like to point out two phases of cryosurgery of cataract which are less well known, and which are familiar to me through personal experience.

Cryoextraction makes it possible to apply enzymatic zonulolysis selectively; that is, when it is really necessary. The decision to make use of zonulolysis can be made intraoperatively when a considerable resistance of the zonule is encountered. In such cases the operation can be interrupted at any moment, zonulolysis can be carried out, and cryoextraction resumed. The question is not to prevent the breaking of the capsule (because there is no risk of such an accident), but to eliminate the possibility of secondary complications, which can follow excessive traction or pressure.[5]

From a total of more than 4,000 cryoextractions, over 500 operations were performed in this way; in this recent series zonulolysis proved necessary in only 4.05% of the cases.

We are now also aware of the fact that the original cryoextraction technique caused an unnecessary difficulty resulting from the very active part which the assistant had in performing the operation. It was the assistant who lifted the corneal flap and pushed the iris aside, and both manipulations required a highly trained hand. Complaints were occasionally heard that highly qualified and skillful assistants were not always available. There are also operators who prefer to depend on as little extraneous help as possible.

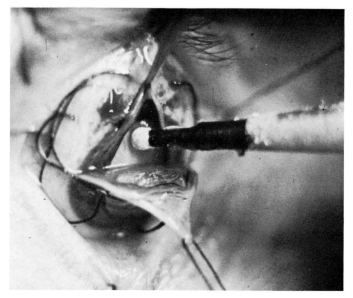

Fig. 24-1. An additional suture lifts the corneal flap. This iris is grasped with a smooth forceps and pulled upward in the form of a tent. The instrument is applied to a sufficiently large exposed part of the lens.

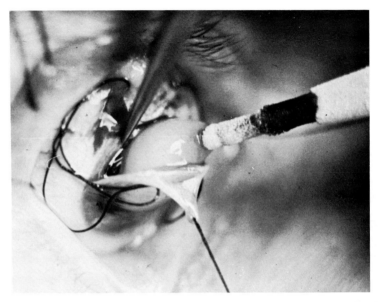

Fig. 24-2. The cataract is removed with rotating movements; the iris is still lifted.

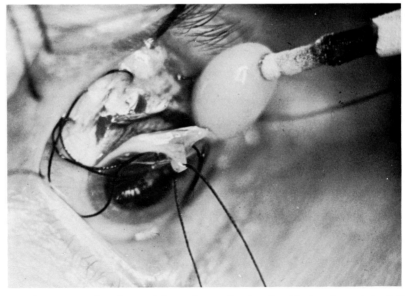

Fig. 24-3. The cataract has been delivered completely; the iris is allowed to fall back into position.

It now appears that this inconvenience can be easily removed, thanks to a slight modification of the operative procedure.[5]

The introduction of a thin long auxiliary suture to lift the corneal flap makes it unnecessary for an assistant to attend to this step. The operator himself grasps the iris near its pupillary border with a smooth forceps, lifts it in the form of a tent (Fig. 24-1), and exposes a sufficiently large part of the lens so that the tip of the instrument can be safely applied to it. The cataract is removed with rotating movements (Fig. 24-2). The iris is adjusted and the corneal flap is allowed to fall back into position (Fig. 24-3). In this way the role of the operative assistant becomes smaller than that assigned to him by the traditional methods of cataract surgery.

The modification just described is undoubtedly one of the many advantages cryoextraction of cataract can offer. It is my belief that the constantly growing popularity of this method will bring about further developments and improvements.

REFERENCES

1. Krwawicz, T.: Experimental studies using a cryosurgical device, Presented at the Twenty-seventh Congress of the Polish Ophthalmological Society, Poznan, Klin. Oczna 30: 129, 1960.
2. Kelman, C. D., and Cooper, I. S.: Cryogenic ophthalmic surgery, Amer. J. Ophthal. 56:731, 1963.
3. Kelman, C. D., and Cooper, I. S.: Cryosurgery for cataract extraction and the treatment of other eye diseases, Highlights Ophthal. 7(1): 181, 1964.
4. Kelman, C. D., and Cooper, I. S.: Cryoextraction (letter to ed. with extensive data), Arch. Ophthal. 74:145, 1965.
5. Bellows, J. G.: The application of cryogenic techniques in ophthalmology, Amer. J. Ophthal. 57:29, 1964.
6. Bellows, J. G.: Indications and technique of cryoextraction of cataracts, Arch. Ophthal. 73:476, 1965.
7. Bellows, J. G.: Cryoextraction by torsion and traction, Amer. J. Ophthal. 61:113, 1966.
8. Sudarsky, R. D.: Thermodynamic considerations in ocular cryosurgery, Proc. Roy. Soc. Med. 59:1053, 1966.
9. Krwawicz, T.: Arch. Soc. Amer. Oftal. Optom. (In press.)

Glaucoma

Andrew de Roetth, Jr.

The primary method of treating glaucoma consists of lowering the intraocular pressure by improving the outflow facility. As a secondary procedure the intraocular pressure can be lowered by decreasing the aqueous inflow. Medically this is done with the use of a carbonic anhydrase inhibitory agent, such as acetazolamide (Diamox), and surgically in the past this was accomplished by the diathermy procedure. Unfortunately diathermy has many drawbacks and complications. For this reason cryosurgery has recently been advocated as a replacement for diathermy. In essence, cryosurgery can be used as an antiglaucomatous procedure; it lowers the intraocular pressure by decreasing the aqueous inflow.

Mechanism of action

Animal experiments done mainly on rabbit eyes helped us to understand the mechanism of action of this new antiglaucomatous method. The cryosurgical probe applied over the ciliary body region produces an ice ball in the eye, including the ciliary body. The freezing of the ciliary body results in a vascular reaction; within a few days after freezing one can see considerable edema, engorgement of all the blood vessels, and hemorrhages in the ciliary processes. This vascular reaction reaches its peak within 2 or 3 days following treatment. At this point, some destruction in the epithelial cells of the ciliary processes can also be seen; both the pigmented and nonpigmented cells are affected. This vascular lesion can be demonstrated best in albino rabbit eyes. The fresh hemorrhage stands out well against the white background. In pigmented eyes, both rabbit and human eyes, it is more difficult to demonstrate this vascular reaction, because the blood cannot be seen against the black background of the pigment.

Approximately 1 week after treatment healing begins, the vascular reaction subsides, and most of the blood is absorbed. In the stroma of the ciliary processes healing will result in fibrous tissue formation. The epithelial layers of the ciliary processes show some tendency for regeneration during healing. However, some of the ciliary processes will heal without the epithelial regeneration, while in others a pigmented scar will take the place of the epithelial layers. Within 6 weeks the eye will be completely healed except for these changes in the ciliary processes (the fibrous tissue formation in the stroma and the damage to the epithelial layers). This damage in the ciliary processes will result in decreased rate of aqueous humor formation and, consequently, in lowered intraocular pressure. At the same time it is important to realize that the overlying tissues, the conjunctiva and the sclera, are not affected by the freezing. There is minimal conjunctival chemosis which usually lasts for a few weeks, but no permanent damage will result. In all the treated eyes, both animal and human, this vascular reaction is considerably greater in pigmented eyes. As far as the final result is concerned, there is more destruction of the epithelial layers in the pigmented eyes as compared to the albino rabbit eyes or the lightly pigmented human eyes.

Technique

Cryosurgery for glaucoma can be done as an out-patient procedure in a glaucoma clinic; hospitalization of the patient is not necessary. The Linde cryosurgical unit, produced by the Union Carbide Corporation, is the best unit for this procedure. The tip of the cryosurgical probe is a circle with a diameter of 4 mm. Under local anesthesia the probe is applied directly on the conjunctival surface over the ciliary body region. The optimum temperature is $-80°$ C.; six 1-minute applications constitute a treatment. The lower half of the globe is usually treated, thus saving the upper half in case the procedure has to be repeated. The underlying ice ball that forms in the eye is larger than the tip of the probe. For this reason, it is important to place the tip of the probe far enough back from the limbus in order to prevent freezing the cornea.

Indications

Clinical experience of the past few years has shown that not all types of glaucomatous eyes react equally to cryosurgery. In general, elderly patients whose glaucoma has been present for a number of years do considerably better with this new treatment. Children and young adults or patients whose glaucoma has been present for only a few months do not benefit from cryosurgery.

For this reason cryosurgery is indicated mainly in the treatment of advanced chronic simple glaucoma, particularly in elderly people who have had the disease for many years. Many of these patients had filtering procedures in the past, but in spite of such surgery and maximal medical therapy, their glaucoma is still not adequately controlled. In such eyes, cryosurgery often is of considerable help. In addition, cryocautery can be employed successfully in elderly patients with aphakic glaucoma whose disease cannot be controlled medically.

Recently a racial difference was observed concerning the results of cryosurgery in the treatment of advanced chronic simple glaucoma; Negro patients with this disease had much better results following freezing than a similar group of white patients. This became particularly obvious when cryosurgery was repeated on a number of eyes. Because of the innocuous nature of this new procedure, cryosurgery has been repeated on a number of eyes within a few months when the first treatment appeared unsuccessful. In the repeated treatment group there was even more difference in the results between Negro patients and the corresponding group of white patients.

Complications

The main complication of cryosurgery is actually an extension or exaggeration of the vascular reaction. The hemorrhage that normally occurs in the ciliary body following freezing occasionally becomes very severe. In these cases the blood is not confined to the ciliary body only, but can be seen in the anterior chamber and the vitreous. Occasionally such a severe hemorrhage can produce a choroidal separation and considerable visual loss. Fortunately this is a rare occurrence; only 4 to 5% of the treated eyes have these severe hemorrhages.

A moderate amount of iris atrophy has been observed in a small number of eyes following cryosurgery for glaucoma. This atrophy is not extensive; the loss of tissue is minimal and, therefore, does not interfere with the function of the eye. Another complication that is more important, although rare, has been the appearance of corneal opacities. The reason for this complication is usually faulty positioning of the cryosurgical probe. If the tip of the probe touches the cornea, a small amount of corneal tissue will freeze during this procedure. In most eyes the cornea can withstand this minimal freezing quite well; occasionally, however, this will result in a mild keratitis and finally in opacities of the limbal cornea in the area of the application.

Postoperative iritis was first considered a complication of cryosurgery. However, this occurs in practically every eye treated and, therefore, cannot really be considered a complication, but should be looked upon as part of the normal postoperative reaction. It should be treated with topical application of steroids and mydriatic drops; otherwise it may result in posterior synechiae and even in secondary cataract. However, this is a so-called second cataract and is caused by the iritis, not the freezing procedure. Apparently the cryosurgical procedure has not produced cataracts thus far; this is true both for the human eyes and for the laboratory animals.

Advantages and disadvantages

Since cryosurgery was developed as a procedure to take the place of diathermy, it should be compared to diathermy. The main difference between these two techniques is in the nature of tissue response to the treatment. Cryosurgery is less damaging to ocular tissues. The overlying tissues, the conjunctiva and the sclera, are not affected at all by the freezing procedure. However, with the use of diathermy, scar tissue will form between conjunctiva and sclera, and the conjunctiva will be bound down to the underlying sclera.

Furthermore, cryosurgery is more of a quantitative method, and diathermy is more of a qualitative procedure. In cryosurgery the vascular reaction remains confined within the ice ball. Therefore, one can tell exactly how much of the ciliary body is involved, since the size of the ice ball is known. With diathermy it is not known exactly how far the electric current or heat will extend from the tip of the diathermy needle or even in what direction it will travel. For this reason, many eyes have been either under-treated or over-treated, and globes have been lost following diathermy because of too much damage to the ciliary body. So far this has not been the case with cryosurgery; it is a considerably less damaging procedure and very few eyes have been over-treated with this new method.

This safety factor, favoring cryosurgery over cyclodiathermy, is of considerable importance because of the advanced nature of glaucoma in most of these eyes. These eyes often have only minimal vision; thus it is all the more important to treat them with the safest and least damaging method. Cryosurgery may not always help the patient, but the surgeon is reasonably certain that it will not do any more damage to the involved eye.

Summary

Cryosurgery is an adjunct in the treatment of glaucoma; it lowers intraocular pressure by decreasing the aqueous inflow. The best results are seen in patients with advanced chronic simple glaucoma; in such eyes cryosurgery often is of considerable help.

Retina

Donald M. Shafer

Low temperatures have become the latest destructive methods for treating many diseases of the retina. The word "destructive" may seem too strong for some people, but all the agents that are now used or have been used in the past, are destructive. They destroy cells or entire structures to accomplish the desired results. Through the years it has always been a tissue-damaging agent that was used—the famous igni-puncture with red hot steel, sodium hydroxide, cauterization, diathermy, and now, freezing. The search has always been for a selectively destructive agent, and freezing has become the best agent available today.

Reasons for using cryosurgery

Retinal adhesion. Cryosurgery is used because it has a selective effect on the choriocapillaris and the retina at probe temperatures of –35° to –70° C., yet does not appreciably destroy the sclera or vitreous at these temperatures. The subsequent natural repair of the damage to the choriocapillaris and retina produces a strong adhesion between the retina and choroid, as indicated by Bietti, and improved by Lincoff and Kelman.

Selective tissue response. At temperatures between –35° and –70° C., the clinical effect on the vitreous and sclera has thus far proved to be minimal. This selective tissue response is desirable and suggests that freezing is an improved agent for retinal detachment surgery.

Cell destruction. Another capability of low temperature application is actual cell destruction in the retina. This is used in other retinal diseases. Lower temperatures, such as –60° to –100° C. may be used. This usage is more effective with the procedure called refreezing, in which a tissue that is edematous from a first freezing and thawing, is refrozen to fracture and destroy cell walls. This is useful in Lindau-von Hippel disease, and possibly in retinoblastoma.

Cryosurgery is used in retinal detachment because it produces strong retinal adhesion, with little vitreous and scleral damage. Cryotherapy may be used in some retinal tumors, because it can be cell destructive with apparently little other damage.

When to use cryosurgery

In addition to increasing use in detachment of the retina, there are three other areas in which cryosurgery of the retina is now used.

Retinal tears without detachment. Most frequently cryosurgery is used for retinal tears without detachment. These may properly be considered under retinal detachment, yet they are somewhat different. To many this automatically brings to mind photocoagulation. In our experience, however, there has been more cryotreatment of these flap tears and less photocoagulation. In many tears without detachment there is already hemorrhage in the vitreous, and there is probably less vitreous reaction to the cryotreatment than from the heat of the photocoagulator. In addition, the cryoapplication, without opening the conjunctiva for anterior tears, is almost as easy as photocoagulation, and reaction is minimal. In an eye 10 days after transconjunctival cryoapplication for anterior tear, there is often no visible response. The most important advantage of cryotreatment is that it is much more surely applied than photocoagulation can be, especially if there are problems such as small pupils, cataracts, hazy vitreous, or a far anterior hole.

Lindau-von Hippel disease. A second retinal condition in which cryosurgery should be considered is Lindau-von Hippel disease. Various methods have been used to treat hemangiomas of the retina including diathermy, and more recently, photocoagulation. The use of diathermy has been largely stopped, because of scleral destruction and the vitreous traction bands that can occur after treating large hemangiomas. Photocoagulation is an effective agent in treating smaller hemangiomas of less than 1 disc diameter in size. But in our experience the repeated applications necessary to ablate larger lesions can be followed by hemorrhage and vitreous band formation, and the tumor may not be destroyed. Using the freezing-thawing-refreezing procedure, cryosurgery has been the most successful way to treat Lindau-von Hippel hemangiomas in our experience.

Retinoblastoma. A third condition in which cryosurgery may possibly be considered is in treatment of retinoblastoma. Admittedly, the long-term results of such treatment are not yet definite, and the procedure must still be considered on trial.

Surgical techniques

The success of cryosurgery depends upon rapidly producing low tissue temperatures, sustaining these temperatures dependably, and rapidly bringing those temperatures back to normal levels. Liquid nitrogen, Freon, and carbon dioxide are the only substances so far that can be made to perform as the retinal surgeon desires. I have used all of them, but, of the commercially available units, I most frequently use the Freon or the carbon dioxide unit. Both can rapidly deliver $-65°$ C. or slightly lower probe temperatures and can warm the probe to zero in a few seconds.

The surgical techniques of using these machines are many. Some are carry-overs from the days of scleral resection and dia-thermy. However, to use cryosurgery to its best advantage we must use its selective tissue response, securing a good chorioretinal adhesion without significant scleral or vitreous damage. If selective tissue response is accepted as a fact, then there is no need for scleral surgery. The creation of a selective scleral bed, whether it is called undermining, lamellar resection, or trapdoor, is not required, because the basic need for this surgery was the scleral destruction by diathermy.

If the sclera is not destroyed by cryoapplication, why should the surgeon do a tedious dissection of a scleral flap? A tremendous advantage of cryosurgery is this ability to secure good chorioretinal adhesion through full-thickness sclera. It lessens operative time, anesthesia time, and the surgeon's time. Most importantly, it gives a relatively safe sclera in the event of reoperation. I say "relatively safe sclera," because it is somewhat softer than untreated sclera 3 or 4 days after cryosurgery. However, it is still much safer to work on than the thin, undermined, diathermized scleral bed.

In the practical management of cryosurgery in retinal detachment, there is a problem of securing a cryoapplication that will dependably produce chorioretinal adhesion. The variability of response to cryosurgery has led to some frustration. Generally, this has not been the result of cryosurgery itself, but rather to the way in which it was applied.

A pure chorioretinal adhesion is secured if ice is visible for 3 seconds in the detached retina at the point of cryoprobe application. This may someday be considered an overdose, but for the present it is the most reliable sign of a good clinical application.

Certainly cryosurgery will fail in those cases in which there is high balloon that never shows ice in the detached retina. In giant tears that have been previously treated, there is no retina in that area to show ice. However, if ice has been seen for 3 seconds in the detached retina, the surgeon can be reasonably certain that a good chorioretinal adhesion will occur in 6 to 21 days.

At the operating table the problem comes down to the question of how the surgeon knows that he has secured 3 seconds of visible ice in the detached retina. As the word "visible" indicates, he knows only by looking at the retina as the cryoprobe is used. This so-called monitoring of the cryoapplication is the most positive way to be sure of the response to the treatment. It is true that making a test application and monitoring it will give a general clue to the time–temperature requirement on that eye, but the variations in scleral thickness and nearness to the retina, the distance from the venae vorticosae to carry off the cold, and other factors, make any subsequent unmonitored application a calculated risk at best. Each application with an unknown response reduces the likelihood of a successful repair of the eye. It is felt, therefore, that monitoring through the indirect scope is the more efficient method.

The all-important question of localization of tears and of drainage will not be discussed. I personally have been using cryosurgery for more than 3 years and have probably averaged 5 cases a week, and I have not had to use diathermy.

Summary

The technique used in cryosurgery for detached retina is designed to utilize its great specific advantage—selective tissue response. There is a minimum of scleral surgery needed. However, with cryosurgery one still has all the other requirements of efficient retinal detachment surgery: complete work-up, accurate localization of tears, closure of all tears with a buckle, and drainage, if necessary, of the subretinal fluid. The method used is really the Custodis technique modified to the usage of cryosurgery. Because a good chorioretinal adhesion can be secured with little scleral damage, no scleral undermining is required. The tear is surrounded by cryoapplication. Each application should show 3 seconds of visible ice through the indirect scope. A buckle is produced after localization by indenting a solid or sponge silicone implant under mattress sutures through full-thickness sclera. After the buckle is produced, subretinal fluid may be drained. Most cases do not require drainage, but this has nothing to do with the cryotechnique itself. The cryosurgical approach makes most retinal detachment surgery much briefer.

The technique of treating retinal tears without detachment is also simplified by cryosurgery. The retinal tears may be divided into two categories: those reached by a cryoprobe through intact conjunctiva, and those so posterior that the conjunctiva and Tenon's capsule must be incised to slip the probe back to the necessary position. The tear is treated all the way around with the cryoprobe. Each 3-second iceball should be touching its neighbor. Without detachment, of course, no drainage is required. If there is any subretinal fluid, the eye should be treated using a buckle.

The treatment of Lindau-von Hippel angiomata requires the entire tumor to be obliterated by ice, thawed, and again engulfed in ice, all under indirect ophthalmoscopic monitoring. Because the treatment of retinoblastoma is still to be completely proved, its technique will not be discussed.

The disadvantages of cryosurgery in retinal detachment are in most instances similar to those of diathermy but occur less frequently. However, four disadvantages are distinctly those of cryosurgery. First, the chorioretinal adhesive time is shorter; if the retina is not bonded to the choroid within 5 to 6 days, it probably will not adhere. Second, a probe frozen to the sclera should not be removed until it has warmed to 0° C.; otherwise thin or damaged sclera can be avulsed by the probe. Third, because a cryoprobe application leaves only a very indefinite edema in the retina, it is easy for the surgeon to get "lost" as he is surrounding a tear. Only concentration on the landmarks while monitoring can prevent this. Fourth, cryotherapy causes the release of subretinal pigment that can clump anywhere under the retina, even under the macula. I have seen only one instance of this. Fortunately the first three of these disadvantages are rarely of significance if understood and evaluated.

There are three advantages of cryosurgery of the retina over diathermy. First, the reduced damage to the sclera makes scleral undermining unnecessary. Second, the less-ened effect on the sclera makes reoperation less hazardous. Third, the lessened effect on the vitreous makes vitreous complications less frequent. These three advantages alone make it a definite advance over the use of diathermy.

Herpesvirus keratitis

John G. Bellows

Over the past 5 years 1,242 compiled cases of herpesvirus keratitis were treated with the freezing technique by a number of ophthalmologists. Results revealed that 96% of the 1,242 cases recovered promptly (Table 24-1).

As frequently happens in medical history, the use of a new and effective form of therapy has been adopted before the modus operandi is completely understood. However, three observations made by independent investigators in different scientific disciplines have helped me to form a working hypothesis to explain the remarkable effectiveness of cryotherapy of herpesvirus keratitis.

These three factors are as follows. (1) Greiff and his co-workers demonstrated, using the influenza virus, that rapid successive freezing and thawing reduces sharply the concentration of the virus.[1, 2] (2) Spiegelman reported that the activities of DNA and RNA are reduced by a factor of 20 with each 10° C. drop in temperature, whereas under similar circumstances chemical reactions are reduced by a factor of 2.[3] (3) Reim and Schmidt found that after a brief freezing of the cornea with a cryoprobe, the concentration of the ATP/ADP ratio drops from 12 to 0.9 in the cornea. This very low concentration of energizing enzymes persists over 50 hours.[4]

All these factors following the freezing of the herpesvirus lesion of the cornea have an

Table 24-1. Cryotherapy of herpesvirus keratitis

Source*	Number of cases	Resolution by one or more applications		Failures
		Number of cases	*Percent*	
Krwawicz	464 (Early)	462	98 (3 days)	2
Krwawicz	204 (Early†)	204	100 (3 days)	0
Krwawicz	256 (Chronic‡)	241	95 (8.2 days)	15
Fanta	150	135	90	15
Hill	30	30	100	0
Anonymous	50	45	90	5
Oelis	15	13	87	2
Cornelius	10	8	80	2
Adest	20	18	90	2
Shechter	15	15	100	0
Pritikin	5	5	100	0
Bellows	23	21	91	2
	1,242	1,197	96	45 (4%)

*I wish to express my deep gratitude to the above-named ophthalmologists for their assistance in this project.
†Previously received traditional therapy.
‡Unresponsive to traditional therapy (7 days or more).

adverse effect upon the activities of the virus. However, the action of intracellular interferon produced in response to the infection is not influenced by freezing. Thus, when the aforementioned effects of freezing have dissipated, the herpesvirus, which have been reduced in number, are prevented from replication by the presence of a substantial intracellular concentration of interferon in the epithelial cells.

Because of the widespread use of safety glasses and the effectiveness of antibiotics and chemotherapeutic agents, the former etiologic factors—injuries and bacterial infections—play a minor role in causing corneal scarring. Herpesvirus keratitis is now the leading cause of corneal scar formation and loss of sight therefrom.[5, 6]

In recent years, IDU and other antiviral agents have been the treatment of choice for herpesvirus keratitis with a cure rate of 55 to 70%.[7] Failures with antiviral therapy are attributed to deep involvement of the cornea, hypersensitization to the drug, or resistance of certain strains of herpesvirus to these agents.

This report of 1,242 compiled cases of herpesvirus keratitis treated with cryogenic techniques over the past 5 years with a 96% recovery has never been equaled before either in the number of cases or in the rate of recovery. The remarkable uniformity of effectiveness in results of cryotherapy in so large a number of cases of herpetic keratitis is particularly significant because they were treated by different ophthalmologists in various parts of the world.

Etiology

Herpesvirus keratitis is of growing concern. The incidence of permissiveness leading to herpetic eruptions in this country is related to the return of increasing numbers of military personnel from malaria-infested areas, to the increased leisure time for exposure to sunlight and wind, and to the widespread use of eyedrops containing solutions or suspensions of chemotherapeutic agents or anti-

biotics with corticosteroids. Another possibility not mentioned before is the use of antibiotic and chemotherapeutic agents, which, by destroying the normal bacterial flora of the conjunctiva, may alter the natural ecologic relation and may result in the undesired and unexpected findings such as activation of the herpesvirus keratitis. Finally, the increased use of contact lenses has amplified the incidence of herpesvirus keratitis because slight trauma to the cornea acts as a precipitating factor.

The skin manifestations of herpes have been described as far back as the time of Hippocrates. However, it was not until 1912 that the virus was discovered. The development of the electron microscope revealed the submicroscopic structures of the herpesvirus. It is possible to distinguish a central core (virion) containing viral DNA. A study of the submicroscopic structures revealed that the core was covered by a protein capsid. Upon its eruption from a cell, the herpesvirus is frequently enveloped with an additional sheath derived from the membrane of the host cell.

The abode of the herpesvirus up to recent years has been thought to be in the nuclei of the epithelial cells or in those of the motor or sensory ganglion cells. Recent studies using fluorescein-labeled antibodies have demonstrated herpesvirus antigen in the lacrimal and salivary glands and in the infected conjunctiva and cornea.[8, 9]

However, as pointed out by Pavan-Langston and Nesburn, the "relatively high adnexal susceptibility [to herpesvirus] does not preclude the possibility that these glands are *not* the reservoirs of the agent but are simply the first to reproduce virus once infected from some as yet undetermined source."[10]

Lysogeny

Virologists have demonstrated that certain bacteria may harbor DNA viruses. In this state (lysogeny), the DNA virus seems to merge with and become a part of the chromosomal ring of the bacterium. In lysogeny the loss of identity of the DNA virus is apparent rather than real because it still possesses the capacity to break out of the bacterial nucleus when exposed to the sunlight, corticosteroids, and high temperatures. It may be more than mere coincidence that these same factors (high temperatures, exposure to sunlight, and corticosteroids) that destroy the repressor substance that inactivates the viral DNA in the chromosomal ring of the bacteria are also the very same factors that have been named as producing a state of permissiveness. (Permissiveness has been considered as a prerequisite for the outbreak of herpesvirus keratitis.) Therefore, permissiveness, which is considered by virologists as a change in the state of the *host cells* that allows a virus to penetrate into a cell and produce a herpesvirus keratitis, may actually result from a destruction of the repressor substance in the bacterium. This frees the virus from the lysogenic state and precipitates an infection.

Another factor is that the normal bacterial flora of the conjunctiva may be altered by the action of antibiotics and chemotherapeutic agents so that the herpesvirus is released from the lysogenic state and attaches itself to the epithelium of the cornea. Therefore, I propose the hypothesis that the lysogenic state in the normal bacterial flora of the conjunctiva may be another habitat of the herpesvirus.

Pathogenesis

Precipitation of an attack of herpesvirus keratitis depends upon a state of permissiveness in the cells of the host or, as proposed in this report, an attack may follow the destruction of the suppressor substance in the conjunctival bacterial flora that house the herpesvirus. This would disrupt the suppressor-viral equilibrium in the bacteria (lysogeny). The modern concept is that the herpesvirus, freed from its habitat, attaches itself to the epithelial cells of the cornea in a place termed the acceptor area. Here the herpesvirus DNA disassociates itself from its protein coat and enters into the cell nucleus as a single strand of DNA.

In the nucleus the single strand viral DNA replicates itself and becomes a double helix similar to the DNA normally present in the nucleus. During the interval of viral DNA multiplication, the original parental particle undergoes an eclipse period in which the parental particle breaks down and releases its chromosome. The free viral chromosome serves as a template to direct the synthesis of new viral components. The viral DNA takes command and directs the RNA to form protein for its capsid instead of the normal protein synthesis.

It is obvious that viruses cannot replicate outside of the cell, because they depend upon the host cell for the precursors and the ribosomes that are essential for multiplication. During the height of virus multiplication, significant concentrations of interferon are formed in the cell reaching a peak in 96 hours. It is quite likely that high concentrations of interferon may halt the spread of the herpesvirus corneal infection.[11] However, when the concentration or virulence of the herpesvirus is too great for the interferon to halt replication, the virus spreads by direct extension from cell to cell.

In some instances, an equilibrium within the cell is established between the interferon and the herpesvirus, and a period of latency develops. Under these circumstances the virus replication ceases and reduces the stimulus to form interferon. Later, when the concentration of interferon falls to a low level, the virus resumes its replication. This in turn again stimulates the formation of interferon within the cell and again the virus replication is halted. This condition in which interferon formation first increases and then decreases, followed by a corresponding decrease and increase in the virus multiplication, may be repeated over an extended period. This alternating cycle is now believed to be the explanation for the tendency of herpesvirus keratitis to recur and become chronic.

Technique for cryotherapy of herpesvirus keratitis

Except in children, cryotherapy for superficial herpesvirus keratitis is a simple office procedure. The cornea is first stained with sodium fluorescein, and the cryoprobe is refrigerated by filling it with solid carbon dioxide ($-79°$ C.). The cornea is anesthetized with 2% solution of tetracaine hydrochloride. The upper eyelid is raised with a finger or lid elevator, and the patient is directed to fix his gaze on a distant object.

The cold tip is applied to a diseased portion of the cornea for 7 to 10 seconds and is then thawed with a stream of saline. This freezing–thawing cycle is repeated rapidly 3 times at each point. It is essential that all parts of the infected cornea, as revealed by the stain, be treated similarly.

The procedure is painless, but the patient is told to expect a slight-to-moderate degree of discomfort lasting 12 to 24 hours. The pain is readily controlled with a simple analgesic. Examination of the cornea the next day will reveal an area of staining that corresponds to the multiple points of application, but it no longer shows the characteristic dendritic outline.

After 72 to 96 hours, the cornea will usually appear normal; it will no longer stain, and it will have regained its luster. If any portion of the cornea shows staining after 4 or 5 days, that portion is again treated at the recommended subzero temperature. Rarely is a third application necessary, but if a small area still stains 5 days after the second freezing treatment, the cold probe should again be applied to it.

Clinical results of cryotherapy

A correct evaluation of a new form of therapy must be made either on the basis of a statistical study in which controls were used, or a large number of cases must show an extraordinarily high percentage of cures. Adding to the validity of the results of cryotherapy is the fact that cryotherapy was usually effective even when used as a last resort after other methods had failed.

The 1,242 patients infected with herpesvirus keratitis that comprised this report received cryotherapy in various parts of the world. Ninety-six percent of the patients (1,197 cases) recovered in a few days after one or more treatments. Only 4% (45 cases) did not respond to cryotherapy. While the reasons were not given for the 45 cases which did not respond to freezing, I can conjecture from my own experience that complications of herpesvirus keratitis, such as iridocyclitis, secondary glaucoma, or thinning of the cornea (which precludes intensive freezing therapy) were some of the reasons for failure.

Summary

This report demonstrates that cryotherapy is by far the most effective method of treatment of herpesvirus keratitis. Cures were obtained in 96% of 1,242 compiled cases. In contrast, treatment with IDU and other antiviral agents is usually only 55% to 70% effective. Older methods of curettage (with or without chemical cauterization) are even less effective than treatment with antiviral agents.

The explanation for the effectiveness of cryotherapy is based on reports by investigators that show that ultrafreezing reduces the concentration of the titer of some types of viruses, the activity of DNA and RNA, and the ATP, the energizing substance required for virus replication. All these factors produced by cryotherapy have an adverse effect upon the herpesvirus, but do not impair the antiviral action of interferon produced intracellularly, which is stable in freezing temperatures. While it is true that extracellular interferon is not active against herpesvirus, it is a very effective antiviral agent intracellularly. It prevents the few active viruses remaining after cryotherapy from replicating. Healing of the lesion then follows.

Conclusions

This report proposes a working hypothesis to explain the remarkable uniformity in the effectiveness of cryogenic procedures in the treatment of herpesvirus keratitis. A new hypothesis is offered: that the habitat of the herpesvirus causing corneal infection may be in the lysogenic state in which the herpesvirus is merged with the choromosomal rings of the normal flora of bacteria that is found in the conjunctiva.

REFERENCES

1. Greiff, D., and Rightsel, W.: Freezing and freeze-drying of viruses, In Meryman, H. T., editor: Cryobiology, New York, 1966, Academic Press, Inc.
2. Greiff, D., and Rightsel, W.: Personal communications, 1968.
3. Spiegelman, S.: Personal communications, 1968.
4. Reim, M., and Schmidt, F.: Biochemische Veranderungen bei der Vereisung der Hornhaut in vivo. Ein Beitrag zur Kaltetherapie, Klin. Mbl. Augenheilk. **150:**96, 1967.
5. Bellows, J. G.: Cryotherapy of dendritic keratitis, Canad. J. Ophthal. **3:**19, 1968.
6. Bellows, J. G.: The changing picture of herpesvirus keratitis, Eye Ear Nose Throat Monthly **46:**717, 1967.
7. Duke-Elder, S.: System of ophthalmology; diseases of the outer eye, vol. 8, St. Louis, 1965, The C. V. Mosby Co.
8. Kaufman, H., Brown, D., and Ellison, E. D.: Herpesvirus in the lacrimal gland, conjunctiva and cornea of man, Amer. J. Ophthal. **65:**32, 1968.
9. Dawson, C., Togni, B., and Moore, T.: Structural changes in chronic herpetic keratitis, Arch. Ophthal. **79:**740, 1968.
10. Pavan-Langston, D., and Nesburn, A. B.: The chronology of primary herpes simplex infection of the eye and adnexal glands, Arch. Ophthal. **80:**258, 1968.
11. Force, E., Stewart, R., and Haff, R.: Development of interferon in rabbit dermis after infection with herpes simplex virus, Virology **25:**322, 1965.

Complications

R. David Sudarsky

Basically, all cryosurgical techniques in ophthalmology can be divided into two groups: those that utilize the adhesive effect of a cryogenic probe (which is strongest between $-2°$ and $-75°$ C.), and those that use the penetrating effect of the cold which increases as the temperature of a cryogenic apparatus is lowered. Complications may result from either of these two effects, as well as from simple mechanical factors.

Cryoextraction of cataract

Complications during cryoextraction of cataract may result from inadvertent adhesion to the surrounding tissues of either the probe tip itself or the ice mass that has formed in the cataract. Adhesion may take place to the conjunctival flap (particularly when it is based at the limbus), to the corneal edge or the endothelium of the cornea, to the limbal incision, to various points of the iris (especially during round pupil extrac-

tion), to the zonules of Zinn, to the vitreous body itself, and to the preplaced corneoscleral sutures. Most of the above complications can be readily and quickly handled by defrosting the probe or separating the probe by one of three methods. The first method is *selective defrosting* by controlled irrigation of the probe tip. This would permit, for example, separating an adhesion to the iris or to the pillar of an iridectomy without loosening the hold on a lens capsule.[1] *Mechanical rupture* of the ice bond at the point of ice adhesion to the tip of the metal probe is the second method which was first utilized by Krwawicz and most recently by Worst.[2, 3] The third method is to use the *internal defrosting mechanism* that is incorporated into most of the console cryosurgical instruments. The latter results in a total separation of the probe from all tissue and can be duplicated by continuous irrigation with room temperature saline.

Specific cryogenic effects of complications. In the conjunctiva usually only small ecchymoses will occur, which generally vanish after a week or so. Changes in the cornea have been described by Taylor.[4] However, a very large series of Krwawicz and another by Worthen and Brubaker fail to duplicate the complications reported by Taylor.[5, 6] In our own research we found it necessary to reduce the temperature of the cornea of a rabbit to $-196°$ C. for over 1 minute in order to produce even microscopic vascularization and alterations in the cornea. Corneal alterations, therefore, as a complication of specific cryogenic effect do not appear to be serious. As with any other method of cataract extraction, mechanical trauma to the corneal endothelium as a result of the surgical maneuver can result in striate keratitis. Bending the cornea does not appear to be harmful according to Paton,[7] but prolonged drying of the endothelial surface by exposing it to the air in the operating room without sufficient moisture can be harmful. The treatment of inadvertent adhesion to the zonules is prompt total separation of the zonules from the probe. If this is not properly done, vitreous loss may ensue. Likewise, adhesion to the vitreous must be treated by separation of this adhesion or total defrosting of the probe. If an adhesion to a suture results, separation of the suture from the cryoprobe is usually not necessary, unless the suture is insufficiently long and there is danger of pulling it out. The suture can easily be separated after the cryoextraction has been completed.[1, 8]

Capsular rupture as a result of intense freezing has been reported when using cryogenic probes that operate below $-40°$ C. I do not feel that capsular rupture can occur in the $-20°$ to $-30°$ C. zone in which most Freon-cooled cryogenic probes are employed for cryoextraction. Mechanical rupture of a delicate capsule can also result when a warm cryoprobe is applied to the lens and then chilled. It is very difficult to hold a cryoprobe sufficiently still during these moments, and I believe that this rare complication can be avoided by applying the previously chilled cryoprobe to the capsule, in which case immediate adherence will take place. The complication of capsular rupture, which has been noted during cryoextraction of cataract, has been shown by Krwawicz and Worthen and Brubaker to occur less frequently than by any other method of lens extraction.[5, 6] Vitreous loss as a complication of cryoextraction appears to be associated with the surgical technique employed. Cryoextraction most frequently necessitates that the lens be slid from its position in the iris–lens diaphragm or gently raised in the direct sky approach advocated by Barraquer.[9] Surgeons trained entirely by tumbling techniques must relearn the technique of sliding extraction to effectively employ cryoextraction of the lens.

With respect to the iris, small but definite areas of permanent iris atrophy, including pigment atrophy of the iris, can be noted. Anterior chamber hemorrhages are occasionally encountered during the first week following cryoextraction, but there is no statistical evidence to indicate that anterior chamber hemorrhage, as a direct consequence of cryoextraction, is more frequent than by other techniques.

Some have advocated the use of the cryoprobe to remove fragments of lens material following rupture of the capsule. I have not been impressed that this is a useful technique. However, the closure of a capsular rupture and successful intracapsular extraction following inadvertent rupture of the capsule early in cataract surgery is without doubt one of the great advantages of cryoextraction.

Most of the complications I have described above, with the possible exception of the specific type of iris atrophy, are in large measure a direct function of the surgeon's own dexterity at lens extraction.

Retinal tears and retinal separation

The second most widely used application of ocular cryosurgery is the treatment of retinal tear and retinal separation. Transconjunctival treatment of peripheral retinal tear is one of the most important uses of this technique and has been widely accepted even by those surgeons who are opposed to the cryosurgical management of retinal separation as a primary technique. Extensive treatment can usually be performed at one sitting. There are few, if any, complications. There may be some conjunctival ecchymoses that persist for a week or so. In my own experience during the past 5 years, I have had only one case of a slightly dry eye following extensive transconjunctival prophylactic cryopexy. The xerophthalmia did not require any further treatment and spontaneously improved after several months.

With respect to cryosurgical management of retinal separation, the following complications have been noted. Rupture of the sclera occurs, but seems to be less frequent than with diathermy techniques. I have encountered rupture of the sclera when applying a cryoprobe beneath the medial and lateral rectus muscles, particularly over areas of the sclera that have been thinned in the region of the long posterior ciliary vessels, where there is frequently a small dehiscence of the sclera. By taking special care in these areas, I have recently avoided this complication, and in 3 cases in which I experienced this complication, an excellent result has been obtained.

Amoils has shown that the net result of the penetrating cold on the choroid is hemostasis and alteration in the endothelium of the blood vessels with increased permeability of the endothelium.[10] Although my initial impression was that perforation for the drainage of subretinal fluid through this treated choroid was likely to yield an increased incidence of hemorrhage from this site, this initial impression has not been confirmed in my experience. I will frequently drain for subretinal fluid through a bed that has been treated with cryopexy, and I have not found an increased incidence of bleeding from the choroidal site. When extensive cryotherapy is applied to the choroid for treatment of numerous retinal breaks and extensive detachment, I have seen an immediate exudation of a clear aqueous type fluid from the choroid, which produces small areas of clear

choroidal separations. This fluid can also be seen when dissecting to drain through an area of sclera and choroid treated by cryopexy. The fluid persists for 4 or 5 days and is then apparently absorbed by the choroid.

Pigment migration, both direct and through the subretinal fluid, appears to me to be a significant complication of cryosurgical management of retinal separation that has not been sufficiently stressed. The paths of pigment migration may be direct through the retinal tear and into the vitreous with dispersion as far as the optic nerve head, or through the subretinal fluid to the region of the macula. The pigment may accumulate in a line at the lowest level of the retinal separation. This pigmented line observed immediately following the drainage of subretinal fluid could be termed a cryomarcation line. A cryomarcation line (Fig. 24-4) differs from the well-known retinal demarcation line, because the pigment is deposited between the retina and the pigment epithelium and is formed immediately after cryopexy, particularly with drainage of subretinal fluid. The line is thickest at the posterior portion of the globe and at its most inferior point; it becomes thinner as it is traced toward the periphery. In contrast, the classical pigmentation line is thickest at the periphery and the pigment is dispersed into the substance of the retina itself and exists both before and after retinal separation surgery.

Fig. 24-5 is a photograph of the macula of a patient who had undergone cryosurgical management of retinal separation 1 year previously. Pigmentary migration to the macular area was noted immediately following the treatment in the operating room and seemed to be unchanged after more than 1 year. Considerable increase in large vitreous floaters is frequently noted following the cryosurgical management of retinal separation and appears to be more severe and more troublesome to the patient than those which occur after classical radio-frequency diathermy techniques. The amount of treatment necessary for cryosurgical management of

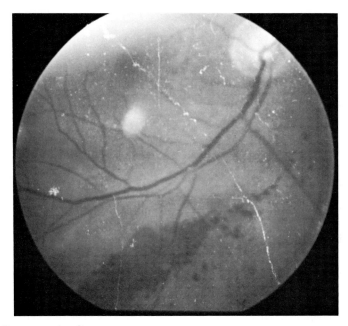

Fig. 24-4. Cryomarcation line.

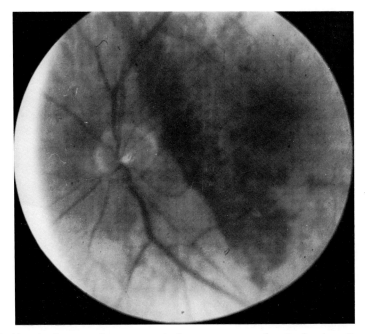

Fig. 24-5. Macula 1 year after cryosurgical management of retinal separation.

retinal separation is usually more extensive than equivalent diathermy applications, principally because each application of retinal cryopexy involves a much larger area of pigment epithelium of the choroid.

New hole formation at the posterior limit of treatment has been described by some, although I have not personally encountered this complication in several hundred treated cases of retinal separation and retinal tear.

Most of these complications are also seen following extensive diathermy treatment. Except for the vitreous floaters and pigment migration that have been shown, the complications appear to be more severe in the radio-frequency diathermy techniques.

Glaucoma

Complications of the cryosurgical management of glaucoma are hard to evaluate, because there appears to be a very thin line between the intensity of the treatment of the ciliary body required to produce a prolonged lowering of the intraocular tension and the amount of treatment which may result in phthisis of the globe. At the present time the cryosurgical management of difficult types of glaucoma is of doubtful value and must be carefully evaluated before any definite conclusions can be drawn.

Herpes simplex keratitis

The proper cryosurgical management of herpes simplex keratitis rarely results in any corneal change. As the keratitis becomes more of a metaherpetic variety, it becomes difficult to evaluate whether it is the disease process itself or attempted cryosurgical management which may result in permanent corneal scarring. Kaufman is of the opinion that the cryosurgical management of acute herpes simplex keratitis is equivalent to simple mechanical debridement.[11] There is no doubt, however, that it is a highly effective method of treating acute epithelial cases.

Summary

During the past 5 years the cryosurgical management of cataracts, retinal separation, herpes simplex keratitis, and glaucoma has been utilized by a large number of ophthalmologists. As our experience becomes larger and the total number of treated cases grows, it becomes increasingly necessary that the statistical method be applied to accurately evaluate the complications as well as the benefits that accrue from these methods of treatment. Only after a surgeon becomes thoroughly familiar with cryogenic techniques can he make a valid analysis of this type of therapy.

REFERENCES

1. Sudarsky, R. D., and Hulquist, R.: Biophysical aspects and instrumentation in ocular cryosurgery, Trans. AMA Sec. Ophthal. June, 1964.
2. Krwawicz, T.: Intracapsular extraction of intumescent cataract by application of low temperature, Brit. J. Ophthal. 45:279, 1961.
3. Worst, J. G. F.: New instruments and technique for cataract cryosurgery, Amer. J. Ophthal. 65:587, 1968.
4. Taylor, D. M., and Dalburg, L. A., Jr.: Corneal complications from cryoextraction of cataracts, Arch. Ophthal. 79:3-8, 1968.
5. Krwawicz, T.: Recent developments in cryogenic ocular surgery, Amer. J. Ophthal. 60: 231, 1965.
6. Worthen, D. M., and Brubaker, R. F.: An evaluation of cataract cryoextraction, Arch. Ophthal. 79:8-9, 1968.
7. Paton, D., and Martinez, M.: Corneal tissue preservation for penetrating keratoplasty; past, present, future, Intern. Surg. 49(5):428, 1968.
8. Sudarsky, R. D., and Hulquist, R.: Cryogenically induced iris atrophy, iridectomy, and cataract in rabbits, Amer. J. Ophthal. 60:217, 1965.
9. Barraquer, J.: Keratophakia for the correction of high hyperopia, J. Cryosurgery 1:39, 1968. Society of Cryosurgery, Miami, Jan. 1968.
10. Amoils, S. P., and Smith, T. R.: Cryotherapy of angiomatosis retinae, Arch. Ophthal. 81: 689, 1969.
11. Kaufman, H.: Society of Cryosurgery, Miami, Jan. 1968.

Discussion

Moderator:

Charles D. Kelman

Dr. Kelman: Dr. de Roetth, without casting any doubt on the validity of your work, how do you account for the virtually consistent failure of others to duplicate your results?

Dr. de Roetth: One can only answer those who publish their results in the literature. It is easy enough to get up and say I don't agree with a person. It is much more difficult to amass a great number of patients, treat them, follow them for years, and publish the results in scientific publications. I think the proof of the pudding is in the cases that are still to be published.

Dr. Kelman: Professor Krwawicz, in cataract extraction, especially with a round pupil, the cryoprobe will occasionally touch the iris. Are there any complications that result from temporary freezing of the iris?

Prof. Krwawicz: I must say that accidental touching of the iris is rather a rare complication. In the material quoted by me (about 4,000 cases), it occurred only eight to ten times. The adhesion is easily released by a stream of saline. Sometimes, of course, a circumscribed area of iris atrophy remains.

Dr. Kelman: What are the effects of the cryoprobe on the corneal endothelium?

Prof. Krwawicz: This accident occasionally happens, but the endothelial cells regenerate in a few days. In the long view it is usually harmless.

Dr. Kelman: Dr. Sudarsky, in a second application of cryothermy to an area of sclera which a few minutes earlier had had its first application, is there a danger because of weakening of the sclera by the first application?

Dr. Sudarsky: I am not certain that there is any greater danger. No doubt the sclera is stronger weeks later than sclera that had been treated with diathermy, but it is weaker than normal sclera. I would not be afraid to reapply, if necessary, in the same area.

Dr. Kelman: Dr. Shafer, under what circumstances should undetached retinal holes be cryopexied if the patient has never had a retinal detachment?

Dr. Shafer: We have to evaluate each different type of tear. If it is a superior tear, I tend to treat it. If there is no pigment, I tend to treat it. If there is definite evidence of vitreous traction, the edge of the tear being slightly everted, or a little tip of retina standing up, or if there is a viterous band, I definitely treat it. Conversely, if the tear is perfectly flat, if it is anterior, and if there is some pigmentation already, I tend not to treat it.

Dr. Kelman: Dr. Bellows, have you considered treatment of vaccinial corneal ulcers with cryosurgery?

Dr. Bellows: I haven't had any experience with vaccinial virus. I would assume, however, that the organism might very well yield to cryotherapy, as might trachoma, adenovirus, and other types of viral ocular infections.

Dr. Kelman: Dr. de Roetth, what has been the experience with cryosurgery in the treatment of active chorioretinitis unresponsive to steroids?

Dr. de Roetth: I have no experience with that. Others have done it. Some of my colleagues have had very minimal, if any, results. I would say the response is poor.

Dr. Kelman: Would you comment on the use of cryosurgery for rubeosis and for hemorrhagic glaucoma?

Dr. de Roetth: That has been one of the disappointments for me. I thought that it would be one of the best indications for cryosurgery in glaucoma, and it has not worked well in our hands. That type of patient did not respond at all, in our unit.

Dr. Kelman: Dr. Sudarsky, what is the incidence of massive vitreous retraction following cryosurgery for retinal detachment?

Dr. Sudarsky: I can only give a guess that it occurs possibly less frequently than if diathermy is used, but it is not statistically significant.

Dr. Kelman: Prof. Krwawicz, have you had experience with cryotherapy for iritis?

Prof. Krwawicz: Oh, yes. In chronic cyclitis, cryoapplication proved to be very useful. In my experience (80 cases), the precipitates disappeared frequently, and the vitreous cleared up.

Dr. Kelman: Where do you apply cryotherapy with your apparatus?

Prof. Krwawicz: Mine is a normal applicator. The ball-shaped tip is 2.5 or 3 mm. The temperature is –60° C. We touch either the upper or the lower hemisphere conjunctiva, and each touch lasts 10 seconds. We use about 12 applications in one procedure, approximately 1 mm. from the limbus.

Dr. Kelman: Dr. de Roetth, do you see any cataract production as a complication of cryosurgery for glaucoma?

Dr. de Roetth: No. The cold itself, as far as I know, has not produced cataract. That is one of the complications we have looked for, and we thought that it would be rather common, but this has not been the case. We have seen cataracts produced secondarily, caused by uncontrolled iritis. Cryosurgery in glaucoma always produces a mild iritis that lasts for a few weeks. At first we didn't realize this and didn't treat the patients adequately, so the first few months to a year we did produce cataract secondary to the iritis, but it was not due to the cold itself.

Dr. Kelman: What is your technique in the treatment of glaucoma?

Dr. de Roetth: We have tried many temperatures and all sizes of applicators, and we still go back to the original one. The surface area of the applicator is about 12 square millimeters. The temperature is –80° C. We use about 6 applications of a minute each over approximately half the globe, let us say the lower half, so we can leave the upper half or repeat if necessary. We do this as an out-patient procedure with local anesthesia, usually in our glaucoma clinic.

Dr. Kelman: Dr. Bellows, you mentioned repeated freezing and thawing in treating dendritic ulcer. Do you do this all in one session?

Dr. Bellows: Yes. The treatment, in order to be successful, should be a repetitive, rapid succession of thawing and freezing to accomplish the results—to get the same results that were obtained by Dr. Greiff with influenza virus. I use a total of 21 seconds—7 seconds, three times. I find that adequate, and if by the fourth or fifth day there are still some staining spots, I treat those separately.

Dr. Kelman: Another question for Dr. Bellows. Has herpes simplex virus been shown to enter a lysogenic state in the conjunctiva?

Dr. Bellows: That is just conjectural, and a possible explanation for the marked increase in the incidence of herpes virus keratitis. If the normal bacterial flora are destroyed, we know that lysogenic conditions do exist and that a bacterium will harbor a virus in a condition that is not an apparent infection, then, under certain conditions, pop out. Now whether this will occur in conjunctiva or not, I do not know.

Chapter 25

Microsurgery of keratoconus*

Richard C. Troutman

The use of the dissecting microscope in surgery of the eye has increased during the past 5 years. In another decade, few, if any, procedures on the anterior segment will be performed without it. Those who have employed a microscope routinely, some for as long as fifteen years, now find it impossible to perform adequate surgery under loupe magnification alone. However, few new procedures have been developed through its use, and its major contribution has been in the refinement of existing procedures to better retain the physical structure and optical properties of the eye and to reduce the morbidity of the operative procedure.

There is still much controversy as to which procedures lend themselves most readily to surgery under the higher magnification ranges available with the operating microscope. There can be little doubt, however, that its use is essential to the improved performance of keratoplasty. The more critical the anatomic and optical requirements of the individual keratoplastic procedure, the more necessary is the increased accuracy afforded by the microscope. Optical keratoplasty, primarily keratoplasty for keratoconus (Fig. 25-1), lends itself best to this new modality.

This presentation shall therefore, deal with microsurgery of keratoconus, since this disease can be considered the prime indication

for the use of higher magnification and for the use of the improved surgical instrumentation now becoming available as a result of 15 years of experience and development.

Characteristics of the disease

The optical-anatomic deformation of the cornea characteristic of keratoconus exhibits a random distribution as to sex and race. It has its onset from puberty to approximately 20 years of age. It usually has no identifiable etiology, although, in some cases, a hereditary pattern has been established. It is progressive and, with few exceptions, is almost always bilateral.

Pathologically, keratoconus is central in

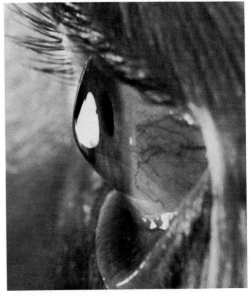

Fig. 25-1. Moderately advanced keratoconus.

*Supported in part by a grant from The John A. Hartford Foundation, Inc., Stereotactic Ophthalmic Microsurgery and also in part by National Institute of Neurological Disease and Blindness, Research Training Grant No. 5-RO1-NB-02861.

the cornea in its early stages (Fig. 25-2). It is characterized by fragmentation of the epithelial basement membrane and fibrillation of Bowman's membrane and anterior stroma. Later in the course of the disease, there is centrifugal and posterior extension (Fig. 25-3) with consecutive degeneration of Bowman's membrane and degeneration of stroma, leading to rupture of Descemet's membrane (Fig. 25-4) followed by acute or chronic edema (Fig. 25-5). The patient is usually a teenager who complains of photophobia, and

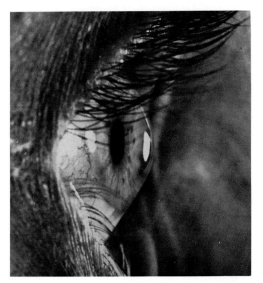

Fig. 25-2. Central thinning of cornea, early keratoconus.

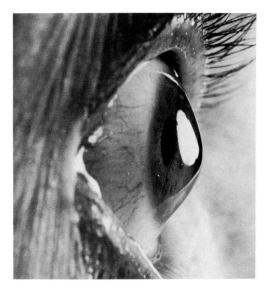

Fig. 25-3. Centrifugal and posterior extension of keratoconus.

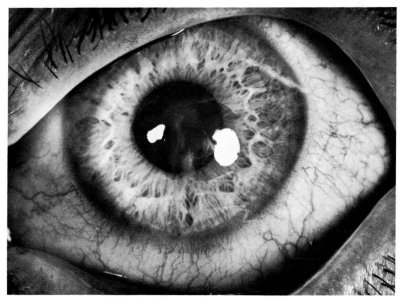

Fig. 25-4. Rupture of Descemet's membrane.

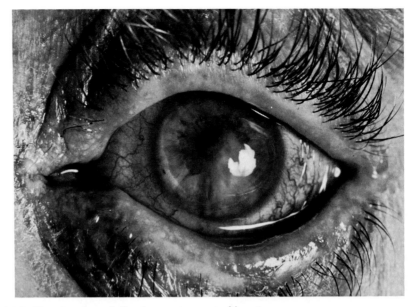

Fig. 25-5. Chronic edema following acute onset of keratoconus.

is often addicted to chronic rubbing of the eyes, which may have been attributed to allergy. The diagnosis is rarely made on the first examination. However serial examinations will show progressive unsymmetrical ametropia accompanied by a moderate to high degree of astigmatism; the axis changes randomly and eventually becomes irregular. The patient has difficulty in seeing, even with maximally correcting spectacles, and eventually can be corrected only with contact lenses. The differential diagnosis is relatively easy. Keratectasia (Fig. 25-6), which may occur secondarily to central corneal ulcer, stromal disease, or contusion may simulate keratoconus but can almost always be differentiated by the history. Megalocornea (Fig. 25-7) has an earlier onset and a definite hereditary pattern. Descemet's membrane always remains intact, even into the late stage of this disease, and the patient often has arachnodactyly. Keratoglobus (Fig. 25-8) is a rather anomalous condition, which, according to some, is an exaggerated megalocornea; others consider it a diffuse keratoconus.

Once the diagnosis has been made, the pa-

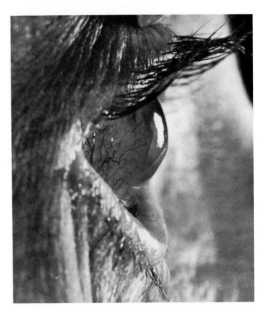

Fig. 25-6. Keratectasia.

tient can often be managed clinically for a number of years. Too frequently the ophthalmologist gives up too early on spectacle correction, which may be adequate until late in the course of the disease and even secondarily after the patient can no longer wear

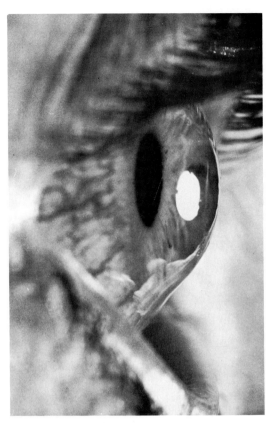

Fig. 25-7. Megalocornea.

contact lenses comfortably. Early in the course of the disease, a simple spherical correction suffices; astigmatic correction is added as indicated. When the astigmatism becomes irregular, a spherical equivalent may continue to provide useful and comfortable correction. Contact lenses should always be tried after the failure of spectacle correction and before surgery is advised. A carefully fitted corneal contact lens is usually more comfortable than a haptic scleral lens. Ordinarily, the scleral lens should be used only if the corneal lens can no longer be tolerated because of the height of the cone or if there is persistent central erosion of the cornea. When haptic lenses are fitted correctly, the patient can often wear them during his entire working or waking hours. The ability to wear a haptic lens, however, is not nearly as consistent as it is with the corneal type. Some patients are unable to wear haptic lenses at all. Others are able to wear them for no longer than 2 or 3 hours at a time, after which the lenses must be removed, the solution replaced, the lens cleansed and then reinserted for an additional short period of time. When this point has been reached, the

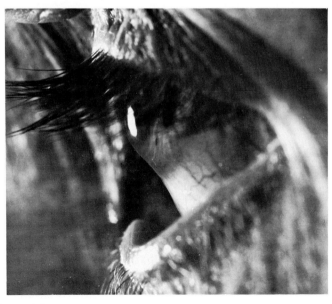

Fig. 25-8. Keratoglobus.

patient is ready for penetrating keratoplasty, since during the period when he cannot use his contact lens correction he is unable to function at all, and when he wears it, he is able to function only intermittently and with continuous discomfort. I do not advocate the use of lamellar keratoplasty because of interface scarring and the resulting decreased acuity.

Until very recently, the late stage of keratoconus was feared by the ophthalmologist because of the relatively high incidence of operative complications. Even when the graft was successful, the eye often had such a high astigmatic and myopic error following the keratoplasty that it was again mandatory for the patient to wear a corneal or haptic lens. Thus, the optical potential was not necessarily improved at all, except possibly for a small increase in corrected acuity with contact lenses.

Aims of surgery

The aims of keratoconus surgery are the restoration of spectacle corrected acuity to 20/30 or better; the preservation of the pupillary aperture by the avoidance of operative complication to the iris; the regularization of the astigmatism below the 3-diopter level; and the reduction of the myopia to the astigmatic error only or emmetropia, to allow minimal, comfortable, optical correction of the eye, preferably by spectacles, if required.

Indications for surgery

Surgical indications are keratometry readings exceeding 60 D in the highest meridian, and vision of less than 20/40 in the better eye with the best possible correction (spectacles or contact lenses). This disease most often occurs in young people who must drive a motor vehicle in the pursuit of their livelihood. In most states a person must have a corrected vision of 20/40 before he is allowed to operate a motor vehicle. Continual contact lens irritability, even when there is good vision, can prevent effective

use of the eyes and this is another indication for surgery.

Increased thinning of the peripheral cornea to biomicroscopic examination indicates rapid extension of the disease. If allowed to progress too far, there would be a tendency to complicate the surgical procedure and make it less possible to obtain low astigmatic errors and a good reduction of the myopia postoperatively. Edema that is chronic or acute and recurrent limits the vision and may lead to a descemetocele or even rupture of the globe. In these cases, immediate surgery is always indicated.

Preparation for surgery

Graft. One of the prerequisites of surgery is the preselection of the diameter of the graft. Eleven millimeters is the maximum I have used. This graft was used in a cornea that could have been called diffuse keratoconus or megalocornea, and it still had a good rim of clear recipient cornea following excision for graft. On the average, however, to obtain a mixed astigmatism or emmetropia, an 8 mm. circular graft is sufficient.

There has been much ado about selection of donor material. It is my feeling that, in the majority of cases, graft rejection is the result of poor technique or the use of defective or old donor material (not necessarily donor material from an older patient). I prefer to use graft material not more than *24 hours old,* and essentially no graft material from the eye of a donor older than *65 years.* Fresh donor material that has been carefully cut and carefully handled so the endothelium is not abraded during cutting, transfer, and suture is the best insurance against graft failure.

Anesthesia. I believe that general anesthesia is mandatory to the performance of good microsurgery, and I have been using this exclusively for the past 8 years. The preparation of the patient is essentially the same as for other intraocular surgery. One must verify the absence of infection and

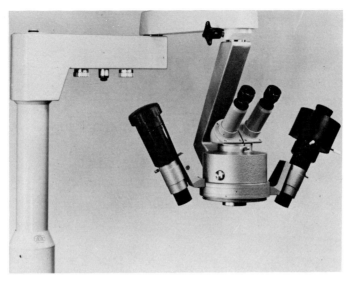

Fig. 25-9. Zeiss zoom ophthalmic surgical microscope.

lacrimal obstruction. If general anesthesia is used, there is no necessity to constrict the pupil preoperatively, but if local anesthesia must be used, then pilocarpine should be given just prior to the operative intervention, since the retrobulbar anesthetic injection will dilate the pupil.

Instruments. In my opinion, the use of microsurgery is essential in the performance of keratoplasty, and therefore the routine use of this modality is very important. The surgeon should have an operating microscope, preferably specifically designed for ophthalmic surgery. A number of models are now available, manufactured by Zeiss (Fig. 25-9), Keeler (Fig. 25-10), Moller-Wedel, and Edward Weck and Co. For keratoplasty, one does not necessarily need the variable magnification that is essential for other anterior segment procedures, particularly for cataract operation. Therefore, the original Zeiss culposcopic microscope, or the new Barraquer-Zeiss microscope at a magnification of 10 or 12 times, will suffice. However, if the microscope is to be used for other anterior segment surgery, one of the several zoom microscopes is more universally useful. Even with keratoplasty, variable magnification will considerably ease the procedure by

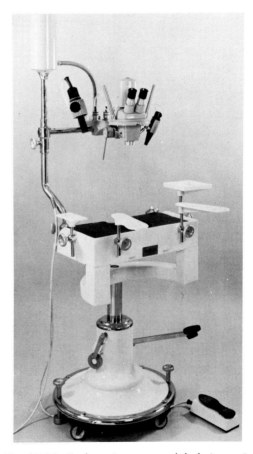

Fig. 25-10. Keeler microzoom ophthalmic surgical unit.

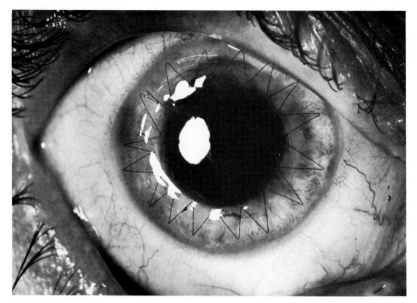

Fig. 25-11. Ethilon suture (22 μ) fixing corneal graft.

allowing the surgeon to select with facility the optimum magnification for various parts of the procedure, without the necessity of losing his field of view during changes of magnification.

The microsurgery instruments* that I use for corneal surgery are divided into five groups.

1. Instruments for exposure and fixation
   a. Barraquer wire speculum
   b. Flieringa ring
   c. Superior rectus forceps, which is used also for donor eye transfer
   d. Llovera fixation forceps
2. Tissue, needle, and suture instruments
   a. Colibri forceps for manipulation of the conjunctiva
   b. Bonn forceps for manipulation of the cornea and iris
   c. Pair of Harms forceps for tying the Ethilon suture
   d. Pointed suture handling forceps
   e. Microneedle holder
3. Cutting instruments
   a. An angled razor knife

*Available in the United States from Edward Weck and Co. and Storz Instrument Co.

   b. A set of trephines, 7 to 11 mm. in diameter in 1-mm. steps
   c. Scissors, 1 pair of microcorneal scissors, right and left (9 mm. curve)
   d. Barraquer, DeWecker iris scissors used also for cutting the Ethilon suture
   e. Heavy curved conjunctival scissors used also for cutting heavier silk sutures
4. Auxiliary instruments
   a. Standard instruments
      (1) A graft transfer spatula
      (2) A pair of 1 mm. wire iris spatulas
      (3) A No. 30 blunt angled needle for air implacement
      (4) An irrigation tip and bulb
   b. Special instruments for lamellar keratoplasty
      (1) A microkeratome of the Barraquer type or of the standard Castroviejo type
      (2) Three lamellar dissecting spatulas of different lengths and curvature, for dissection of the host cornea

5. Sutures, drapes, and sponges
   a. Sutures: No. 4-0 silk for the superior rectus, No. 6-0 silk for fixation of the Flieringa ring, 22.1 μ Ethilon suture (Fig. 25-11) for fixation of the graft, for both interrupted and continuous sutures
   b. Drapes and sponges: the Weck-Sel sponge, a lintfree sponge for use in the operative field, and a 3M aperture drape for isolation of the field from surrounding lint-bearing drapes.

Surgical procedure

The surgical procedure is divided into a *preparatory stage,* the first part of which is carried out under relatively low magnification ($\times 6$ to $\times 10$). The second part of the preparatory stage and the *graft insertion stage,* is done under the highest operating magnification ($\times 10$ to $\times 20$).

Preparatory stage. The speculum is inserted, a No. 4-0 silk is placed beneath the superior rectus, and a No. 6-0 silk is used to fix the Flieringa ring to the sclera at four points. A 4 mm. fornix-based flap is prepared at the 12 o'clock position so that, at a later time, a peripheral iridectomy may be performed through a secondary incision. The donor button is excised by trephine and completed with scissors. Care must be taken to produce a button with vertical sides. From the host, an identically sized button is cut by partially penetrating the cornea with an unguarded trephine. Any attempt to use the guard to limit the depth of the trephine cut will cause an irregular incision, since the cone will tend to displace the trephine. A razor knife is used to enter the eye at the 9 o'clock position, from which right- and left-curved corneal scissors can more readily complete the excision of the diseased cornea. Prior to the razor penetration, a secondary incision may be made at the surgical limbus at the area of the preformed flap and a small peripheral iridectomy performed. In an 8 mm. or larger graft, a mid-peripheral iridectomy can be performed through the trephine opening. However, when this is done, care must be taken not to damage the lens or to create an iridodialysis with accompanying bleeding, as a result of attempting to make the iridectomy too peripheral. The donor button, which has been transferred from the donor eye to a Petri dish where it is kept moistened by a buffered solution, is then carefully transferred with a spatula to the host.

Graft insertion stage. The donor button is sutured to the host with 8 interrupted sutures of 22.1 μ Ethilon. The anterior chamber is filled with saline, which it should retain, and a continuous suture is begun at the inferior temporal quadrant, progressing clockwise in the left eye, or counter-clockwise in the right eye, until it is completed and can be tied to itself. The continuous suture has been customarily inserted from the donor button to the recipient in a radial direction. Fig. 25-12 illustrates this radial insertion, the lower figure demonstrating the "cumulative moment of forces"* induced by this method of suture placement. This method tends to cause graft rotation which results in the direction of the crossover limb of the suture to its next insertion. The radial continuous suture, therefore, has the disadvantage that a very acute angle is formed between the suture emerging from the recipient to the donor. This acute angle results in a moment of forces that tends to unbalance the even distribution of thread tension. This results in graft rotation by producing a lateral deformation at the circumference of the graft. One advantage, of course, is that radial introduction of the needle makes it easier to align the edges of the graft.

Recently we have been using a symmetrical continuous suture as illustrated in Fig. 25-13. Because of the equal angles, the moment of force is minimized; no graft rotation should result, thus permitting a balanced distribution of thread tension.

---

*Terminology suggested by J. Elstein.

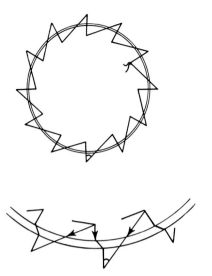

Fig. 25-12. Radial continuous suture; arrows indicate cumulative moment of forces inducing graft rotation (after J. Elstein).

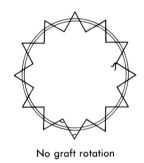

No graft rotation

Fig. 25-13. Symmetrical continuous suture; equalization of moment of forces by equalization of angles, indicated by arrows (after J. Elstein).

The symmetrical continuous suture has the disadvantage of a technically more difficult introduction of the needle at an oblique angle. This can be minimized by first placing radial interrupted sutures to fix the graft in position, and then placing the symmetrical continuous suture. The knot of the continu-

ous suture is tied over the donor material, since this causes the least discomfort. The knot size is so small that it does not cause necrosis or faceting of the cornea. The interrupted sutures may be removed; the anterior chamber is formed by forcing a stream of buffered solution between the apposed edges of the wound. A drop of fluorescein is placed on the cornea and pressure is applied to the dome of the graft and around the suture line on the recipient cornea. A flush of brilliant green indicates an area that is not well closed. Any slightly gaping area that permits the loss of fluid is closed by additional interrupted sutures, placed more superficially than the continuous suture. In both the donor and recipient corneas, the continuous suture should be placed with bites of approximately 1.5 mm. in length, and at a maximum depth of three-quarters. With a special suture forceps at each loop, it is pulled up gently but firmly two or three times before tying. The additional interrupted sutures, if any, are placed with bites of approximately 1 mm. in length and at about one-half thickness. During the suturing, the donor button is grasped at its anterior half with the Bonn forceps, double teeth down, and the needle is passed through the anterior cornea beneath the tip of the forceps to emerge at its posterior quarter. The depth of the secondary penetration into the host cornea is adjusted with the eye fixed by grasping the Flieringa ring. This eliminates the necessity to grasp and possibly tear the host cornea during this passage of the needle.

When the ring, superior rectus suture, and speculum have been removed, 2% pilocarpine is instilled, and a dressing is applied to the operated eye.

Postoperative care

Twenty-four hours postoperatively the dressing is removed, and a unilateral protective shield is applied to protect the operated eye. No patch or pressure dressing is applied to the eye once the operative dressing is removed. However, the patient wears

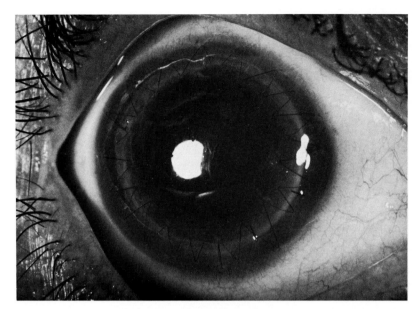

Fig. 25-14. Symmetrical continuous suture at twenty-first day postoperative.

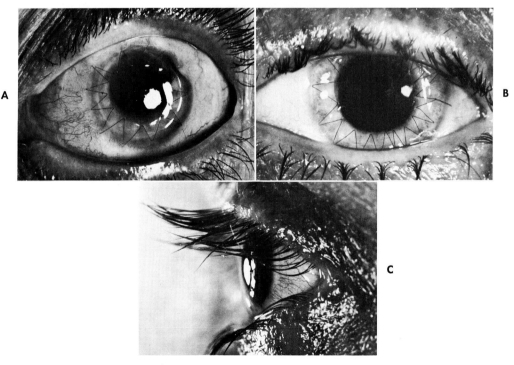

Fig. 25-15. A, Symmetrical continuous suture at 6 weeks postoperative. **B** and **C,** Symmetrical continuous suture at 12 weeks, anterior view and lateral view.

a shield or protective glasses continuously for three months.

From 48 hours to discharge (5 to 7 days) the patient is given 0.2% hyoscine hydrobromide daily, a hydrocortisone 1% suspension (prednisolone acetate) twice daily, and Ophthocort ophthalmic ointment at bedtime.

From 7 to 42 days, local medication is discontinued gradually; first the hyoscine, then the hydrocortisone, and finally the ointment. The patient is seen at 2-week intervals, and the progress of the healing is followed by biomicroscopy and keratometry (Fig. 25-14).

At the end of six weeks, the interrupted sutures are removed.

From 6 weeks to 3 months, the patient is subjected to serial keratometry at 2- to 3-week intervals. When the keratometry readings become constant, the eye is corrected with a spectacle lens. Should the graft become cloudy in the immediate postoperative period and fail to respond to steroids, it will usually be necessary to replace it within this period (Fig. 25-15).

Some time between 3 to 6 months, the continuous suture is removed by cutting every

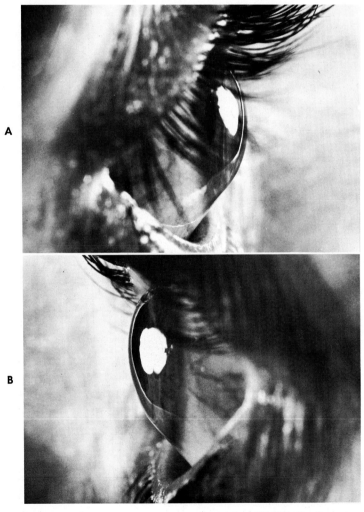

A

B

Fig. 25-16. A, Six months postoperative; visual acuity is 20/20. **B,** One year postoperative; visual acuity is 20/20.

other loop, and then removing each section with the special pointed suture handling forceps. After removal of the sutures, serial keratometry is continued and when it becomes stable, a final spectacle correction is given. No type of contact lens should be worn for 1 year or until corneal sensation returns. The fellow eye may be grafted 6 months after the first eye. At the final bilateral correction, it may be discovered that some minor vertical muscle imbalance exists, and a prism correction for this should be incorporated in the final spectacle correction. This imbalance tends to disappear 1 to 2 years following the surgery. Although one may speculate as to its origin, it is difficult to determine it precisely (Fig. 25-16).

Summary

I believe that the use of the dissecting microscope for surgery of the anterior segment will become an essential part of the surgical armamentarium in the next decade. I believe, further, that the use of the operating microscope is mandatory at the present time for all keratoplasty procedures, particularly in those procedures in which the primary aim is the improvement of the optics of a pathologic cornea. By far the most commonly performed and the most important of this group is the operation for keratoconus.

REFERENCES

 1. Barraquer, J. I.: The microscope in ocular surgery, Amer. J. Ophthal. **42:**916, 1956.
 2. Barraquer, J. I.: Autokeratoplastie avec surfacage pour la correction de la myopie (queratomileusis)—technique et résultats, Ann. Oculist (Paris) **198:**401, 1965.
 3. Barraquer, J. I.: Personal communication, 1966.
 4. Barraquer, J. I.: Personal communication, 1967.
 5. Barraquer, J. I., Barraquer, J., and Littmann, H.: A new operating microscope for ocular surgery, Amer. J. Ophthal. **63:**90, 1967.
 6. Durham, D. G.: Diamond knives in ocular surgery, Amer. J. Ophthal. **62:**16, 1966.
 7. Elstein, J.: Personal communication, 1968.
 8. Harms, H.: Augenoperationen unter dem binocularen Mikroskop., Ber. dtsch. ophthal. Ges. **58:**119, 1953.
 9. Harms, H.: Indikationen zur Linsenextraktion bei Glaukom, Klin. Mbl. Augenheilk. **126:**410, 1955.
10. Harms, H.: Erfahrungen mit der fortlaufenden Naht bei der Keratoplastik, Marhold, Halle (Saale), 1957.
11. Harms, H., and Mackensen, G.: Ocular surgery under the microscope (Translated and edited by Blodi, F. C.), Chicago, 1966, Year Book Medical Publishers, Inc.
12. Littmann, H.: Ein neues Operations—Mikroskop, Klin. Mbl. Augenheilk. **124:**473, 1954.
13. Mackensen, G., Roper-Hall, M. J., and Troutman, R. C., editors: Microsurgery of the eye, New York, 1968, S. Karger.
14. Perritt, R. A.: Mitteilung, National Assembly, United States Chapter, J. Coll. Surg., 1948.
15. Perritt, R. A.: Recent advances in corneal surgery, Amer. Acad. Ophthal. Otolaryng., Course No. 288, 1950.
16. Pierse, D.: Microsurgery, Presented at the annual meeting of the Ophthal. Soc. U. Kingdom, Edinburgh, April, 1966, Trans. Ophthal. Soc. U. K. **86:**281, 1966.
17. Troutman, R. C.: Personal interview; microsurgery, Highlights Ophthal. **7:**162, 1964.
18. Troutman, R. C.: The operating microscope in corneal surgery. In King, J. H., Jr., and McTighe, J. W., editors: The Cornea World Congress, Washington, D. C., 1965, Butterworth & Co., Ltd., pp. 424-434.
19. Troutman, R. C.: High magnification in surgery of cataracts. In Symposium on Cataracts, St. Louis, 1965, The C. V. Mosby Co., pp. 115-136.
20. Troutman, R. C.: The operating microscope in ophthalmic surgery, Trans. Amer. Ophthal. Soc. **63:**335, 1965.
21. Troutman, R. C.: International Symposium of Microsurgery of the Eye, Amer. J. Ophthal. **63:**869-877, 1967.
22. Troutman, R. C.: The operating microscope; past, present, and future, Trans. Ophthal. Soc. U. K. **87:**205, 1967.
23. Wiener, N.: Cybernetics, Cambridge, Mass., 1961, The M.I.T. Press; New York, 1961, John Wiley & Sons, Inc.
24. V. Mueller & Co., Chicago, Catalogue.
25. Symposium on Stereotactic Surgery, J. Neurosurg. **15**(3):217, 1958.

Old dyes—new
views

Fluorescein dyes

A. Edward Maumenee

I would like to review the use of fluorescein in the diagnosis of fundus lesions. As early as 1930 this dye was used in ophthalmology by Dr. Sorsby in the examination of the fundus, but he tried to use it for the study of retinal detachments to see if the holes in the detachments could be outlined.

Fluorescein was neglected from that time until 1954 when we at the Wilmer Institute used it to try to determine whether a hemangioma in the choroid would fluoresce. By using a cobalt blue filter to activate the dye, we were able to see fluorescence in the fundus in hemangiomas. It was not until Novotny and Alvis were able to photograph this fluorescence that this technique gained popularity with ophthalmologists.

I would like to review some of the lesions that we think we understand a little better from the use of this dye.

Serous detachments of the macular area

By carefully examining patients with serous detachments of the macular area with a slit lamp and contact lens, plus fluorescein, one should have no difficulty in breaking these lesions down into various categories for purposes of specific treatment.

Serous detachment of sensory epithelium. The first group is composed of those patients with serous detachment of the sensory epithelium of the retina (in contrast to detachment of the pigment epithelium). There may be a large area of serous detachment of the sensory epithelium, but there is practically always a small spot of pigment epi-

thelium detachment as well. After fluorescein (10 ml. of 5% fluorescein, or 5 ml. of 10% fluorescein) is given intravenously, one may watch with a cobalt blue filter, with a Wrattan No. 47 filter, or with a Baird Atomic Interference Filter No. 5 for the characteristic fluorescence. Leakage will occur at the spot of the pigment epithelial disturbance, and in certain patients leakage may continue as the patient is observed over a period of time (5, 10, 15, or 30 minutes). After the leak has been documented, it may be treated by photocoagulation, using the Zeiss photocoagulator or the laser beam. By merely causing some reaction around the small spot of pigment epithelium detachment, the large area of serous detachment will disappear, usually within a matter of 3 or 4 days. If the patient has not developed cystic degeneration of the retina in the macular area, the visual acuity will return to normal.

It has been our preference at the Wilmer Institute to periodically observe most of these lesions for 3 to 4 months for presence of cystic degeneration before we elect to photocoagulate them. There have been a number of ophthalmologists around the world who have treated their patients in this fashion. They have discovered that because the retina is elevated in the area of the lesion, a light photocoagulator or laser beam can destroy the area of leakage without damaging the nerve fiber layer; normal visual acuity is restored even in regions on the nasal side of the macula. Dr. Donald Gass reports that it makes no difference whether the lesion is on the nasal or the temporal side of the foveal area in deciding whether treatment should be done or not.[1]

Serous detachment of pigment epithelium. One patient had a serous detachment which was rather unusual in its appearance. When he was given fluorescein, it was noted that there was one small spot of leakage initially, and then the whole area became diffusely filled with fluorescein. The one small spot was photocoagulated and the entire process subsided within a matter of a week, although the lesion had been elevated for over a year and a half. Unfortunately, the patient had a large amount of pigment disturbance under the epithelium. When the leakage was obliterated and the detachment subsided, it left a disturbance in the pigment epithelium and his visual acuity was permanently reduced to 20/100. This patient had a serous detachment of the pigment epithelium. The lesions of the pigment epithelium have a more solid appearance than lesions of the sensory epithelium. Following intravenous injection of fluorescein, the entire lesion fluoresces.

Gass-Irvine syndrome. Another important distinction in studying the macular lesions has come from the work of Donald Gass, who observed a different fluorescein pattern in patients who have had cataract extractions and subsequent macular lesions.[2] Dr. S. R. Irvine had previously described this condition as occurring many weeks or years following cataract extraction.[3] It occurs more frequently when the hyaloid face is ruptured in the postoperative period, or when there is peaking of the pupil caused by vitreous in the wound. However, the condition can also occur with an intact face of the vitreous and a relatively quiet eye. In nearly all of the approximately fifty patients I have seen with this lesion, minimal irritation of the eye, such as instilling a drop of any medication, results in circumcorneal injection. Also, 100% of the patients have had increased vitreous opacities in the postoperative period, which suggests that this is probably an inflammatory process. Following intravenous injection of fluorescein, these patients are noted to have intraretinal edema and cystic cloverleaf-like changes. The leakage of fluorescein is not from the pigment epithelium or posterior to it, but is from the tips of the capillaries in the macular region. The leakage of fluorescein then goes on to the characteristic star-shaped figure.

As far as the treatment of these patients is concerned, I think the first principle is a proper diagnosis. The patient has usually had good vision during the immediate postoperative period, but 2 months later his vision is 20/50 or less. The detachment of the macula is very flat and difficult to see. If fluorescein is given, however, the detachment can be detected immediately because the macular lesion will fluoresce. Dr. Iliff has reported, and we have confirmed that if the patient has a peaked pupil, the release or cut of the strands out of the pupillary area will allow the pupil to become round again.[4, 5] I have found that by using a Barkan knife that has a blade smaller than the shaft, the surgeon can maintain the anterior chamber by pressing the blade of the knife up against the posterior part of the cornea. These strands can be cut with one or two sweeps at the most. The pupil is restored to its completely round shape again, even if the peaked pupil has been present for a matter of a year or more. Following this procedure the irritation will subside and the macular lesions can improve.

We have learned relatively recently that our dose of steroids was almost in the homeopathic range. We originally thought that 20 to 50 mg. of prednisone per day was a fairly good dose. We have now found by talking to colleagues in other branches of medicine that considerably more prednisone than this can be given. By using 100 to 125 mg. of prednisone per day, the macular lesions in these patients have subsided and visual acuity has improved within a matter of a week. Of course, if the patients have had cystic degeneration of the macula, then one cannot expect the steroid therapy to cure this completely.

Contraction of internal surface of retina. A condition that can be confused with the

Gass-Irvine syndrome is contraction of the internal surface of the retina. The vessels are usually quite tortuous in the macular area. There may be little or no leakage of fluorescein into the macular region noted on examination, even though there is often a serous detachment or intraretinal edema present in the region of the macula.

Vitreous adhesion to the macular area. Dr. Schepens[6] has reported that vitreous adhesion to the macular area is a cause of the Gass-Irvine syndrome. I disagree. Dr. Gass also disagrees and most of the people who have tried to find vitreous attachment in these cases disagree with this theory.[7] However, in phakic eyes of patients in the age range from 40 to 60, a very common cause of intraretinal edema is vitreous adhesion to the macular area. The vitreous may extend to the macula, producing an operculum where the vitreous has pulled the macula off, resulting in a hole in the macula. Usually these patients do not develop retinal detachments. As a matter of fact, that is a rare complication. Again, fluorescein is helpful in differentiating these cases, because they seldom have any staining following intravenous injection of fluorescein. This is not 100% true, because some of the patients can and do have a small amount of fluorescein leakage in the macular area.

I am not aware of any way of treating these latter two conditions, but I can say that in contraction of the internal surface of the retina, occasionally there will be a spontaneous cure and the visual acuity can improve.

Another point to remember is that if a patient has vitreous adhesion to the macula in one eye with intraretinal edema or a macular hole, and if in the opposite eye the vitreous is already detached, I think it is unlikely that he will develop the same lesion in the second eye. If the vitreous is still attached, however, the condition can occur bilaterally, usually some months after the onset of the condition in the first eye.

Other lesions of the macula

I would like to discuss some other lesions of the macula for which fluorescein is of some value in establishing a diagnosis.

Best's familial macular degeneration. In cases of Best's familial macular degeneration, the vitelliform-type of lesion has not revealed leakage of fluorescein. The only fluorescein that shows through is in places where there is a disturbance in the pigment epithelium such as one would see with drusen.

Macula flavilatus. Macula flavilatus or the fleck macula syndrome, which has been described by Alex Krill,[8] is a condition with a macular disturbance and loss of central visual acuity when the macula appears to be quite normal. These lesions fluoresce very much like the lesions of drusen and when seen grossly have small fishlike figures distributed in a lacelike pattern. No leakage is seen after intravenous injection of fluorescein. Dr. Krill has been fortunate in obtaining one eye with this syndrome and has been able to show that the pathology is an accumulation of a polysaccharide in the pigment epithelium. There is some fluorescence overlying the lesions because of defects in the retinal pigment epithelium in these areas.[8]

Pits of the optic disc. Another condition that we thought might lead to treatment with fluorescein guidance is pits of the optic disc. Patients with this condition frequently develop serous detachment of the macula. Following intravenous injection of fluorescein, we could find no specific leak of fluorescein into the serous detachment. Dr. Andrew Ferry studied the histopathology of a pit and noted that the retina was tucked down into the pit with serous detachment of the sensory epithelium.[9] Because of this, we thought that if it were possible to photocoagulate along the margin of the detachment at the pit to produce a chorioretinal adhesion, the recurrent episodes might cease. This was done; however, photocoagulation failed, and serous detachment of the sensory epithelium is still as high as it has ever been in the past. On several occasions I used both the laser and the Zeiss photocoagulator to try to produce chorioretinal adhesions in this area. Dr. Donald Gass has recently tried this procedure in a similar case and he has also been unsuccessful in the treatment of this condition.[10]

Hemangioma of the choroid. Hemangioma of the choroid is frequently associated with serous detachments of the macula. If the surface of a hemangioma is photocoagulated rather lightly the serous detachment of the macula will disappear. We thought initially in 1954 that fluorescein would be the ideal method of differentiating a hemangioma from a melanoma, but this has not turned out to be true. All hemangiomas I have ever seen have fluoresced. Fluorescein is not of much value in differentiating a hemangioma from a melanoma, unless the melanoma does not fluoresce. However, there should not be much trouble in differentiating these entities because they generally do not even look alike.

Inflammatory lesions. Sometimes we have patients with inflammatory lesions that are confused with melanomas. I do think that fluorescein is helpful to some extent in differentiating these from melanomas, because in the active stage of inflammatory choroiditis, the inflammatory lesion does not fluoresce during the choroidal flush. Both hemangiomas and melanomas fluoresce during the choroidal flush because they have choroidal vessels. However, during a choroidal flush, the inflammatory lesion is actually a little darker than the surrounding normal choroid. In time there is leakage of fluorescein into the inflammatory area. During the active stage of the inflammation, no distinct blood vessels leak.

Histoplasmosis. The final condition that I wish to discuss is the inflammatory lesion in the macular area of histoplasmosis. These patients have positive histoplasmin skin tests but, of course, it is not certain whether these lesions are actually caused by the organism of histoplasma.

We had a patient with this condition who had lost one eye, and had a lesion very close to the fovea in the other. Her visual acuity had been dropping because of a serous detachment of the macula, and, following photocoagulation, she has done very well.* The fluorescing lesion no longer fluoresced as much as it did prior to photocoagulation. It is extraordinary how close one can come to the macula with the photocoagulator without destroying its function. The patient is now $4\frac{1}{2}$ years post-photocoagulation and her visual acuity is 20/30; however, she can only see half of the 20/30 line because of destruction to the macula.

Summary

In summary, I think fluorescein is extremely helpful in studying posterior lesions. It can give some clue as to the method of therapy that should be used for some of the conditions mentioned.

---

*Since this chapter was presented at the Symposium, the serous detachment has completely disappeared.

REFERENCES

1. Gass, J. D. M.: Personal communication.
2. Gass, J. D. M., and Norton, E. W. D.: Fluorescein studies of patients with macular edema and papilledema following cataract extraction, Trans. Amer. Ophthal. Soc. 64:232, 1966.
3. Irvine, S. R.: A newly defined vitreous syndrome following cataract surgery. Proctor lecture, Amer. J. Ophthal. 36:599, 1953.
4. Iliff, C. E.: Personal communication.
5. MacLean, A., and Maumenee, A. E.: Hemangioma of the choroid, Trans. Amer. Ophthal. Soc. 57:171, 1959.
6. Tolentino, F. I., and Schepens, C. L.: Edema of posterior pole after cataract extraction, Arch. Ophthal. 74:781, 1965.
7. Gass, J. D. M.: Personal communication.
8. Ernest, J. T., and Krill, A. E.: Fluorescein studies in fundus flavimaculatus and drusen, Amer. J. Ophthal. 62:1, 1966.
9. Ferry, A. P.: Macular detachment associated with congenital pit of the optic nervehead, Arch. Ophthal. 70:346, 1963.
10. Gass, J. D. M.: Personal communication.

Survey of ocular dyes*

**Miles A. Galin and
Richard Robbins**

A dye is a colorant that combines in some way with the substance to which it is applied. Natural dyes, such as safflower, indigo, and alizarin from plants, kermes and cochineal from insects, and Tyrian purple from shellfish, have been known for millenia, but no organic colorant was produced until almost the end of the eighteenth century. In 1856, 9 years before the ring structure of benzene (C_6H_6) came to Kekulé in a vision,[1] William Perkin, an 18-year-old English boy, produced and recognized the first aniline dye while trying to synthesize quinine from the benzene derivative aniline ($C_6H_5NH_2$). He named it mauve from the French word for the mallow plant.†

By the end of the nineteenth century, prototypes of each of the major dye groups (triphenylmethane, oxazine, and thiazine) existed and had completely displaced both natural and inorganic dyes.

Although the mechanisms by which dyes stain tissues are still obscure, the distinctions made by histologists have practical value. Dyes used in tissue staining are classified as:

1. Acid—the charge on the coloring ion is negative (cationic)
2. Basic—the charge on the coloring ion is positive (anionic)
3. Neutral—a complex salt of a dye acid with a dye base (such as eosinate of methylene blue)

Acid dyes generally stain basic cell components and basic dyes generally stain acidic cell components. The process of staining may involve ion exchange reactions between the

stain and active sites at the surface or within the cell. Other mechanisms, such as chelation to chromatin, have been suggested for certain dyes as well.

Vital staining presupposes the ability of an agent to stain a tissue (making it more readily visible) without altering or destroying the cell. At the beginning of this century, acid dyes were generally employed for vital staining because they stained all tissues except those of the central nervous system. Staining of the cornea and bulbar conjunctiva was first done in the 1890's. Although fluorescein is the most widely used ocular dye, many others have been tried, among them escorin, gentian violet, methylene blue, toluidine blue, trypan blue, eosine, mercurochrome, Bismarck brown, scarlet red, alcian blue, Sudan III, bromthymol blue, litmus, and rose bengal.[2] Rose bengal and fluorescein have had the most extensive application opthalmologically. (It should be pointed out that fluorescein is an indicator dye and does not stain cells. Its use is dependent on its visibility in dilute concentrations primarily due to its fluorescence. It is not a vital stain.)

Although few investigations of dyes have appeared in ophthalmic literature as to the mechanism of vital staining,[3] this subject has been actively studied in other tissues with a variety of dyes. For example, the acridine dyes bind nucleic acids, and their metachromatic properties make it possible to distinguish DNA from RNA; DNA fluoresces green and RNA fluoresces red with acridine orange. Thus mitosis can be followed in certain tissues from metaphase to telophase with this vital stain. One may even follow tissue invasion by organisms, such as the agent of psittacosis, by the color transformation from green to red to green as the invasive particles are formed.

The vital stain most frequently used in ophthalmology, rose bengal, stains damaged cells and leaves normal cells unstained. Simultaneous staining with a mixture of rose bengal and fluorescein helps determine the presence of degenerating cells. Counterstain-

*Aided, in part, by Grant #NB07162 from the United States Public Health Service.

†That same year, J. Natanson discovered an aniline dye later called fuchsin or magenta. By not giving it a trivial name he relegated himself to this footnote; mauve was in use for but ten years while magenta is still used today.

ing with alcian blue shows the presence of mucus.

Vital staining of the retina has also been tried. Basic dyes that stain nervous tissue are decolored by normal retina. Kiton-fast green V can stain the edges of retinal tears (where retinal metabolism is presumably poor), outlining them in green to facilitate their identification.[4]

Areas of different enzymatic activity may be vitally stained with a variety of dyes (such as styryl quinoline), but such methods have had limited application.[5] Methylene blue also has limited application as an ocular vital stain, although it will dye nerve fibers and filaments. This dye has been used more as an indicator dye than as a vital stain in ophthalmology.

Indicator dyes (such as fluorescein) have had the most extensive use in ophthalmology. Recently, high molecular weight dextrans with covalently bonded chromagens have been used to study the movement of fluid through the eye. It has been demonstrated using dextran-red that after a successful cyclodialysis, aqueous passes from the suprachoroidal space directly through the sclera.[6] Studies in our laboratory on corneal transfer have been performed with dextran-blue 2,000, a macromolecule with a blue chromagen. It was postulated that the corneal transfer of certain macromolecules (such as viruses) might be traced by such an indicator dye. The effect of various drugs, such as steroids, on the passage of dextran-blue 2,000 was also investigated. It was found that steroids significantly enhance the passage of this dye into the deeper layers of the corneal stroma. The nonsteroid-treated cornea is quite resistant to the passage of dextran-blue 2,000. This indicator dye is a polymer consisting of repeated glucose units joined through alpha $(1{\rightarrow}6)$ glycosidic linkages. The blue chromophore is cibachrome C. There is one chromophore molecule present for every 20 to 30 glucoses. Because of the nature of the linkages, there is virtually no potential for the chromophore to migrate independently of the parent molecule. On the basis of the known diameter of the molecule and its elasticity in solution, it was felt that this dye approximated the molecular size of herpes simplex virus (1,800 Å). The steroid effect, therefore, on the passage of this dye through the cornea may have clinical significance in determining why herpes simplex virus can become a fulminating disease on the steroid-treated cornea.

Any survey of ocular dyes would be incomplete without mention of the extensive use to which fluorescein has been put in ophthalmology. Contact lens fitting, tonometry, foreign body detection, lacrimal patency evaluation, corneal surgery, detection of neoplasia, determination of aqueous flow, retinal and choroidal circulating patterns, differentiation and classification of posterior polar lesions, antibody studies and aniline dye detoxification all have been enhanced by the use of this agent.

Work is continuing in our laboratory in vital staining and indicator dyes for ophthalmic use. The investigative potential of these may prove to be enormously fruitful.

REFERENCES

1. Selye, H.: From dream to discovery, New York, 1964, McGraw-Hill Book Company, p. 50.
2. Duke Elder, W. S.: System of ophthalmology, Vol. 7, St. Louis, 1962, The C. V. Mosby Co., p. 243.
3. Norn, M. S.: Vital staining of the cornea and conjunctiva, Amer. J. Ophthal. 64:1078, 1967.
4. Sorsby, A.: Vital staining of the retina. In Ridley, F., and Sorsby, A., editors: Modern trends in ophthalmology, London, 1955, Butterworth and Co., p. 238.
5. Ballintine, E. J., and Peters, L.: Effects of intracarotid injection of a basic dye on the ciliary body, Amer. J. Ophthal. 38:153, 1956.
6. Bill, A.: Movement of albumen and dextran through the sclera, Arch. Ophthal. 74:248, 1965.

Diagnostic dyes in superior limbic keratoconjunctivitis and other superficial entities

Frederick H. Theodore

The term "vital staining" for the diagnosis of external disease is largely incorrect; the cells that are stained are, in most instances, dead or devitalized. Actually, this chemopathic affinity is essentially what the ophthalmologist wants when he utilizes dyes for this purpose; that is, to demonstrate, if possible, foci of diseased, necrotic, or absent tissue. While some dyes, such as methylene blue, may be used to delineate normal structures such as nerve-endings, these are usually research procedures. What the ophthalmologist is basically interested in for clinical practice are chemical aids in the recognition and differentiation of external disease processes.

Over the years a large number of dyes have been tried and employed for this purpose. These have been well summarized by Passmore and King.[1] Certain water-soluble dyes have proved to be of value for corneal and conjunctival staining. Included in this group are sodium fluorescein, merbromin (mercurochrome) and the sodium salt of rose bengal, all xanthene or acid chromophore dyes, as well as quinone imide or basic chromophore dyes, such as the thiazines (methylene blue, polychrome methylene blue, and azure II) and the oxazines (Nile blue sulfate and brilliant cresyl blue). Scarlet red, an azo dye which is soluble in olive oil, has also been used. In addition, many other chemicals both old and new have been, and are being, studied by investigators in this field.

However, for practical purposes two products, fluorescein (apparently the first chemical to be used for diagnostic staining) and rose bengal (now in use for 50 years) still appear to be the most widely used and, in general, the most satisfactory, by virtue of their effectiveness, stability, and relative lack

of irritation, allergic reactions, or discoloration of the surrounding skin. This discussion will therefore be limited to the application of these dyes to the diagnosis of superficial external disease entities. Actually, these drugs are not true dyes, but are classified as such because fluorane contains a xanthene ring.[1]

Use of fluorescein

Fluorescein preparations are available both as solutions and as sterilized fluorescein papers. Solutions generally are most active, stable, and least irritating at pH 8.6, and are easier to use. However, the apparently peculiar affinity of *Pseudomonas aeruginosa (Bacillus pyocyaneus)* for fluorescein makes contamination with this bacterium a serious hazard, despite precautions as to sterile preparation and the addition of effective preservatives such as thiomersol (Merthiolate) and chlorobutanol. Benzalkonium (Zephiran) is not a safe preservative.

The dangers of such contamination have been well documented by Theodore, largely in collaboration with Feinstein.[2-5] This work was instrumental in the enactment of governmental regulations requiring that all eye drops be prepared sterilely and contain suitable preservatives. In investigating the source of a severe *Pseudomonas* corneal ulcer from fluorescein staining, Theodore cultured 26 bottles of fluorescein in one hospital. All were heavily contaminated with *Pseudomonas*. Of 15 bottles checked in the offices of opthalmologists, 10 were likewise contaminated. Almost all of the remaining 5 had been prepared sterilely with suitable preservatives.

Thus fluorescein solutions require careful preparation and care during use. Opened bottles, even of preserved sterile solutions, should be discarded very quickly once used. In fact, it is best to use small disposable individual containers if a solution is required. Moreover, allergy from the mercurial preservative may occur, even though the major ingredient, fluorescein, appears virtually non-allergenic.[6] Largely because of the danger of contamination, fluorescein is best used as sterilized fluorescein-impregnated papers as first introduced by Kimura.[7] These papers should be wrapped in cellophane until used. Uncovered matchbook types of fluorescein papers provided with applanation tonometers create an unnecessary hazard, although they are dry.

To prevent irritation and to ensure sufficient dye to stain thoroughly, fluorescein papers should be moistened with sterile water, saline, or irrigating solution, immediately before use. Usually, the wet paper is applied to the lower fornix. However, when profuse tearing is present, such as with an extensive corneal abrasion, no staining (a false negative) may occur. In general, therefore, it is safer to place the paper on the upper bulbar conjunctiva and allow it to wash over the cornea in a downward direction. This should not be done if superior limbic keratoconjunctivitis is suspected (see pp. 262 to 264), as false positive staining may occur. Generous staining requires copious secondary irrigation to eliminate all excess dye. All this is bothersome and time-consuming, but "micro-staining" with dry papers may give false negatives as regards the cornea, and false positives as regards the conjunctiva.

The great value of fluorescein for surface staining is well known. The precorneal film is clearly stained and delineated. Contact lens points of contact and erosions are demonstrable. Corneal epithelial defects stain bright green. Foreign bodies are outlined. In the treatment of corneal ulcers both the outlines of the epithelial staining and the intensity of staining in the base of the ulcer are valuable indications of the healing tendency. Fluorescein is often of value in indicating postoperative leaks, especially after cataract extractions or glaucoma filtering procedures. The dye is seen to wash away rapidly from the center of an otherwise stagnant lake of fluorescein.

Although rose bengal is superior to fluorescein for staining the conjunctiva, fluorescein is also of value in studies of the conjunctiva. Instead of giving a green appearance as in the corneal disease, in the conjunctiva the stain is yellow or orange where the epithelium is denuded or destroyed as in a chemical burn or injury. With the blue filter of the slit lamp both corneal and conjunctival defects show the same well-known fluorescent appearance.

Use of rose bengal

Kleefeld, a pioneer in biomicroscopy and in vital staining, was the first to use rose bengal in ophthalmology.[8, 9] An excellent paper on rose bengal in English by Forster[10] is also recommended.

Rose bengal, used in a 0.7 to 1.0% aqueous solution (Table 26-1), has a special affinity for devitalized conjunctival and corneal epithelium. The staining consists of fine pinpoint rose-colored dots as seen under the slit lamp. Using a green filter the dots stain purplish blue. (This is important where extreme redness or hemorrhage would otherwise mask a pink stain.) The corneal epithelium also takes the stain, especially in the limbal region. Corneal staining is less intense than with fluorescein, but in certain conditions is positive where fluorescein is negative. As first pointed out by Kleefeld, rose bengal is of value in investigation of corneal ulcers in which fine differentiation and study of the margins is important, as in herpetic keratitis. Fluorescein diffuses into the cornea too readily, obscuring such details; rose bengal does not.

Rose bengal appears less apt to be contaminated than fluorescein,[11] but sterile pre-

Table 26-1. Formula for rose bengal solution* (Courtesy Barnes-Hind Pharmaceuticals, Inc.)

Ingredients	Percent
Rose bengal	1.0
Chlorbutanol (hydrous)	1.05
Polyvinylpyrrolidone	10.0
Boric acid reagent in sodium hydroxide q.s. (pH 6.7)	1.9
Distilled water q.s.	100

*Incorporate the PVP into water followed by the chlorbutanol. The other ingredients can then be added. Sterilize by Millipore filter (0.45 μ) aseptically under pressure.

served solutions should be prepared. Unless specially compounded, the dye is apt to be much more irritating to the eye than fluorescein, and preliminary local anesthesia is often necessary. Although such anesthetic drops do not generally alter the basic staining pattern, it is best not to use them. The solution prepared for me by Barnes-Hind causes no significant irritation and no anesthesia is needed.

Since the use of rose bengal may cause skin staining persisting for many hours, it is advisable to spread ophthalmic ointment on both lids before it is instilled. This, and the use of wet cotton to absorb excess dye spillage from the conjunctival sac, will prevent lid discoloration after irrigation of the conjunctiva.

Norn recommends a mixture of rose bengal and fluorescein because there are pathologic conditions in which only one component stains and other conditions in which only the other component works.[12]

Superior limbic keratoconjunctivitis

Superior limbic keratoconjunctivitis is a new clinical entity of significant and increasing occurrence that appears to have arisen in the past 15 years.[13-16] This rather unique and easily recognizable recurrent disease is characterized by a number of distinctive features: (1) marked inflammation of the tarsal conjunctiva of the upper lid; (2) inflammation of the upper bulbar conjunctiva; (3) fine punctate fluorescein or rose bengal staining of the cornea at the upper limbus and the adjacent conjunctiva above the limbus; and (4) superior limbic proliferation. In approximately one-third of all attacks there are filaments situated at the superior limbus or in the upper part of the cornea. Although the filaments, when present, constitute the most outstanding feature of the entity, they are essentially only a complication. The underlying process is believed to be the peculiar keratoconjunctivitis. The fact that the upper corneal limbus appears to be the focal point of the process was the basis for the name "superior limbic keratoconjunctivi-

tis" (SLK), which I have used for the past 12 years in describing this entity.

From the onset, the occurrence of superior limbic keratoconjunctivitis appears to have been nationwide. At the beginning, however, because its multifaceted picture was not generally recognized, many instances of the disease, in which filaments did not develop or were only transient, appear to have been overlooked. This is due to the fact that the unique keratoconjunctivitis, which is the primary process, is often subtle and requires careful slit lamp observation, specific staining, and repeated examinations for proper diagnosis. Without this background, the observer, suddenly confronted with the dramatic appearance of filaments which overshadow the rest of the ocular findings, is apt to catalogue the disease merely as another instance of filamentary keratitis and thus disregard less obvious instances of SLK.

At present, with better appreciation of the entire SLK syndrome, the entity has been recognized in various phases by many ophthalmologists as a not infrequent occurrence. A number of observers have studied fairly large groups of such cases and are in agreement as to the importance of SLK in terms of incidence, occurrence, recurrence, severity, disability, and chronicity. Furthermore, there is now evidence that the condition is even more widespread and occurs in other countries. An American who developed the disease while in Indonesia was understandably given intensive antitrachomatous therapy both in the Orient and in Europe for over 6 months without improvement. Instances of the disease have been observed in Australia as well.

The major characteristics of superior limbic keratoconjunctivitis are outlined below. Fig. 26-1 depicts the objective findings.

Major characteristics of superior limbic keratoconjunctivitis
1. Age incidence: 4 to 81 years
2. Sex incidence: slightly higher in women
3. Duration: 1 to 10 years with remissions and recurrences
4. Prognosis: eventual clearing

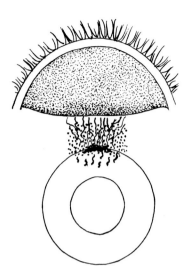

Fig. 26-1. Superior limbic keratoconjunctivitis. Schematic drawing showing upper lid palpebral conjunctivitis; injection of the superior bulbar conjunctiva; specific pinpoint staining with rose bengal or fluorescein of the involved bulbar conjunctiva and limbic cornea; proliferative changes of the cornea at the superior limbus; and corneal filaments. (Modified from Theodore, F. H.: Further observations on superior limbic keratoconjunctivitis, Trans. Amer. Acad. Ophthal. Otolaryn. **71:**341, 1967.)

5. Usually bilateral: often unilateral or much worse in one eye than other; recurrences may vary from eye to eye
6. Papillary inflammation of upper tarsal conjunctiva; remainder of conjunctiva less inflamed
7. Injection of superior bulbar conjunctiva
8. Fine punctate fluorescein staining of conjunctiva above the limbus and of the cornea just below the limbus; best seen with blue filter of slit lamp
9. Distinctive rose bengal staining of same area; appears purplish blue with green filter
10. Superior limbic proliferation of varying degree
11. Occurrence of filaments at superior limbus or upper cornea in approximately one-third of the cases; filaments inconstant; symptoms aggravated when they are present
12. Impaired tearing in some patients
13. Area of localized conjunctival dryness above limbus, more marked than in normal eyes; hyalinized epithelium demonstrated on conjunctival scrapings of the involved bulbar conjunctiva
14. Corneal hypesthesia occasionally present
15. Favorable response upon application of 0.5% silver nitrate to conjunctiva in almost all patients

Staining in SLK

Staining with fluorescein or rose bengal offers great help in the diagnosis of SLK. With fluorescein, superficial punctate staining of the bulbar conjunctiva (often involving the entire segment from the 10:30 to the 1:30 o'clock position and extending above the limbus for 4 or 5 mm. or more) and staining of the cornea in a zone 1 to 2 mm. at the limbus are best seen utilizing the blue filter of the slit lamp, although they are also visible with ordinary illumination. Such staining may occur fortuitously following the mildest trauma, such as the touching of a Fluor-i-Strip to the bulbar conjunctiva. To avoid the production of a false positive finding, the ophthalmologist should apply the stain to the inferior fornix in enough quantity to fill the entire conjunctival sac; then the sac should be thoroughly irrigated. Unless irrigation is complete, irregularly sized tiny lakes of fluorescein remain and may simulate stains. The actual stains of SLK are fine and uniform, and stand out sharply. While such positive bulbar conjunctival staining varies in degree with the severity of SLK, it is found routinely in some measure in all cases and appears to be an essential part of the clinical picture.

Similar selective staining of the involved bulbar conjunctiva and adjacent limbic cornea is afforded by the use of rose bengal. In cases of SLK of average severity a discrete area of superior bulbar staining is immediately visible to the naked eye; in mild or receding cases fine punctate staining can be seen on biomicroscopy. Such fine rose bengal staining also involves the superior limbic area of the cornea. The stains of rose bengal, if obscured in ordinary light by hemorrhage or conjunctival injection, become readily apparent in green light (assuming a dark purplish blue color).

Other findings in SLK

The etiology of SLK is at present unknown. Viral cultures have been negative. Bacterial cultures show nonpathogenic staphylococci. Epithelial scrapings of the upper lid conjunctiva reveal a predominantly polymorphonuclear response. Scrapings of the involved superior bulbar conjunctiva show degenerated hyalinized epithelium.

A significant percentage of cases show impairment of tearing but not more than in the general population. What is unusual is the high incidence of extreme localized dryness of the involved superior bulbar conjunctiva in eyes with normal Schirmer tests. The upper bulbar conjunctiva is, surprisingly, rather dry in normal patients, but in SLK the filter paper adheres like a suction cup.

Tenzel has called attention to the possible relationship of SLK to hyperthyroidism.[17] My own experiences do indicate some instances occurring in patients with evidence of thyroid hyperactivity, but also include patients with thyroid hypofunction as well.[18] Furthermore, the majority of patients appear to have normal thyroid function.

Treatment of SLK

Treatment is nonspecific. There is no response to sulfonamides, antibiotics, or idoxuridine, and little, if any, to steroids. The local application of silver nitrate 0.5% to the conjunctiva of the upper and lower lids by means of cotton-tipped applicators is the best single treatment available at present. The results are usually dramatic. Where filaments are present, they often disappear in a matter of minutes after such treatment. Where filaments are not present, symptoms are relieved greatly by the next day, and the objective findings of superior bulbar hyperemia and the characteristic bulbar staining diminish in degree. The last to clear is the limbic staining, but this, too, improves somewhat in the course of several weeks. I can only recall one patient who was not helped by silver nitrate treatments. The home use of a sodium propionate–naphazoline mixture (Neo-Propisol) is also prescribed.

Diagnosis

Generally SLK is easily differentiated from other superficial entities. However, if fila-

ments are not present, the following conditions may require differentiation: (1) trachoma; (2) superficial punctate keratitis (Thygeson); (3) marginal infiltrates situated at the 12 o'clock position; (4) limbic lesions of vernal conjunctivitis; (5) phlyctenulosis; (6) other undescribed forms of keratoconjunctivitis involving the upper palpebral conjunctiva; (7) limbic tumors; and (8) self-induced keratoconjunctivitis.

In none of these conditions except the last is there bulbar conjunctival staining of any significance. Corneal staining may occur in early trachoma, a condition always to be borne in mind in these days of widening horizons for both the American traveler and the American military forces. However, the presence of inclusion bodies and the response to sulfonamides and broad spectrum antibiotics in trachoma do not occur in SLK.

Superficial punctate keratitis (Thygeson) stains diffusely over the entire cornea in a punctate fashion. There is no real bulbar staining. Moreover, there is a dramatic response to topical steroid treatment. The disease generally occurs in young adults, usually boys.

Marginal infiltrates, limbic vernal conjunctivitis, and phlyctenulosis all may stain with fluorescein. However, the staining is not like that of SLK. The response of these diseases to steroids is dramatic. Limbic tumors might be confused with SLK, but the staining is different.

Self-induced conjunctivitis may show conjunctival staining with both fluorescein and rose bengal very similar in character to that of SLK, but the staining occurs in a different location. While it is entirely conceivable that lesions of the superior limbic and superior bulbar conjunctiva might be caused in this manner, my experience has been limited to self-induced lesions of the medial, lateral, or inferior portions of the limbus and conjunctiva.

Diseases causing corneal filaments

Filaments appear to be a complication of corneal disease, altered corneal physiology, tear abnormality, or corneal edema. The major causes of corneal filaments are listed below:

1. Keratoconjunctivitis sicca (Sjögren's syndrome) —lower or central cornea
2. Superior limbic keratoconjunctivitis—upper cornea
3. Secondary keratoconjunctivitis sicca—trachoma; ocular pemphigoid; erythema multiforme; membranous conjunctivitis; chemical burns; post-radiation; lacrimal gland disease
4. After ocular surgery—cataract; detachment; glaucoma or muscle (occlusion a factor)
5. After loss of corneal epithelium—recurrent corneal erosion; herpes; contact lens; allergy; topical drug reactions (especially proparacaine)
6. Keratopathy—bullous; neuropathic; conjunctival carcinoma
7. Conjunctivitis—gram-negative (*Proteus*); epidemic keratoconjunctivitis; pharyngoconjunctival fever

Dye staining is needed diagnostically in only relatively few of the conditions noted. In most of the entities in which filaments occur, general examination is enough for diagnosis. Staining is, of course, helpful but only as an adjuvant method.

Keratoconjunctivitis sicca. The use of diagnostic dyes in the diagnosis of primary keratoconjunctivitis sicca (Sjögren's syndrome) is very valuable. Corneal staining with fluorescein often shows diffuse punctate lesions and the filaments are highlighted. However, bulbar conjunctival staining with fluorescein is far less pronounced than in SLK; in fact, it is usually absent. Moreover, the involved areas are the exposed medial and lateral portions of the bulbar conjunctiva. Rose bengal is more valuable for staining the involved bulbar conjunctiva and the adjacent limbic areas, as well as any filaments present. It is, however, far less valuable than the Schirmer test; in my experience, definitely positive staining occurs in only about one-third of those patients with complete dryness of the filter papers used. This should not be surprising since conjunctival devitalization is the result of impaired tearing and is ordinarily less common. I cannot agree with the findings of Forster, who feels that a positive rose bengal test occurs more often than a positive Schirmer test.[10] These observations are also valid to some extent in

instances of secondary keratoconjunctivitis sicca.

Fluorescein staining is, of course, of recognized value in the diagnosis of many other entities as listed previously, such as recurrent corneal erosions, herpes simplex, contact lens lesions, and drug reactions. It is less well appreciated that conjunctival neoplasms may masquerade as chronic keratoconjunctivitis, and are associated with punctate staining, corneal lesions, and epithelial desquamation.[19] The importance of *Bacillus proteus* as a not infrequent cause of chronic keratoconjunctivitis is also generally overlooked.[14] Here, too, epithelial staining and spotty desquamation are best demonstrated by fluorescein staining; rose bengal staining is less valuable.

The occurrence of severe necrotizing reactions of the corneal epithelium with filament formation after the instillation of only a single drop of proparacaine (Ophthaine or Ophthetic) has been noted by me over the past four years.[14, 20] Such occurrences are often considered traumatic in origin if tonometry or gonioscopy is performed in these patients.

Summary

Vital staining is essentially an incorrect term; for the diagnosis of external ocular diseases dyes are employed to stain diseased, devitalized, or denuded areas. For clinical purposes two dyes, fluorescein and rose bengal, have maintained their popularity over the years. Fluorescein is better for corneal staining; its use in conjunctival disease is more limited. Rose bengal is preferable in conjunctival lesions, although it has some value in superficial corneal staining. Fluorescein has a peculiar affinity for contamination with *Pseudomonas aeruginosa*, and must be used with care.

Both dyes are of special value in superior limbic keratoconjunctivitis, a newly recognized entity, as well as, at times, in other superficial entities that require differentiation from this interesting and easily overlooked condition.

REFERENCES

1. Passmore, J. W., and King, J. H.: Vital staining of the conjunctiva and cornea, Arch. Ophthal. **53:**568, 1955.
2. Theodore, F. H., and Minsky, H.: Lack of sterility of eye medicaments, J.A.M.A. **147:** 1381, 1951.
3. Theodore, F. H.: Contamination of eye solutions, Amer. J. Ophthal. **34:**1764, 1951.
4. Theodore, F. H., and Feinstein, R. R.: Practical suggestions for the preparation and maintenance of sterile ophthalmic solutions, Amer. J. Ophthal. **35:**656, 1952.
5. Theodore, F. H., and Feinstein, R. R.: Preparation and maintenance of sterile ophthalmic solutions, J.A.M.A. **152:**1631, 1953.
6. Theodore, F. H., and Schlossman, A.: Ocular allergy, Baltimore, 1958, The Williams & Wilkins Co., p. 75.
7. Kimura, S. J.: Fluorescein paper, Amer. J. Ophthal. **34:**446, 1951.
8. Kleefeld, G.: Une nouvelle coloration des ulcères cornéens, Bull. Soc. belge d'ophtal. **41:** 58, 1920.
9. Sjögren, H.: Zur Kenntnis der Keratoconjunctivitis Sicca (Keratitis filiformis bei Hypofunktion der Tränendrüsen, Acta Ophthal. (Supp. 2), pp. 1-151, 1933.
10. Forster, H. W.: Rose bengal test in diagnosis of deficient tear formation, Arch. Ophthal. **45:**419, 1951.
11. Norn, M. S., and Frølund Thomsen, V.: Contamination of eye drops used for vital staining, Acta Ophthal. **45:**650, 1967.
12. Norn, M. S.: Vital staining of the cornea and conjunctiva, Amer. J. Ophthal. **64:**1078, 1967.
13. Theodore, F. H.: Superior limbic keratoconjunctivitis, Eye Ear Nose Throat Monthly **42:**25, 1963.
14. Theodore, F. H.: Further observations on superior limbic keratoconjunctivitis, Trans. Amer. Acad. Ophth. Otolaryng. **71:**341, 1967.
15. Thygeson, P.: Observations on filamentary keratitis, Transactions of the A.M.A. Section on Ophthalmology, 112th Annual Meeting, 1963, pp. 49-55.
16. Corwin, M.: Superior limbic keratoconjunctivitis (SLK), Amer. J. Ophthal. **66:**338, 1968.
17. Tenzel, R. R.: Comments on superior limbic filamentous keratitis. Part 2. Arch. Ophthal. **79:**508, 1968.
18. Theodore, F. H.: Comments on findings of elevated protein-bound iodine in superior limbic keratoconjunctivitis. Part 1. Arch. Ophthal. **79:**508, 1968.
19. Theodore, F. H.: Carcinoma of the conjunctiva masquerading as chronic conjunctivitis, Eye Ear Nose Throat Monthly **46:**1419, 1967.
20. Theodore, F. H.: Idiosyncratic corneal reactions from proparacaine, Eye Ear Nose Throat Monthly **47:**286, 1968.

Orbital radiology in unilateral exophthalmos

Judah Zizmor

Orbital radiology deals with a very wide spectrum of disease. Those diseases which produce unilateral exophthalmos are of particular interest as problems in radiologic diagnosis.

Among the causes of unilateral exophthalmos are thyroid dysfunction, infections, infestations, tumors (whether benign or malignant; primary, secondary, or metastatic), bone dysplasias, vascular malformations, congenital anomalies, fractures, foreign bodies, and even autoimmune diseases.

The routine roentgenographic examination of the orbit is still basic and indispensable in the investigation of unilateral exophthalmos. Positive signs of abnormality are provided in approximately 50% of patients with unilateral exophthalmos on routine film study. Pfeiffer, in his study of 200 cases of unilateral exophthalmos, stated that positive roentgenographic signs indicated the diagnosis in 42% of cases, and in another 20% the findings led to the specific diagnosis if correlated with other clinical findings.[1]

The roentgenographic signs of unilateral exophthalmos on routine films are:[2, 3]

1. Increased soft tissue density
2. Calcification
3. Expansion of orbital margins
4. Fossa formation
5. Dehiscence of bone
6. Osteolysis
7. Hyperostosis and osteoblastosis
8. Thickened bony walls
9. Diminished orbital volume
10. Expansion of optic canal
11. Orbital gas

In my experience, all of these signs have been associated with orbital tumors, except for the sign of orbital gas. Orbital gas has been associated either with fractures or with orbital infection secondary to sinus disease.

During the past 35 years more complicated roentgenographic diagnostic procedures have been introduced for use in those cases of unilateral exophthalmos that show no positive signs of abnormality on routine films.

The roentgenographic study of the orbit for orbital tumors and unilateral exophthalmos may include the following procedures:

1. Complete routine skull study with stereoscopic or nonstereoscopic roentgenograms, including Caldwell, Waters, right and left optic foramen, base, and lateral views[1]
2. Tomography of the orbits and antra
3. Air orbitography[4]
4. Opaque orbitography with 20% aqueous iodide solutions[5]
5. Arteriography of the carotid and ophthalmic arteries with 50 to 60% organic aqueous iodide solutions[6, 7]
6. Orbital phlebography via the angular vein, or via retrograde, jugular vein, inferior petrosal, or cavernous sinus route with aqueous organic iodide solutions[6-8]
7. Subtraction technique of Ziedses des Plantes, a photographic method for diminishing overlying bone density to enhance the visibility of angiograms of the orbits and brain[9]

These more complicated radiographic procedures will often contribute important evidence of orbital mass lesions not demonstrable on routine films, and thereby will increase the percentage of cases with positive radiographic findings.

Positive radiographic signs of unilateral exophthalmos

Increased orbital soft tissue density. Increased orbital soft tissue density is a sign of unilateral exophthalmos, but is not specific or diagnostic of the pathologic cause.

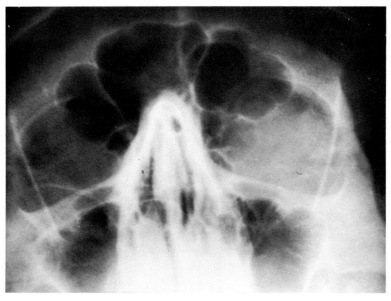

Fig. 26-2. Rhabdomyosarcoma of the left orbit. The patient (H. F.), a 42-year-old male, developed exophthalmos over a 6 month period. The roentgenogram shows an increase in soft tissue in the left orbit without evidence of bone destruction or expansion of the orbit.

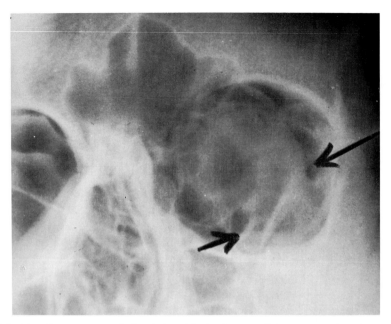

Fig. 26-3. Myofibrosarcoma of the left orbit (a firm modular encapsulated tumor). The patient (H. D.) is 20 years old. The globe is displaced upward and forward. Progressive onset over 18 months. The roentgenogram shows an increase of soft tissue; the tumor is profiled by air. The tumor profile extends from the posterior inferior margin almost to the anterior inferior margin of the left orbit. The air orbitogram profiles a posterior inferior soft tissue mass in the left orbit.

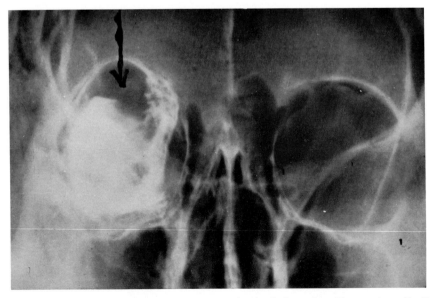

Fig. 26-4. Neurilemmoma of the superior one-third of the orbit. The patient (J. C. S.) had right exophthalmos over a 2 year period. Opaque orbitography with 20% Diodrast injected into the muscle cone profiles a mass in the upper right orbit. (Courtesy Dr. Daniel Silva, Mexico City.)

Increase of orbital soft tissues is associated with hyperthyroidism, trauma, hemorrhage, edema, cellulitis, cysts, granuloma or pseudotumor primary orbital tumors (both benign and malignant), secondary orbital tumors by extension from adjacent tissues, or metastatic tumors from remote primary tumors (Figs. 26-2 to 26-4).

Emphysema of orbital soft tissues. Emphysema of the orbital soft tissues frequently accompanies fractures of the common bony walls between the orbit and the sinuses, and is presumptive evidence of fracture even if the exact fracture line is not demonstrated (as is frequently the case with a fracture of the medial orbital wall). Orbital cellulitis

and abscess may result in the formation of gas within the orbital soft tissues caused by the metabolism of the infecting organism, or the gas may enter the orbit through a fistulous communication with an infected sinus in which the bony margins are made dehiscent by osteomyelitis (Figs. 26-5 and 26-6).

Expansion of orbital margins. Expansion of orbital margins is associated with benign tumors of the orbit, such as hemangioma, neurofibroma, lacrimal gland tumors, dermoid cysts, and meningioma. In infants, orbital enlargement in response to a benign tumor develops after 1 to 3 months of exophthalmos and increased intraorbital pressure.

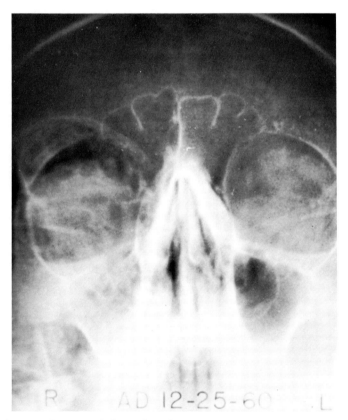

Fig. 26-5. Blow-out fracture of the right orbit with emphysema. The patient (A. D.) was struck in the right eye by a fist on the previous night. The roentgenogram shows emphysema and increased soft tissue density in the right orbit. The cloudy right antrum is caused by hemorrhage. The right orbital floor is depressed.

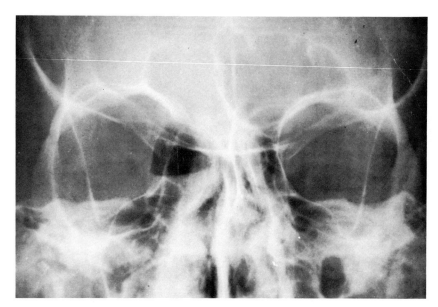

Fig. 26-6. Ethnoidal mucocele with air and fluid level. The patient (J. W. H.), an 11-year-old boy, had had an acute upper respiratory infection with purulent nasal discharge, headaches, and development of progressive right orbital swelling, unilateral exophthalmos, and fever. The roentgenogram shows cloudy right frontal and ethnoidal sinuses with a 20 × 18 mm. area of gas and fluid level in the plane of the medial aspect of the right orbit and the superior ethnoid cells. Oval bone dehiscence is present.

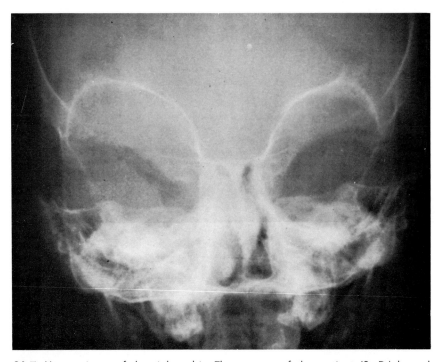

Fig. 26-7. Hemangioma of the right orbit. The parents of the patient (S. D.) have been aware of right exophthalmos since the child's birth. Roentgenograms were taken at the age of 16 months. The roentgenogram shows expansion of the right orbit with an increase of soft tissue.

In adults, orbital enlargement develops after unilateral exophthalmos of 1 to 3 years' duration (Fig. 26-7).

Fossa formation. Fossa formation is a local expansion of the bony orbital wall caused by the persistent pressure of a small cyst, such as an orbital dermoid, or by an encapsulated benign or malignant tumor of the lacrimal gland. The bony cortex is intact (Fig. 26-8).

Dehiscence of bone. Dehiscence of bone may be congenital or acquired. It is associated with meningocele, encephalocele, dermoid and epidermoid cysts, mucoceles, aneurysms, fractures, neurofibroma, and lacrimal gland tumors (Fig. 26-9).

Osteolysis of the bony orbit. Osteolysis of

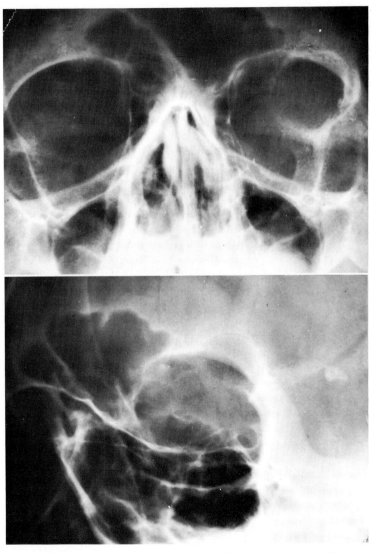

Fig. 26-8. Dermoid of the left orbit. The patient (F. R.), a 34-year-old male, has had progressive exophthalmos over a 4 year period. The roentgenogram shows a 2.5 × 2.5 cm. elevation of the roof of the outer half of the left orbit. The margin is demarcated by a white mucoperiosteal line. This is highly suggestive of orbital dermoid.

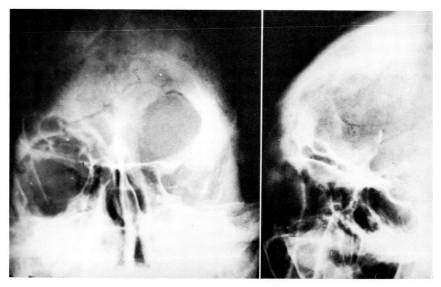

Fig. 26-9. Expanding left frontal mucocele. The patient (A. F.) has had a 5 year history of left exophthalmos. There is a long history of sinusitis and frontal headaches. Mental retardation of unknown duration. The roentgenogram shows a very large oval bone dehiscence and expansion of all borders of the left frontal sinus with invasion of the left orbit. There is posterior expansion of 7 cm. into the frontal lobe with a piece of displaced frontal bone at the posterior extension of the mucocele.

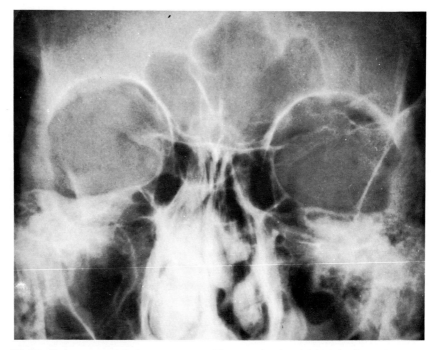

Fig. 26-10. Right retro-orbital meningioma. The patient (A. S.) has had gradual onset of exophthalmos for 6 months. The roentgenogram shows extensive osteolysis of the greater and lesser wings of the right sphenoid and the lateral orbital margin.

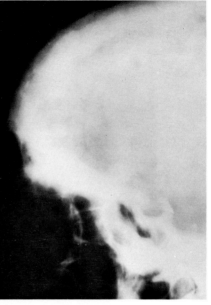

B

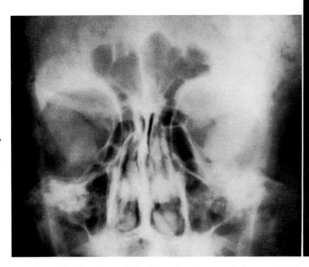

A

Fig. 26-11. A and **B,** Paget's disease (phase 2). The patient (I. D.), a 64-year-old male, has left exophthalmos associated with Paget's disease. The roentgenograms show hyperostosis of the greater and lesser wings of the left sphenoid, roof of left orbit, and cranial vault.

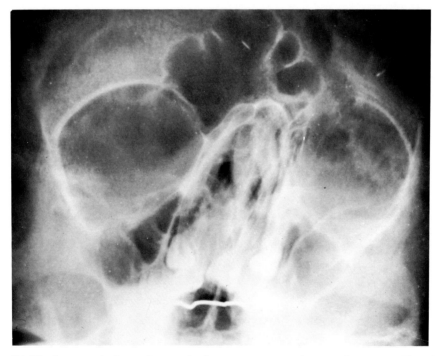

Fig. 26-12. Asymmetrical craniostenosis from premature closure of sutures. The child (K. H.) has had a deformed cranium and face, a small left orbit, and left exophthalmos since infancy. The roentgenogram shows asymmetry of the facial bones with a small left orbit, left maxilla, and zygoma. The anterior frontal portion of the cranial vault shows evidence of increased convolutional markings on the left side, with an asymmetrical cranial vault caused by unilateral craniostenosis.

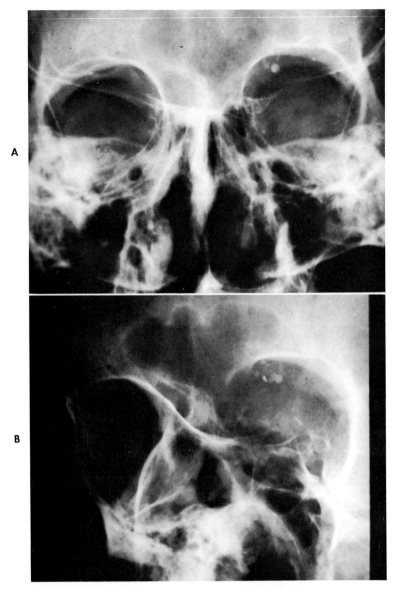

Fig. 26-13. A and **B,** Hemangioma of the left orbit. The patient (C. J.) has had left exophthalmos of 8 years' duration. The roentgenograms show multiple calcific phleboliths in the superior medial quadrant of the left orbit with expansion of the orbit.

the bony orbit may result from primary orbital disease of infectious, neoplastic, or cystic nature; from hyperparathyroidism and the reticuloendothelioses; by secondary extension of infectious or neoplastic disease from adjacent sinuses, brain, skin, bone, and nasopharynx; or by metastases from remote primary neoplasms; and from autoimmune diseases such as Wegener's granulomatosis (Fig. 26-10).

Hyperostosis of the bony orbit. Hyperostosis of the bony orbit may be secondary to Paget's disease, fibrous dysplasia, infantile cortical hyperostosis, mixed tumors of the

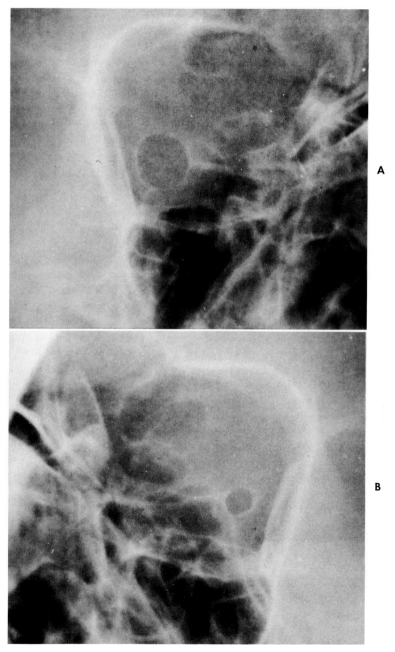

Fig. 26-14. A and **B,** Glioma of the right optic nerve. The patient (M. D.), 29 years old, has had progressive right exophthalmos with gradual loss of vision over a period of 2 years. The roentgenogram shows the right optic canal is expanded in all diameters. It measures 10 × 11 mm. The left optic canal measures 5 × 4.5 mm.

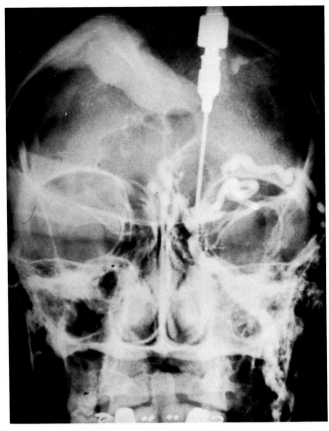

Fig. 26-15. Left arteriovenous aneurysm. The patient (A. C. M.), an adult male, was hit over the left eye 4 months previously. The blow caused unconsciousness. He subsequently developed left pulsating exophthalmos with conjunctival hyperemia. Left retrograde angular vein orbital phlebography illustrates the venous engorgement and vascular hypertrophy caused by an arteriovenous fistula. (Courtesy Dr. Daniel Silva, Mexico City.)

lacrimal gland, transitional cell carcinomas of the nasopharynx, prostatic malignancy, neuroblastoma, meningioma, osteoma, and osteopetrosis (Fig. 26-11).

Diminished orbital volume. Diminished orbital volume is concomitant with hyperostotic thickening of orbital walls caused by Paget's disease, osteoma, fibrous dysplasia, osteopetrosis, and infantile cortical hyperostosis. Diminished orbital volume may also be secondary to fracture, early enucleation of the eye, radiation injury of bone, craniostenosis, and osteogenesis imperfecta. It may be caused by lateral displacement of the medial orbital wall by hypertrophic polypoid disease of the accessory nasal sinuses, or by

other diseases of the nasal passages and sinuses such as fibrous dysplasia, rhinoscleroma, and dentigerous cysts. Hypoplasia of the maxilla associated with chronic maxillary sinusitis may result in a smaller orbit (Fig. 26-12).

Calcification. Calcification within orbital soft tissue may be associated with infections, neoplasms (either benign or malignant), retinoblastoma, mucocele, parasitic infestations, aneurysms, hematoma, and trauma. Smooth, round, or oval phleboliths are diagnostic of hemangioma, but are seen in only 20 to 25% of cases. Calcifications of more irregular configuration and texture have been seen with plexiform neurofibroma, tubercu-

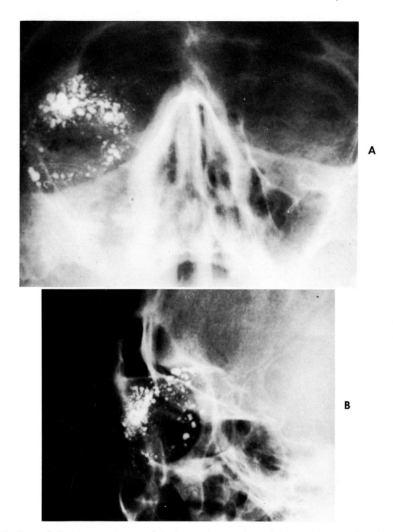

Fig. 26-16. A and **B,** Iatrogenic exophthalmos due to lipoidol granuloma of right orbit. The patient (A. B.) had a mucocele removed from the right frontal sinus 4 years previously. For an unknown reason lipoidol was injected into the right nasofrontal duct. The lipoidol entered the right orbit and caused granuloma formation, which subsequently caused prop-tosis. The roentgenogram shows dehiscence of the floor of the right frontal sinus. There is a typical smooth erosion of the floor of the right frontal sinus and roof of the right orbit caused by the mucocele. There are many droplets of oil in the right orbit.

losis, toxoplasmosis, cysticercosis, and orbital hematoma. Calcification of the lens, iris, retina, and choroid may result from inflammation and trauma (Fig. 26-13).

Expansion of the optic canal. Glioma, neurofibroma, and meningioma of the optic nerve, retinoblastoma, and sarcoma of the choroid may expand the optic canal. Erosion of the optic canal wall is seen with aneurysms of the ophthalmic and internal carotid ar-teries, arteriovenous aneurysms, pituitary adenoma, and carcinoma, mucocele and carcinoma of the sphenoid (Figs. 26-14 to 26-16).

Causes of unilateral exophthalmos

In 1962, Ira Jones, reporting on unilateral exophthalmos from the Eye Institute of the College of Physicians and Surgeons, Columbia University, listed their more recent experience with unilateral exophthalmos.[8] Thy-

Table 26-2. Analysis of causes of expanding lesions of the orbit (230 cases from the Eye Institute of the College of Physicians and Surgeons, Columbia University)

Cause	Percent
Thyroid	16
Hemangioma	12
Lymphoma	10
Granuloma	8
Lacrimal gland tumor	7
Meningioma	5
Lymphangioma	4
Glioma	3
Metastatic tumor	3
Peripheral nerve tumor	3
Dermoid cyst	3
Mucocele	3
Rhabdomyosarcoma	2
Aneurysm	2
Angiosarcoma	2
Osteoma	1
Eosinophilic granuloma	1
Sarcoid	1
Fibrous dysplasia	0.5
Liposarcoma	0.5
Encephalocele	0.5
Tuberculosis	0.5
Myxoma	0.5
Dacryadenitis	0.5

Table 26-3. Analysis of causes of unilateral exophthalmos (200 cases from the Manhattan Eye, Ear and Throat Hospital)

Cause	Percent
Mucocele	15
Orbital cellulitis and abscess	14
Extension of nasal sinus and nasopharyngeal malignancy	11
Thyroid	5
Acute orbital fractures	5
Hemangioma	5
Granuloma	4
Glioma	4
Neurofibroma	4
Fibrous dysplasia	4
Paget's disease	4
Lymphoma	4
Metastatic tumor	3
Reticuloendothelioses	3
Dermoid cyst	3
Osteoma	2
Retinoblastoma	2
Meningioma	2
Rhabdomyosarcoma	2
Aneurysm	1
Craniostenosis	0.5
Lipiodol granuloma	0.5
Dentigerous cyst	0.5
Tuberculosis	0.5
Neuroblastoma	0.5

roid disease, hemangioma, lymphoma, granuloma, and lacrimal gland tumor were the five leading causes of unilateral exophthalmos comprising 53% of their cases (Table 26-2).

The following is a listing of the common causes of exophthalmos by age groups.*

Infancy
  Infantile hemangioma
  Lymphangioma
  Neurofibroma
Childhood
  Glioma
  Sarcoma
  Blood dyscrasias
  Extension of sinus disease
Adulthood
  Thyroid disease
  Cavernous hemangioma
  Lymphoma
  Granuloma
  Lacrimal gland tumor
  Meningioma
  Extension of sinus disease

---

*Modified from Jones, I.: Unilateral exophthalmos, Highlights Ophthal. 5(1):3, 1962.

Although thyroid dysfunction is the commonest cause of unilateral exophthalmos in the general population, the frequency of different causes of unilateral exophthalmos in different hospitals will vary with the relative number of patients seen in the thyroid, ophthalmologic, otolaryngologic, neoplastic, neurosurgical and plastic services.

In the x-ray department at Manhattan Eye, Ear and Throat Hospital, our experience with unilateral exophthalmos is weighted by the very large active otolaryngologic service. Mucocele, orbital cellulitis from the extension of nasal sinus infection, and neoplastic invasion of the orbit are the three leading causes of unilateral exophthalmos, and account for 40% of the cases.

Summary

Routine radiological examination of the orbit will disclose positive signs of unilateral exophthalmos in 40 to 60% of the cases.

Orbitography with air or radiopaque solutions, and orbital angiography with the subtraction technique can add significantly to the percentage of patients with unilateral exophthalmos showing positive radiographic signs.

REFERENCES

1. Pfeiffer, R. L.: Roentgenography of exophthalmos, Amer. J. Ophthal. **26**:724, 1943.
2. Zizmor, J.: Recent trends in the roentgenographic diagnosis of orbital tumors, Trans. Amer. Acad. Ophthal. Otolaryn., vol. **70**:579, 1966.
3. Zizmor, J., Fasano, C. V., Smith, B., and Robbett, W.: Roentgenographic diagnosis of unilateral exophthalmos, J.A.M.A. **197**:343, 1966.
4. Dubilier, W., Jr., Von Gal, H., Fremond, A., and Evans, J. A.: Orbital pneumotomogrhaphy, Radiology **66**(3):387, 1956.
5. Lombardi, G.: Orbitography with water soluble contrast media, Acta Radiologica **47**:417, 1957.
6. Krayenbuhl, H.: Diagnostic value of orbital angiography, Brit. J. Ophthal. **42**:180, 1942.
7. Krayenbuhl, H.: The value of orbital angiography for diagnosis of unilateral exophthalmos, J. Neurosurg. **19**:289, 1962.
8. Hanafee, W., Rosen, L. M., Weidner, W., and Wilson, G. H.: Venography of the cavernous sinus, orbital veins, and basal venous plexus, Radiology **84**(4):751, 1965.
9. Ziedses des Plantes, B. G.: Subtraktion, vol. 7, Stuttgart, 1961, G. Thieme, Verlag.
10. Jones, I.: Unilateral exophthalmos, Highlights Ophthal. **5**(1):3, 1962.
11. Duke-Elder, S.: Textbook of ophthalmology, vol. 5, St. Louis, 1952, The C. V. Mosby Co.
12. Reese, A. B.: Tumors of the eye, New York, 1951, Paul B. Hoeber, Inc.

Chapter 27

Phaco-emulsification

Charles D. Kelman

Who would have dreamed 100 years ago that an ophthalmologist in New York could examine the fundus of a patient in Paris without moving from his office? Yet with trans-Atlantic television this is so easily possible that we do not even marvel at its feasibility. It is hard to imagine papers being delivered on accommodative spectacles, electromagnetic visual occipital stimulation, cataract retransparentization, cataract dissolving, transplantation of monkey eyes to human beings, or accommodative pseudophakia. From my own long list of medical incredibles, 4 years ago I chose the problem of dissolving cataracts. In light of what might be on the program in 100 years, dissolving cataracts becomes hardly incredible at all.

Chemical methods of dissolving the opaque lens are still under investigation, but the results are hardly promising. So far, any chemical capable of dissolving a lens also damages the cornea and other structures irreparably.

Physical methods include lasers, electron beams, ultrasonic waves, and mechanical devices. Time does not allow elaboration of the failures I encountered in the early part of this investigation with physical methods. Most could not be made selective enough to affect only the lens. Most mechanical devices to fragment or emulsify the lens were traumatic and extremely dangerous. One approach, supported by the Hartford Foundation, seemed promising and this was followed and developed.

I am referring to the use of an ultrasonic transducer to physically disrupt the cataract structure and to emulsify, fragment, dissolve, and withdraw the material through a needle. This method eliminates the 180 degree incision, and hopefully someday only a needle

puncture will be necessary. The incision has already been reduced to 2 mm., and it will soon be even smaller. The possibility for immediate mobilization and return to normal duties after a cataract extraction as an outpatient is an appealing one, and is not an impossibility. The importance of such a technique in the United States and in underprivileged nations is obvious.

Technique

A small incision is made at the limbus after a 2 mm. flap has been fashioned. The anterior capsule is removed with a dull cystotome and cut with de Wecker scissors without exerting undue traction on the zonules adjacent to the incision. After a good portion of the nucleus is removed, the lens is prolapsed out of the capsule, and the softer portions of the lens are emulsified and aspirated, using either a straight tipped needle, or, toward the end of the procedure, a spoon-shaped tip. The spoon-tipped needle affords maximum protection to the posterior capsule toward the end of the procedure when there is little material to hold the posterior capsule back away from the tip. After the visible lens fragments are removed, there will be small particles of lens material in the capsular fornices. No attempt should be made to remove this material at this time, except perhaps for a very gentle irrigation which may bring the remaining lens material anterior to the iris.

A few drops of alpha-chymotrypsin are introduced posterior to the iris and irrigated from the eye after 2 minutes. It is important to refill the anterior chamber gently with air after introducing the alpha-chymotrypsin to return the posterior capsule-zonular diaphragm to its physiologic backward-bowed position. This position allows the enzyme access to the zonules.

A specially designed forceps is then passed into the eye to grasp one lip of the anterior capsule at the four o'clock position. This is drawn toward the wound until the zonules at the six o'clock position are ruptured. The anterior capsule is grasped at the eight o'clock position, then withdrawn from the eye. No attempt should be made to grasp the posterior capsule directly, as it is not possible to do so without also grasping the vitreous face.

There may be some soft cortical material subjacent to the wound. The emulsifier can again be introduced into the eye, but it should be used only as an irrigating–aspirating device. The ultrasonic action should not be employed. The remaining soft material can be simply aspirated with the two-way irrigation system. The spoon-tipped needle should be employed for this purpose. Leaving a small piece of cortical material after the capsule has been removed is far better than rupturing the vitreous face, as the cortical material will be absorbed in a few days. One absorbable suture is placed in the shelved incision, and the conjunctiva is closed with three absorbable sutures. The postoperative treatment of the eye is the same as for any cataract extraction, except that the patient is allowed unrestricted activity. A contact lens may be worn almost immediately, since corneal sensitivity is not decreased.

I routinely use 1% atropine on alternate days and Maxitrol daily. Acetazolamide (Diamox), 250 mg., is given twice a day for 3 days. The eye may be left unpatched following surgery, or a light dressing may be applied for 24 hours.

This operation was performed in one patient who had malignant melanoma and was scheduled for enucleation approximately a week after cataract surgery. Histologic examination of that eye showed no visible or demonstrable effects of the ultrasonic energy upon the iris, cornea, ciliary body, or any portion of the eye.

Complications

The complications that I have found in this technique include striate keratitis and vitreous rupture. Of the patients I have operated on, none have had their vision compromised by the use of this technique. In all cases the postoperative vision has been at least as good as would have been expected had conventional cataract surgical techniques been used.

The striate keratitis may be caused by stretch of the incision, excessive irrigation, or possibly rubbing of the round lens against the corneal endothelium. Improvements in instrumentation and technique are reducing these hazards. Vitreous loss was probably caused by the unwieldiness of the earlier models of the instrument, or to poor visualization, which permitted the instrument tip to be brought too close to the posterior lens capsule or led to the operator's grasping the vitreous directly with the forceps in removing the lens.

Summary

What the long term results of this operation will be cannot be foretold. There must be a very long follow-up period on these patients before this technique can be unquestionably recommended. It does seem to me that intracameral cataract surgery is a definite possibility and perhaps an important direction for cataract surgery to take. Whether the lens will be dissolved or emulsified by ultrasonic action, or whether some other technique will be developed, remains to be seen. I certainly think the possibility of removing a cataract through a needle puncture exists.

Discussion

Dr. Breinin: We'll have a few questions directed at Dr. Kelman at this time. One of the complications of phaco-emulsification has been severe striate keratitis. Has this complication been corrected or ameliorated?

Dr. Kelman: As the technique been improved and as I have become better at doing this, the incidence of striate keratitis has dropped enormously. In the first 6 or 7 cases, they all had it very badly. In the last 6 or 7 cases only one patient had striate keratitis.

Dr. Breinin: With the perfection of the Kelman phaco-emulsification procedure, do you feel there will be a return to a planned extracapsular technique with preservation of the posterior capsule and zonules in eyes predisposed to retinal detachment?

Dr. Kelman: I think that if we could be certain of removing all the cortex and nucleus, leaving only the posterior capsule, most surgeons would consider this to be the ideal method of cataract extraction. I think that as I progress with this technique, I will be doing more and more planned extracapsular extractions leaving the posterior capsule. The reason that I removed the posterior capsule in the early cases was that I did not want to be confused between any reaction to the lens material remaining and a possible reaction to the ultrasonic energy. As soon as I am convinced, and I think I am now, that the energy is safe and that there is no deleterious effect on the eye, I will start leaving in more and more posterior capsules.

Chapter 28

Packaged donor grafts for keratoplasty*

Miguel Martinez and
David Paton

There are important conveniences and significant technical advantages in having laboratory-prepared donor grafts available in the operating room. Moreover, one variety of experimental graft to be discussed requires advance preparation in the laboratory.

For routine cases of penetrating keratoplasty there is no likelihood that preserved graft tissue will become preferable to fresh donor material. However, fresh tissue is not always obtainable when and where it is needed; present evidence supports the view that deep-frozen corneal tissue will eventually become an acceptable substitute for fresh tissue.[1]

Certain eyes with marked corneal vascularization or otherwise severely altered physiology have a poor chance of maintaining a clear graft if fresh tissue is used. Such eyes account for a sizable portion of the estimated five million persons in the world with corneal blindness. There is now reasonable hope that keratoplasty can successfully restore vision to many of these eyes if an inorganic membrane is substituted for the endothelial cells of the graft.[2] The artificial posterior membrane and the nonviable graft to which it is attached effectively eliminate the homograft reaction as a mechanism of graft failure. Edema of the grafted tissue can be limited by controlling the artificial membrane's permeability, while the proper passage of fluids and gases through the membrane reduces the risk of malnutrition of the graft, which occurs more readily with an impermeable membrane. For severely damaged corneas, therefore, laboratory-prepared nonviable grafts with a semipermeable inorganic membrane that replaces the endothelium may afford the best chance of attaining a good visual result.

Furthermore, lamellar keratoplasty does not require the use of a viable graft, and the successful use of glycerine-preserved corneal material is well known.[3] Surgical technique can be greatly improved by the use of precut lamellar grafts that have uniform thickness and sharply sectioned margins.

In view of the above considerations, donor grafts of the following types are now being prepared and packaged in our laboratory for subsequent clinical trial: (1) Deep-frozen, viable grafts for full-thickness keratoplasty for use when fresh donor eyes are unavailable; (2) nonviable preserved grafts with a semipermeable silicone membrane substituted for the endothelial layer to be used for full-thickness keratoplasty in cases with marked corneal vascularization; and (3) nonviable lamellar grafts of various sizes

*This work is supported by a grant from The John A. Hartford Foundation, Inc. Mr. R. J. Bailey, our engineering consultant, has designed and built the electrical freezing apparatus reported in this paper. Dr. Keith Green has performed the membrane permeability studies to determine, in vitro, the optimal thickness of the various silicone membranes being tested.

We also gratefully acknowledge the counsel of Dr. Karl Meyer; the assistance of Dr. William Casey and Dr. Martin Choy in overseas clinical pilot studies; and the maximum cooperation of Mr. Frederick Griffith in supplying donor tissue from the Medical Eye Bank of Maryland.

and thicknesses for the varied uses of split-thickness keratoplasty. After preparation under contamination-free conditions, each type of graft is packaged and stored for future use. In some instances, preliminary sutures are placed in the graft tissue to further facilitate the work of the surgeon.

Methods

The equipment requisite to preparation of the three types of donor grafts is housed in a series of interconnected, transparent, contamination-free chambers, as shown in Fig. 28-1. The legend of Fig. 28-1 describes the location of the housed instrumentation, not all of which is used for any one particular type of graft to be packaged. Filtered air is pumped into the last of these incubator-type chambers and exits through vents in the first chamber. Although wires, tubes, and even portions of the housed equipment pass through the walls of the chambers, these exit points are hermetically sealed. The technician has no difficulty in transferring the corneal material from one chamber to the next, using long rubber gloves mounted in the diaphragmatic orifices of each separate work station.

Fresh donor eyes are delivered by eye bank personnel to the laboratory's refrigerator and are processed expeditiously if the material is to be used for deep-frozen corneal grafts. For other graft types, several days may have elapsed since the death of the donor before the refrigerated tissue is prepared for packaging.

Nonviable grafts for lamellar keratoplasty

The results of refractive keratoplasty or keratomileusis have demonstrated conclusive-

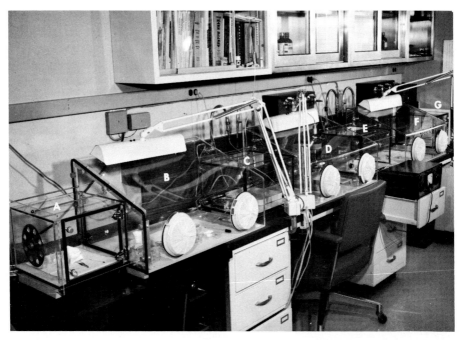

Fig. 28-1. The contamination-free, interconnected, transparent housing in which all three types of precut and preserved corneal grafts are prepared. **A,** initial receiving compartment; **B,** location for placing corneas on molds and for sectioning lamellar grafts (equipment not shown, see Fig. 28-2); **C,** dehydration chamber; **D,** compartment for donor button-cutting instrument (see Fig. 28-4); **E,** rehydration chamber; **F,** location for packaging all types of preserved grafts; and **G,** filtered air source.

ly that interface opacification between donor and recipient tissue is minimized when machine operated keratomes are used to cut the donor and recipient tissues. This is contrary to the opinion of some ophthalmologists that manual separation of the corneal lamellae with relatively blunt instruments is a better way to find the proper plane of cleavage. A machine cut graft is far superior to one cut from the donor eye by hand. For example, glycerine-preserved corneas are now generally stored with a scleral rim, and after rehydration they are mounted in a clamp, and the graft is cut from soft tissue, which is far more difficult to section than fresh tissue.[4] Previous less satisfactory grafts from glycerine-preserved corneas may prove to have resulted from the poor technical preparation of the tissue in the operating room, rather than from any inferior quality of the nonviable tissue as compared to fresh material.

Procedure. The corneal epithelium is removed from the donor eye by rubbing with a gauze sponge. With a hand-held sharp trephine a full-thickness corneal button is cut from the donor eye. Graft diameters of 9 mm. and 11 mm. are standard sizes. This tissue is then mounted with the anterior surface flattened downward onto a thermoelectric module and is frozen in this flattened position in a small pool of sterile saline. The thermoelectric module serves as the stage for a Leitz microtome (Fig. 28-2), and the blade then cuts away one-fifth to one-third of the exposed posterior portion of the graft button, depending upon the desired thickness for the standard graft button preparations. By sectioning the flattened cornea from its posterior aspect (rather than cutting a lamellar graft from the anterior surface of the donor cornea) uniform thickness of the graft tissue is obtained.

The lamellar graft is then thawed and

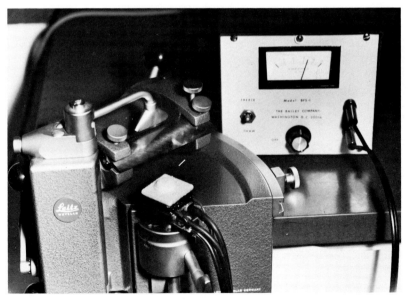

Fig. 28-2. A microtome with thermoelectric module as its stage, upon which is mounted a flattened and frozen corneal button which is ready for lamellar sectioning. The power supply is shown in the background, and the rubber tubes for the module's cooling system are in the foreground. The microtome will be altered to be contained in compartment B of Fig. 28-1.

transferred to glycerine solutions. After routine dehydration, the precision cut button is transferred to a sterile polyethylene-coated Mylar package, which is sealed by heat and placed within a second plastic package that can be stored indefinitely. In the operating room the donor button is rehydrated in balanced physiologic solution containing an antibiotic, and it is ready for use in a matter of minutes.

Deep-frozen (viable) grafts for penetrating keratoplasty

To date, our work with this form of prepared graft is limited to the development of instrumentation for facilitating, and adding accuracy to, existing methods of freezing corneal tissue. Thus, proceeding from the freezing technique reported by others,[5, 6] at present our only modifications are: (1) the use of a precut graft button (not the entire donor cornea) which is frozen and packaged, and (2) the technique of freezing by the use of automatic self-monitored electrical equipment.

Procedure. The fresh donor eye is placed in an open methacrylate container secured within the framework of an ordinary light microscope so that the donor eye can be raised or lowered using the microscope knob designed for adjusting the condenser. At the level of the microscope stage is a horizontal firm plastic strip with a round central opening through which the cornea of the donor eye is introduced upward by elevating the eye in its container. The intraocular pressure in the donor eye can be accurately adjusted to normal by the amount of pressure forcing the sclera of the eye against the plastic strip. The intraocular pressure can be monitored by a pressure transducer system from the eye itself, but we have not found this necessary. The corneal graft button is cut by a rotating motor powered cutting blade mounted in the portion of the microscope originally designed to hold the lens system. The rotating blade is powered by a Kerr dental drill regulated by a foot switch. Graft

diameters of 7 mm. and 8 mm. are routine sizes. The purpose of this automatic trephine-like arrangement is to obtain a precise, sharply cut donor button without the use of corneal scissors and without causing damage to the endothelial cells. The button is cut so rapidly that the anterior chamber does not collapse; the button is then removed by an erysiphake attached to suction, so that the donor tissue is never handled. No forceps are used to grasp the tissue, and nothing but fluid touches the endothelium during the preparations for freezing.

The donor button is then placed (epithelial surface down) in a small plastic saucer, and solutions of sucrose and dimethyl sulfoxide are employed as per methods reported elsewhere.[6] When the button is in the final solution the saucer and button are placed on the thermoelectric freezer, and a microthermistor needle is introduced into the stroma from the graft margin.

The details of the thermoelectric freezer have been described elsewhere.[7] Briefly, our instrumentation for deep-freezing viable cornea is composed of three main components:

1. The thermoelectric freezer has *two* separate modules (one on top of the other, to augment the effect of a single module) and an exhaust fan. Both features are designed to obtain maximal cooling (Fig. 28-3, *A*).

2. The temperature controller consists of a power supply regulating the freezer's temperature according to the required amount of coldness at any specific period of time. The controller changes the tissue specimen temperature in exact proportion to the changes of a simple electrical resistance; the temperature of the specimen is monitored by the thermistor within the corneal button itself, so that the temperature controller adjusts itself (with accuracy within 1° C.), to the desired temperature (from the actual temperature within the tissue as determined by the controller's own feed-back mechanism).

3. There is a program unit to cool the corneal specimen at a desired rate, and this

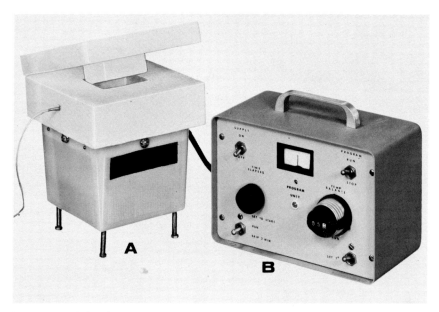

Fig. 28-3. Two of the three electrical components of the system for deep-freezing viable corneal tissue are shown. (The power supply, similar to the one in Fig. 28-2, is not shown; it will eventually be combined in the same container as the program unit.) The freezer **(A)** has an insulated top portion containing cascade-arranged thermoelectric modules upon which the corneal buttons are frozen. The program unit **(B)** has a clockwork mechanism for varying the power supply of the temperature controller according to an optimal freezing curve to maintain viability of the corneal cells.

unit regulates the temperature controller. The program unit (Fig. 28-3, *B*) supplies the variation in the electrical resistance of the controller, thereby freezing the corneal button according to the optimal freezing curve for maintenance of tissue viability. The program unit is an electromechanical device which is preset, so a time/temperature program can be repeated as often as necessary. Whenever required, a quite different program can be set up in a few minutes. Thus, the instrument is very useful for laboratory investigation of the optimal techniques of tissue freezing. The program unit contains 20 electrical resistances, each adjustable and each selected consecutively by a clock mechanism at whatever specific time interval is desired. The instrument produces a change in temperature for each selected interval of time. The total duration of programmed operation is now 40 minutes; the

entire three-part freezing apparatus is operated by turning on a single switch.

Once it is frozen to approximately –50° C., the corneal button and surrounding frozen media are packaged in Mylar polyethylene envelopes and are transferred to a storage tank of liquid nitrogen. In the sterile sealed plastic envelopes the corneal button and its surrounding iceball of preservative can remain in the storage tank until needed for surgery.

Preserved, composite grafts

What we call a composite graft consists of nonviable full-thickness cornea (except that epithelium and endothelium have been removed) integrated with a thin silicone membrane which replaces the endothelium and serves as a semipermeable barrier for fluids entering from the anterior chamber. In vitro and animal experiments indicate that the optimal thickness of this membrane is approximately 10 μ, which is considerably thinner than the impermeable silicone membranes *sutured* to the posterior surface of the cornea by the originators of this concept.[2] The technique of securing a silicone membrane by *bonding* it to a dried cornea has been reported previously.[8]

Procedure. The epithelium of the donor eye is removed by rubbing it off with a gauze sponge, and the cornea is removed from the eye with an 11 mm. trephine. Descemet's membrane is denuded of endothelium by rubbing the posterior surface of the cornea with gauze. The cornea is then placed over

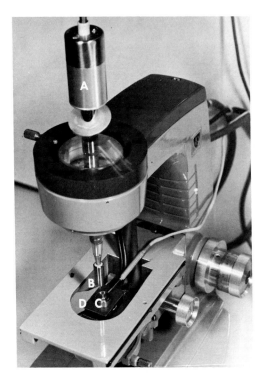

Fig. 28-4. An adapted microscope framework has a mounted electric motor, **A,** and a rotating chip of razor blade for cutting the corneal composite graft buttons, **B** (see text), from a full-sized cornea. A cornea will be mounted on the grooved mold, **C,** which is secured to a thermo-electric module, **D,** located centrally within the microscope stage. The power supply is not shown.

a methyl methacrylate mold with the same curvature as the posterior curvature of the average cornea. The donor cornea is allowed to dry on the mold in a moisture-free and contamination-free environment for several days. Wrinkles that appear in the dried tissue are confined to the stroma; Descemet's membrane remains completely smooth. The cornea acquires the texture of cartilage and becomes slightly discolored. The liquid silicone elastomer is applied to the posterior surface of the cornea as a single drop, which is then spread over Descemet's membrane. The cornea is placed in a clamp that is adjusted to a known distance above the original mold, thus producing the precise thickness of the bonded silicone membrane considered desirable.

After the silicone membrane has been allowed to cure for several days, the cornea is placed in a balanced physiologic solution and rehydrated. The silicone membrane remains permanently bonded to Descemet's membrane. Once rehydrated, the cornea is placed on a grooved mold attached to the surface of a thermoelectric module. In this manner the rehydrated cornea with its silicone membrane is rapidly frozen (not by any programmed system in this circumstance) for the purpose of secure fixation and facility of cutting a 6 mm. central donor button by means of the automatic trephine device described earlier for cutting viable grafts (Fig. 28-4).

The composite donor button is then thawed, and at this stage, initial preplaced sutures can be introduced, using a micromanipulator for accuracy. The button is then dehydrated (with or without the attached sutures) in a glycerine solution within a small Mylar polyethylene container, and this envelope is heat sealed. The envelope is then placed within a larger heat sealed envelope, along with a 2 ml. vial of physiologic rehydrating fluid and a disposable No. 25 needle; the air in the larger envelope is replaced with nitrogen. In this form the pre-cut, presutured, preserved composite graft can be

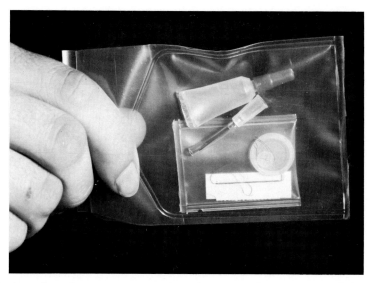

Fig. 28-5. A packaged, precut, preserved, and presutured composite graft button (inner envelope), with disposable needle for injecting reconstituting fluid (from vial) into the inner envelope—all contained for sterility purposes within an outer Mylar polyethylene envelope.

stored indefinitely until ready for use (Fig. 28-5).

Since the graft tissue consists of a nonviable tissue matrix, the substitution of animal tissue for this human tissue is a variation which we are now in the process of exploring. Pig corneas with a silicone membrane replacing the endothelium have been placed within a lamellar pocket in cats' eyes, and the grafts have remained entirely clear. The implications of successful heterografting with nonviable composite grafts and the great assistance this would provide for worldwide corneal surgery, justifies further experiments along this line.

Summary

It is our opinion that ready-to-use donor material will offer technical advantages in the operating room that cannot be equaled with fresh tissue, that such methods will be time-saving for the surgeon, and that they will afford opportunities to improve upon techniques presently used for combining an artificial endothelial membrane with graft tissue for use in cases unsuitable for penetrating grafts with fresh donor material.

REFERENCES

1. Kaufman, H. E., Escapini, H., Capella, J. A., Robbins, J. E., and Kaplan, M.: Living preserved corneal tissue for penetrating keratoplasty; clinical trial, Arch. Ophthal. **76:**471, 1966.
2. Dohlman, C. H., Brown, S. I., and Martola, E. L.: Artificial corneal endothelium, Arch. Ophthal. **75:**453, 1966.
3. King, J. H., Jr.: Current methods of corneal preservation, Surv. Ophthal. **5:**253, 1960.
4. King, J. H., Jr., Chavan, S. B., and Furness, C. W.: An instrument for lamellar keratoplasty, Trans. Amer. Acad. Ophthal. **62:**132, 1958.
5. Mueller, F. O.: Techniques for full-thickness keratopasty in rabbits using fresh and frozen corneal tissue, Brit. J. Ophthal. **48:**377, 1964.
6. Capella, J. A., Kaufman, H. E., and Robbins, J. E.: Preservation of viable corneal tissue, Arch. Ophthal. **74:**669, 1965.
7. Martinez, M., Paton, D., and Bailey, R. J.: Cryoinstrumentation for laboratory-prepared, pre-cut corneal grafts, J. Cryosurg. In Press. 1969.
8. Martinez, M.: Bonded synthetic membrane for corneal grafts, Arch. Ophthal. **79:**357, 1968.

Chapter 29

General anesthesia for intraocular surgery*

Gerald L. Wolf, Cyril Sanger,
Irving Berlin, and Seamus Lynch

Freedom from pain and immobility of the globe are absolute requirements for ophthalmic surgery. These requirements can be achieved by local anesthetic blockade of the pain and motor nerve fibers that innervate the orbital contents and motor blockade of the muscles rimming the orbit. Local anesthesia is not without hazard, however. Among these hazards can be included cardiorespiratory depression from premedicant drugs, reactions to local anesthetic drugs (both relative overdose and allergic reactions), and vomiting with resultant aspiration in an elderly, sedated patient. Some hazards particularly related to local blockade for ophthalmic surgery are incomplete muscle blockade, which permits compression of the globe during intraocular manipulation; retrobulbar hemmorrhage; penetration of the optic nerve meninges with resultant optic nerve trauma; intraocular injection of the anesthetic in the presence of posterior staphyloma; and psychologic trauma to the patient, which may result in acute anxiety reactions intraoperatively or more delayed sequelae.[1]

In an attempt to achieve the requirements of freedom from pain and immobility of the globe, but avoid the aforementioned hazards, a specialized technique of general anesthesia for ophthalmic surgery was developed at the Manhattan Eye, Ear and Throat Hospital in 1960. Since that time it has been utilized with little modification on approximately 7,000 intraocular procedures.

General anesthesia enables the surgeon to work in a relaxed, unhurried fashion. He can be confident that his patient will not move, cough, or sit up during a delicate procedure. He is assured that the globe will not move and the lids will not squeeze. He is also relieved of the total care of the patient, and can focus his entire attention on the operative procedure, knowing that the patient is being well attended by another physician. If a problem should develop, he would then be immediately informed. If a surgical complication develops, he has adequate time available to plan and execute a proper corrective procedure. He feels no urgency other than that related to the particular operative problem at hand.

The psychologic trauma to the awake patient with an open eye, preoperatively, intraoperatively, and postoperatively is indeed profound. When informed of the advisability of general anesthesia for his intraocular surgery, the patient usually accepts with enthusiasm. If a second procedure is necessary, it is not approached with dread.

Modern anesthesia must not be confused with the anesthetic techniques of years ago, just as modern ophthalmic surgical techniques are not to be confused with surgery of years ago. Three important features of present-day anesthesia of specific interest to ophthalmologists are related to induction, maintenance, and emergence. Rapid induction, free of the excitment stage, can be achieved with short-acting intravenous agents

---

*The facilities of the Computing Center of the Downstate Medical Center, Brooklyn, New York (NIH grant No. FR0029) were used.

This work was aided by a Medical Research Grant from Ayerst Laboratories.

that establish surgical levels of anesthesia within minutes. Maintenance of anesthesia with modern inhalation agents is associated with a distinct lowering of intraocular tension. Emergence is virtually free of nausea and vomiting. In the event that nausea and vomiting do occur, there is now available an entire armamentarium of effective antiemetic agents. The low incidence of this complication, coupled with its effective treatment, is validly superimposed on a background of modern surgical technique involving multiple sutures, closely placed, resulting in an effective wound closure that can readily withstand most indirect trauma.

At Manhattan Eye, Ear and Throat Hospital, patients scheduled for surgery under general anesthesia are visited by an anesthesiologist the day prior to their operative procedure. They are interviewed, and examined, and premedication orders are written. These usually consist of secobarbital, a small dose of meperidine (Demerol), atropine, and an antiemetic drug such as trimethobenzamide hydrochloride (Tigan). This results in an awake, but calm, patient. Ocular hypotensive agents, ordered by the ophthalmologist, are administered either before the patient is taken to the operating room or in the operating room. In the majority of cases, the hypotensive used is either mannitol or acetazolamide (Diamox). Oral glycerine is to be avoided prior to general anesthesia, since its effect is that of loading the gastrointestinal tract with fluid, resulting in the danger of regurgitation and aspiration during anesthesia.

Induction of anesthesia is achieved with a short-acting barbiturate. Thiopental sodium (Pentothal) in a dilute 0.4% concentration is administered by intravenous infusion. Once sleep has been produced, 100% oxygen is delivered to the patient via a semiclosed carbon dioxide absorption system prior to insertion of an endotracheal tube. Intubation is utilized in order to assure total accessibility to the globe by the ophthalmologist, and, at the same time, guarantee airway patency of the patient. Total muscular relaxation, necessary to perform endotracheal intubation, is accomplished by intravenous administration of the short-acting muscle relaxant, succinylcholine chloride (Anectine). A topical anesthetic is instilled into the trachea prior to inserting the endotracheal tube, in order to diminish stimulation caused by its presence. The equipment we have chosen has been with particular reference to avoidance of bulk in the vicinity of the operative field. Our preference is for a relatively short, rubber, cuffed Magill endotracheal tube with a snug-fitting curved adapter that lies flush against the lower lip. Alternatively, a longer, non-kinking endotracheal tube, either a Sanders or wire spiral anode tube, can be used. When such a tube is used, it curves around the lower lip and lies flush against the chin. The tube adapter is connected to a lightweight metal Y adapter, then to two 4-foot long corrugated rubber tubes that lead to the anesthesia machine. The necessary one-way valves are positioned at the machine end of the corrugated rubber tubes to avoid bulk of anesthesia equipment adjacent to the operative field and to allow for ready inspection of proper function of the valves by the anesthesiologist.

After endotracheal intubation, spontaneous respiration is allowed to return, and deep general anesthesia is maintained by inhalation of approximately 2% halothane in carrier gas of at least 50% oxygen, the rest nitrous oxide. The operating table is placed in a slightly head-up position to reduce the intraocular tension even further than the expected lowering caused by general anesthesia.

After the completion of surgery, extubation of the trachea is performed while the patient is still deeply anesthetized with halothane, so that reaction to the tube during emergence from anesthesia is avoided. The patient is then taken to the recovery room and returned to his room, when awake, after approximately one hour.

Succinylcholine, the depolarizing muscle

relaxant used to facilitate endotracheal intubation in over 95% of our cases, is of special interest to the ophthalmologist. Structurally similar to acetylcholine, succinylcholine causes prolonged depolarization of the myoneural junction, thereby producing muscle relaxation. The usual dose for intubation is approximately 1 mg. per kilogram of body weight. The duration of the muscle relaxing effect is 5 minutes, since the circulating drug is rapidly metabolized by pseudocholinesterase found in normal serum. If pseudocholinesterase activity is less than normal, however, breakdown of succinylcholine is dependent upon alkaline hydrolysis, a slow process. Pseudocholinesterase activity can be depressed by disease, such as malnutrition or liver disease; by congenital deficiency; and by drugs. Phospholine iodide, an organophosphorus irreversible anticholinesterase used topically in the eye to inhibit ocular cholinesterase, is sufficiently absorbed and sufficiently potent to inhibit serum pseudocholinesterase. Serum pseudocholinesterase activity falls rapidly during the first 2 weeks of administration of phospholine iodide, and continues to fall more gradually thereafter. Levels of activity of less than 5% of normal have been reported. Following cessation of administration a period of approximately 4 weeks is required before normal pseudocholinesterase activity returns.[2]

Prolonged apneas of over 5 hours duration, rather than the usual 5 minutes, have been reported following general anesthesia incorporating succinylcholine to patients receiving phospholine iodide eyedrops.[3] Administration of succinylcholine to these patients, however, was by means of intermittent injection or intravenous infusion to produce relaxation of extended duration for intra-abdominal and genitourinary procedures.

Ideally, phospholine iodide should be withheld for at least 1 month prior to the administration of an anesthetic. If this is impractical, the anesthesiologist should certainly be made aware of the situation so that succinyl-

choline can be avoided entirely, or, if required, its dosage can be reduced.

Our policy is to administer one single half dose of succinylcholine to patients requiring its use who are on phospholine iodide. We have had no clinically significant apneas in our series. We have experimented with the commercially available laboratory tests for the determination of pseudocholinesterase activity, and now have available in our clinical laboratory routine determinations of pseudocholinesterase activity on patients requiring general anesthesia who are on phospholine iodide eyedrops. We feel, however, that the danger of prolonged apnea following succinylcholine administration to patients on phospholine iodide is slight in a specialty eye hospital where both ophthalmologists and anesthesiologists are well aware of its dangers. The greater danger exists for the patient on phospholine iodide who requires a general surgical procedure in which administration of succinylcholine may be necessary for the duration of the operative procedure by continuous intravenous infusion, and for whom the history may not be sufficiently detailed to reveal the use of phospholine iodide, as may certainly occur in an emergency procedure. We, therefore, feel it is wise that patients on phospholine therapy be made aware of this problem and that they carry a medical identification card stating that they are on continuous phospholine therapy.

Our experience at the Manhattan Eye, Ear and Throat Hospital with cataract extraction has been quite extensive. Table 29-1 lists the number of procedures performed per calendar year. These figures include both ward and private cataract patients, and the use of both local and general anesthesia. The total number of extractions to the present time is a little under 13,000. Of these 13,000, approximately 60% of the cataract extractions were performed under local anesthesia and approximately 40% under general anesthesia. This figure has not been a constant one through the years, however. In 1960 only 5% of the procedures were under

Table 29-1. Number of cataract extractions performed from 1960-1967 at the Manhattan Eye, Ear and Throat Hospital

Year	Number of extractions
1960	1,255
1961	1,262
1962	1,422
1963	1,476
1964	1,887
1965	1,769
1966	1,727
1967	1,818
Total	12,616

general anesthesia; 95% were under local anesthesia. During 1967 approximately 1,800 cataract extractions were performed. Of these, 20% were service cases and 80% were private. Of the 400 service cases 10% were performed under general anesthesia and 90% were performed under local anesthesia. Since many of our residents later practice in hospitals were general anesthesia for intraocular surgery is not readily available, the need for extensive training in local blockade is necessary. Of the private cases during 1967, 60% were performed under general anesthesia and 40% under local.

There have been no deaths directly attributed to general anesthesia in the 5,000 cataract extractions performed under general anesthesia since 1960; and there have been no deaths directly caused by general anesthesia in the 2,000 intraocular noncataract procedures performed during that time. There was one cardiac arrest successfully resuscitated that occurred in 1962. The patient was a diabetic woman who arrested after induction. She recovered fully after resuscitation with no sequelae. Anesthesia is implicated as a contributory cause of death in one patient. In this patient intubation was extremely difficult due to a previously undisclosed infantile larynx. Compromise of her airway developed early in the postoperative period and tracheostomy was deemed necessary. During the tracheostomy, performed

under local anesthesia, she became apneic and resuscitation was unsuccessful.

We are presently in the process of statistical analysis of our entire series in an attempt to evaluate the relative merits of general and local anesthesia for intraocular procedures. We have analyzed 200 of these procedures utilizing a random sampling technique suggested by our biostatistician. Certainly many more have yet to be analyzed to lend statistical significance to this study. An interim report, however, can be offered at this time.

The following data refer to the 200 cases randomly sampled from the group of cataract extractions performed under general anesthesia since 1960.

Twenty-two percent of the patients were 50 to 60 years of age, 37% were 60 to 70 years of age, 28% were 70 to 80, and 9% were over 80 years of age. Twenty-one percent of the patients gave a history of cardiac disease of varying severity. Four percent were blind in the unoperated eye. Sixteen percent of this series had both cataracts removed during a single hospital admission.

Of our sampled series, 59% received acetazolamide (Diamox) preoperatively, 7% received mannitol, and 7% received urea. None of the patients required catheterization of the bladder. Our policy is to catheterize the bladder only when retention occurs; we feel that routine catheterization is not indicated.

Only 1% of eyes in this series was reported to bulge. There was vitreous loss reported in 2%. There was no expulsive hemorrhage. Five to 7 interrupted sutures were used to close 70% of the corneoscleral incisions. There was no iris prolapse. There was no wound separation. Flat chamber was reported in 2% of cases.

Seventy percent of our patients remained in the recovery room from 60 to 120 minutes. Two percent of this series developed nausea and vomiting in the recovery room. After the patient left the recovery room, vomiting occurred in 15% of this series. However, approximately 3 years ago it was determined that the greatest incidence of vomiting occurred from 2 to 4 hours postoperatively, and coincided with the first postoperative dose of meperidine (Demerol). It was suggested that the first dose of meperidine be reduced, and that it be combined with an antiemetic tranquilizer, such as prochlorperazine (Compazine). Thereafter, the incidence of postoperative vomiting fell sharply. Our impression is that vomiting now occurs in less than 5% of the patients, but the exact figure must await further sampling and analysis.

The usual duration of hospitalization in this series is 8 days. However, the current stay averages 6 days for both local and general anesthesia.

• • •

General anesthesia for intraocular surgery is a technique requiring meticulous attention to detail and a thorough knowledge of ocular physiology. It varies considerably from the usual techniques of anesthesia for general surgery. It, therefore, should be undertaken by an anesthesiologist properly trained to handle the problems of intraocular surgery.

Our objective is to develop an anesthetic technique that will permit the greatest possible success for ophthalmic surgery, and at the same time be safest for the patient. We hope that this study contributes toward attaining this objective.

REFERENCES

1. Rosen, D. A.: Anaesthesia in ophthalmology, Canad. Anaesth. Soc. J. 9(6):545, 1962.
2. De Roetth, A., Jr., Dettbarn, W., Rosenberg, P., Wilensky, J., and Wong, A.: Effect of phospholine iodide on blood cholinesterase levels of normal and glaucoma subjects, Amer. J. Ophthal. 59:586, 1965.
3. Pantuck, E. J.: Ecothiopate iodide eye drops and prolonged response to suxamethonium, Brit. J. Anaesth. 38(5):406, 1966.

COMPLICATIONS IN OCULAR SURGERY

Presiding Chairman: **Arnold I. Turtz**

Chapter 30

Strabismus surgery

Moderator:
Harold W. Brown

Panelists:
Edward A. Dunlap
Philip Knapp
Marshall M. Parks

Dr. Brown: Dr. Dunlap, what are the causes of postoperative limitation of passive rotation, and what is the treatment for this complication?

Dr. Dunlap: The causes of postoperative restriction and movement are largely or almost invariably iatrogenic. There is a congenital variety with which we're not concerned, and there is the acquired variety. Restriction can arise from orbital fractures and detachment surgery. A very common cause is conjunctival contracture. It can occur from repeated surgical procedures on the same muscle or muscles. Probably the commonest cause is adhesions of one form or another.

The causes of adhesion are almost legion, and include rough handling of tissue, rough sponging, disregard for bleeding or failure of meticulous control in bleeding, or excessive cautery. In other words, slovenly surgery is probably the biggest cause of adhesions. Some occur from suture reaction, and others from postoperative infections.

Treatment of these acquired motility defects is difficult at best. Currently there are five available maneuvers. Transplants are in some disfavor, although they are reported to be 50% successful; they are probably somewhat neglected. The use of Gelfilm is widespread now for preventing adhesions after repeated operations. I don't think it must be used in the virginal case. The disadvantage of Gelfilm is its impermanence. Gordon Cole's conjunctival recession, or bare

sclera closure, is probably one of the most valuable maneuvers for the management of this form of squint.

Another maneuver is Callahan's lid–globe suture, in which the eye is anchored in place with a suture through the lid, which is left in place for approximately a week or two.

Last, along with Gelfilm, are the plastic implants, which, I think, are becoming increasingly popular because they have the advantage of easier maneuverability and permanence. The two available materials at this time are medical Silastic and Supramid Extra. I tend to favor the use of the latter.

Depending on the site of the restriction, the sheet implant can be placed over the muscle, under the muscle, or between the muscle and the adjacent muscle in an effort to prevent conjunctival adhesions. If only one muscle is involved, a Supramid tube can be slipped around the muscle. Usually a combination of these maneuvers must be used. The greatest chance of maximum benefit is from the use of a conjunctival recession, a piece of plastic implant, and the Callahan lid–globe suture.

One last point: By all means do forced duction throughout the surgery. Don't do it ahead of time and then forget to do it after you get into the actual surgery. Constantly test motility of the globe and make sure that it is freed or you're doomed to failure even before you close.

Dr. Parks: I don't think I have anything to add to Dr. Dunlap's complete lecture on this subject.

Dr. Knapp: Two minor points: There is a good reason for extending the conjunctival recession up to the limbus. In these cases there is usually thick, ugly tissue, and if a small area of conjunctiva is recessed, you end up with a white valley between two red hills, which is ugly. If it's a uniform white from the limbus all the way back, it looks much more presentable.

Second, it is very important to anchor these sheets of Supramid with No. 6-0 Merseline sutures. We used to use ordinary catgut to anchor them, but these inert substances tend to extrude unless they are buried under a muscle and anchored with something that's going to be permanent.

Dr. Brown: Thank you, Dr. Knapp. These inert substances sometimes cause cysts and granulomas. The next question has to do with cysts. Dr. Parks, an occasional complication of muscle surgery is the formation of subconjunctival cysts or granulomas in the vicinity of the insertion of the operated muscle. What is the natural course of these and how are they best managed? Should they be operated upon early or late?

Dr. Parks: The cysts are really just one of the many problems that can occur with the absorbable catgut sutures. I will review the entire subject very quickly. One of the principal difficulties with these sutures is immediate hypersensitivity to the animal product that is placed in the human being. It can be quite a virulent-looking affair, especially in repeat surgery. It doesn't have to be specifically eye surgery that is being repeated. Repeated exposure to catgut that was placed in the body for other procedures, such as a hernia, may result in very great reactions, which, in some cases, are present within 24 hours on the second or third exposure.

This immediate reaction has to be differentiated from infection. One of the best techniques to make that differentiation is to have a little piece of catgut buried in the skin of the arm. Therefore, routinely in all cases, I suture a quarter-inch piece of catgut into the surface of the forearm, and as the eye reaction develops, so does reaction in the arm. This procedure gives a very quick, precise diagnosis, the patient is treated for the catgut reaction, not for infection. It is best treated, I have found, with systemic steroids for approximately 5 days. Within 24 hours the reaction subsides. I haven't found topical steroids really adequate. If reaction returns after discontinuing steroids, it usually does so in a matter of 2 to 3 days. The systemic steroids can then be repeated for 5 days. The longest I've had to extend this therapy has been three sessions of 5-day therapy to control this reaction. I have made a point of this because it is one of the ways I think ultimate cyst formation can be prevented—by treating the suture reaction.

The majority of suture reactions are not of the order I've just discussed, but are more subtle and gradual. They may develop in a patient who has had no exposure to catgut, and they come on at a little later period. They may gradually begin to show up 3 to 6 weeks after surgery with chromic catgut, or a little sooner with plain catgut. This seems to be a reaction that develops as a patient develops antibodies to the foreign product on first exposure. Granuloma or eventual cyst formation can come about by two routes, the immediate or the delayed reaction.

Some of these patients will form a pustule (a sterile abscess), principally where the knot has been tied. That means it's related to the quantity of catgut material that is in a very small area. As this subconjunctival sterile abscess or pustule begins to dry up, it converts eventually into cyst formation. Others form a solid nodule, the granuloma, which simply persists and never forms a cyst.

Many years ago I used to think that this cyst was due to an overlapping of the conjunctiva where it was not approximated properly, and a little imbedded tissue formed a buried epithelial cyst. I now make the incision down in the fornix and I've never seen any of these cysts occur in the fornix where this incision has been made and repaired, even though we often simply let the tissue fall together without suturing. In these same cases in which there has been no incision made over the muscle site, I had cysts form where the knot was tied. I am convinced that the cyst we speak about is not due to conjunctival epithelium that has evolved into a cyst, but is a reaction to catgut.

The ideal thing is to try to prevent this. One of the things you can do to prevent a conspicuous cyst, if it is going to form, is to keep it as far away from the cornea as possible. This can be done by a technique that will allow the knot to be made as far away from the limbus as possible. Rather than bringing the suture up through the former insertion site toward the limbus, in a recession procedure, try to keep the knot back away from the limbus along the recessed site of the muscle. If cyst formation occurs, the result is more cosmetically acceptable.

Some of these cysts are large and some are tiny. We usually do not have to do anything for the tiny little blisters, but if they are large, we usually dissect the cyst and remove it. This is not an entirely easy problem. These cysts are usually firmly adherent to the muscle substance and the sclera. I have tried to dissect them out in toto and have been amazed at the extensiveness of this attachment to the tissues. This problem can be corrected as part of a second muscle procedure if the alignment is not satisfactory as a result of the first surgery. It is more difficult to come to a decision to operate on the cyst when the result, from a motility point of view, has been quite satisfactory. The cosmetic appearance then determines whether to proceed with this. Many times in children, the cyst is left intact until they have another anesthetic for perhaps a T and A procedure, and when the child is under anesthesia the cyst can be excised.

For the solid granuloma, when it forms, I usually prescribe topical steroids. This requires rather a long-range type of treatment. Systemic steroids are not effective. Most of these granulomas subside over the years and some disappear entirely.

Dr. Brown: Thank you, Dr. Parks. In removing the cysts, is there any technique you use to prevent recurrence? Do you ever externalize the cyst?

Dr. Parks: I dissect them out in toto, and I do not recall ever having one recur.

Dr. Brown: Dr. Dunlap, what is your treatment?

Dr. Dunlap: I procrastinate on these as long as I can. The superficial variety, which are purely subconjunctival, will often subside of their own accord over a period of time. If they do not, I usually treat by slitting them and laying them wide open. The deep ones are entirely different and much nastier. They usually have to be explored and dissected out as Dr. Parks has described. Occasionally, a large superficial one must be dissected out but most will heal just by slitting and laying them wide open.

Dr. Knapp: I also separate them into superficial and deep cysts. The superficial ones can be treated in the office in a fairly young child. All that is necessary is to marsupialize it with one cut of a scissors under local anesthesia. I have never had any trouble with those. The deep ones, however, can be a real headache, and must be dissected out.

Dr. Brown: Dr. Knapp, how should a surgeon attempt to reattach a muscle which has been lost in the orbit? What would be your approach to a traumatically severed muscle if upon exploration the proximal end could not be recovered or repair was not possible?

Dr. Knapp: When this happens, it is certainly a great temptation to utter an expletive and walk out of the operating room. But actually you've got to gird your loins, and don't go fishing. The first thing you need is good light. I used to use the Behren's illuminated Arruga retractor, but in recent years, Dr. Devoe has developed a modified ear, nose, and throat instrument that looks like a miner's helmet and gives an excellent light. Illumination is essential.

Then the surgeon must search carefully. If the muscle can't be found, all the tissue found should be brought up, including Tenon's capsule, and by reattaching it function may be restored because the muscle may be attached to this mass.

When a muscle is lost in the operating room, it can usually be found. You may be working quite far back in the orbit, but with care the muscle can often be found. I think you have to use your knowledge of anatomy. For instance, if an inferior oblique is cut on the temporal side, it is simple to repair, because it is known how closely adherent it is to the undersurface of the inferior rectus, at which point it can be found and reattached. The inferior oblique is simple, but the superior oblique is another problem. If the two ends of the superior oblique can be found and sewn together, everything is fine. But I think that most of us feel, as Dr. Berke has taught us, that if the superior oblique is cut inadvertently, the simplest thing to do is to cut the inferior oblique. This works beautifully!

The commonest muscle to slip off is the medial rectus, probably because it is the one operated upon most often. It depends on the technique of the surgeon how far back it retracts. In other words, if the muscle is completely freed, including the nasal check ligaments, and the muscle comes off, it goes way back into the apex of the orbit along the nasal wall. This was actually reported by Worth in the early 1900's. Even these can be found with that good light and careful searching.

The lateral rectus is usually not too hard to find, because most people don't free it up and it is usually attached to the bony orbital wall. If the inferior rectus slips, it is not difficult to find because, again, the inferior oblique helps you. But if the inferior rectus is cut inadvertently during an inferior oblique myotomy, then you are in real trouble.

In recent years we have used both No. 5-0 and No. 4-0 plain and chromic catgut, and occasionally the knots seem to untie on the muscles; we have had a regular epidemic of it. If this is discovered on the first or second day postoperatively, the suture will still be attached to the end of the muscle. The longer you wait the harder it is to iden-

tify and the more the muscle gets bound down with scar tissue and postoperative reaction.

I don't know the cause of this. These sutures have good tensile strength, and a nice spatula needle, but I think they are making them slick. Each time I've helped somebody pick up one of these I've been tying an extra knot. Now I'm tying five knots, which is probably unnecessary; in the old days we used only two and never had any trouble. Before the conjunctiva is closed, always look at the muscle. Twice I have actually watched these sutures untie.

Dr. Brown: Thank you, Dr. Knapp. There are men who tie two knots and they are known as two-knotters. There are three-knotters and four-knotters and for many years I have been known as a five-knotter. Dr. Knapp has now joined the five-knotter group! One trouble with the many-knotted catgut suture is that if the knots are buried, they may form cysts. For this reason I try to externalize all knots.

The next question for the panel is: what is the best approach in dealing with diplopia following strabismus surgery in an adult?

Dr. Dunlap: I would think that postoperative diplopia in an adult would be fairly uncommon because of presumed long-standing sensory adaptation. I can not recall any persistent diplopia in an adult that has given me a great deal of trouble. Of course, it is very common to get transient diplopia in an adult after a large horizontal squint correction. But I don't question them about this and if they bring it up I tend to minimize its existence and tell them that it will go away in a relatively short time, and almost invariably it does.

Dr. Brown: There is a possibility that we might be able to determine preoperatively the adult with an old strabismus who probably will have trouble with postoperative diplopia. Dr. Parks, I think I heard you talk about this in Philadelphia.

Dr. Parks: One of the things you should do is to try to anticipate whether this patient is going to have diplopia. We have to fall back on some very well-recognized, basic physiologic facts to come up with this information, which is very helpful from a clinical point of view.

What is the cause of this postoperative diplopia? There are two general causes I would think of. One is the patient who has abnormal retinal correspondence. He has an angle of deviation prior to surgery and he is adjusted to this angle. He has established fusion with the abnormal retinal correspondence system because abnormal retinal correspondence is single binocular vision in the presence of a deviation, which means, of course, refusion. This patient has solved his diplopia with this abnormal retinal correspondence system plus suppression.

When the angle is moved to a different position after surgery, whether it is straight or not, the object of regard is falling in his nonfixating eye outside the suppression scotoma; this patient has diplopia after surgery. you can anticipate this simply by putting prisms in front of his eye before surgery and he will tell you he has diplopia.

The important thing is to realize that this patient doesn't have diplopia without prisms in front of his eyes before surgery. He does have diplopia with prisms of adequate strength vertically or horizontally, since the image is moved out of the suppression scotoma. I think you should tell this patient he is going to have diplopia after surgery. You should also tell him that the diplopia is going to disappear. Secondly, he is going to know which is the correct image and which is the incorrect image. He is going to see the clear image, which is on the fovea of his fixating eye as the correct image, and he is going to know the dull image, which is off the fovea of his nonfixating eye, is the wrong image.

The next thing is to tell him to just overlook it and eventually it will disappear. The reason we know it will disappear is that the patient did develop abnormal retinal correspondence before—when he was younger

and had this deviation. He always retains this capacity to switch around and develop a different sensorial pattern that can adapt for any particular angle of deviation. Older patients take longer, maybe several weeks or a few months. Younger patients take just a day or two before adaptation occurs. But you have to tell the patient to be tolerant.

The other type of diplopia is the kind that is present prior to surgery in a patient who has acquired his deviation after the age (generally age 10) at which he can develop the sensorial adaptation known as abnormal retinal correspondence and suppression. This is an acquired case. This patient has diplopia before surgery and unless you can put him in a position to reestablish fusion with his normal retinal correspondence system, he is going to have diplopia after surgery. So it is just going to be a matter of transferring his diplopia from one region to another. I think you have to make this differentiation.

The patient who has diplopia before surgery has diplopia without putting prisms in front of his eyes. It is just there. You simply have to ask him whether he sees two lights or one. If he says he sees two lights you know this strabismus was acquired at a later date, and you can discuss the possibility of postoperative diplopia with reference to the kind of result you anticipate.

Dr. Brown: Thank you, Dr. Parks. Dr. Knapp, you are a persuasive doctor. How do you talk these people out of their diplopia? You cannot correct it, but you may be able to anticipate it. Do you prepare the patient ahead of time by telling them about it or do you wait until it occurs and work from there?

Dr. Knapp: I think that, as Dr. Taylor brought out, persistent postoperative diplopia always has a psychologic basis. The problems that I have seen occur after the well-meaning surgeon tells the adult that there is nothing to this operation. The patient wakes up and sees double, and is not prepared for it. I find less trouble if the patient has been warned preoperatively that he is going to see double. I tell all adults they are going to see double. Many of them come back and say, "Well, you're absolutely wrong, doctor. I never was bothered by diplopia at all."

The patients that give the surgeon more trouble are the ones that have had 2 or 3 years of ill-advised orthoptic training or visual training or whatever name they like to give to it. Some of them have been stripped of the normal defense mechanism that Dr. Parks described so well, and they can be a real problem because they have been made so binocularly aware. Quite a few years ago when I was working with Dr. Burian, he had me trying to figure out how fast suppression occured, and I got so I was seeing physiologic diplopia at all times. It took several months to learn to get rid of it and it is a real nuisance. It is surprising how bright that second image is.

I think the main thing is to warn patients ahead of time and tell them that they must only judge your surgery by the alignment and that the diplopia is up to them. There should be very little trouble.

Dr. Brown: Thank you, Dr. Knapp. A question from the audience: Years ago I used white linen sutures and can recall no inflammatory reaction. Do any of the panelists have any experience with them? Dr. Parks, you've experimented on sutures. Will you discuss this question?

Dr. Parks: Yes, we have studied just about every suture you can think of and have tried to figure out which would give the best results. Any of the nonabsorbable sutures are going to be visible and this is an objection. There might be a possibility with some of the real fine virgin silk sutures, but I have not had the opportunity of working with these. They might not be sufficiently visible to be detracting from a cosmetic point of view, but certainly the linen suture and related larger sutures were detracting to the point that they were not an ideal solution.

Dr. Brown: What is the panel's opinion regarding collagen sutures for strabismus?

Dr. Knapp: We ran a series of these cases in 1960-1961. Ethicon supplied us with the sutures and we compared reconstituted collagen with regular sutures. We finally came to the conclusion that the collagen sutures offered little advantage. There was statistically a little difference in the amount of hypersensitivity response, but it was not enough to make any clinical difference. We no longer use them.

Dr. Brown: What absorbable sutures do the panelists favor at the present time?

Dr. Parks: Well, we all seem to have our favorites, and mine is the No. 6-0 chromic catgut. I use it stained with a little dye. I like the needle known as the G-6 needle, which is commonly used for cataract work. I use chromic suture and I find that the knot stays nice and tight, whereas with the plain suture there is a tendency for untying.

Dr. Brown: Do you have more reaction with the chromic suture?

Dr. Parks: I don't think there is any difference in terms of reactions except for timing. The reaction occurs sooner with the plain sutures, and a little later with the chromic, simply because the liberation of the antigen is somewhat delayed by the chromic process.

Dr. Brown: Dr. Dunlap, what experience have you had with the nonabsorbable linen or silk suture?

Dr. Dunlap: I have had no experience with linen sutures. I do not like Dacron sutures because they pull through the tissue with a great deal of difficulty and suck tissue into the suture tract. I will use No. 6-0 Dacron to anchor down the Supramid plates, however. The only time I use silk is in a running silk conjunctival closure in an adult where it is easy to pull out.

We tried collagen suture a few years ago when it was on an experimental basis. We found absolutely no practical difference between the two. However, I think there is one point in favor of collagen suture. You can predict absorption time with the collagen suture with complete accuracy, whereas chromic gut sutures have a varying absorption rate. I saw a youngster recently on whom I'd done a squint operation 2½ years ago, and both the recession and re-section chromic suture knots were still there and visible under the conjunctiva. This distressed me a great deal. I think that perhaps collagen is preferable just on the basis of knowing that it is going to absorb in a specific period of time.

Dr. Brown: We have time for just one more question. Someone must have had an unfortunate experience in surgery to prompt this unusual question. Is muscle surgery in highly myopic children accompanied by a higher incidence of complication, including retinal detachment? Dr. Parks, will you comment on this question?

Dr. Parks: I have operated upon quite a few highly myopic children for strabismus, and, of course, many of them have been children with very poor vision in that eye and have simply had a recess-resect procedure. I guess the majority of these have had unilateral surgery with two muscles in one eye, and I have never had a retinal detachment occur as a result of the muscle surgery in any of these patients.

Dr. Knapp: I'm unaware of any retinal changes we've caused.

Dr. Dunlap: I've had no trouble that I can recognize as being specifically due to the myopia. I suppose if you operated upon a myope of minus 30, especially an adult, you might have to worry about the thin sclera and the suture holding, but otherwise I don't think you need anticipate any increased trouble.

Chapter 31

Glaucoma surgery

Moderator:
George Gorin

Panelists:
Maurice Luntz
H. Saul Sugar
Raymond Harrison

Dr. Gorin: What is the treatment for flat chamber after a filtering procedure? What type of surgical intervention is indicated if medical treatment fails and when should it be performed?

Dr. Harrison: This is a serious problem which occurs frequently. Flat anterior chamber may occur early in the postoperative period or many months or even years after surgery.

Late loss of the anterior chamber after a successful filtering procedure is usually caused by a dehiscence in the bleb wall resulting from injury, although it may also occur spontaneously. In my experience the anterior chamber re-forms in such cases after application of a pressure patch for 24 or 48 hours. When the chamber does not re-form, it may be necessary to excise the filtering bleb, undermine the conjunctiva, bring the flap down, and suture it to the cornea 3 to 4 mm. from the limbus.

When the anterior chamber fails to reform following a filtering operation, one should first rule out malignant glaucoma. If the cornea is hazy, tonometry should be done at the first or the second dressing. If the eye is hypotonous, one should first check whether there is a leak, which, if present, should be repaired immediately. The same goes for buttonholing of the conjunctiva, which should be noticed before the end of the operation and repaired before leaving the operating room. Assuming

there is no leak, then one is dealing presumably with aqueous suppression caused by accidental cyclodialysis. Chandler and Maumenee in 1961 reported separation of ciliary body as a cause of hypotony, especially following filtering operations. This is followed by choroidal detachment, which further delays re-formation of the anterior chamber.

Early development of a small bleb, even though the chamber is flat, is a good prognostic sign. The following factors should be taken into account when considering surgical intervention. First, if the eye is very irritated, early formation of peripheral anterior synechiae is to be feared. Second, if there is corneal edema or evidence of Fuchs' dystrophy, the chamber should be reformed immediately. I have seen irreversible bullous keratopathy develop when the chamber was not re-formed before the fourth or fifth day under such circumstances. A third factor calling for early surgical intervention is the presence of contact between the lens capsule and the corneal endothelium, resulting in a localized, milky white subcapsular opacity.

Medical management in the meantime is not neglected. I usually apply a pressure patch over the site of drainage. I avoid Diamox postoperatively in order to encourage aqueous formation. Atropine is a useful drug for flat chamber because it encourages closure of a cyclodialysis cleft, if one is present.

My technique for surgical re-formation of the anterior chamber is as follows. I use a small Wheeler knife, stained with fluorescein to enter the anterior chamber. I use a No. 30 needle for putting in air and saline. I think it is important to use both, because if only saline is used it will leak through the cyclo-dialysis cleft and the chamber will not re-form. An air bubble will prevent that from occurring. Saline also has the advantage of filling the bleb. If there is a choroidal de-tachment, I do not attempt to drain supra-choroidal fluid at the first surgical interven-tion. If the chamber is lost following air–saline injection, drainage of fluid should be carried out. Drainage can be done by a sepa-rate sclerotomy followed by reformation of the anterior chamber through a corneal in-cision, as described above. Another technique described by Dr. Schutz that is used at the Manhattan Eye, Ear and Throat Hospital is very effective and less traumatic. He advo-cates an anterior sclerotomy for drainage of fluid; he fills the anterior chamber with air through a cyclodialysis approach using the sclerotomy opening.

Dr. Gorin: Dr. Sugar, do you have any comments on this question?

Dr. Sugar: I would like to suggest that in the early cases with a soft eye, if there is very little bleb formation, one must first make sure that there is no leak to the out-side. If there is no evidence of this, I would give the patient water to drink in the same manner that one does in a water-drinking test, to stimulate the formation of the an-terior chamber. If there is a large filtering bleb and the chamber is flat, I would not do anything surgically unless there were touch between the lens and the cornea, which would mean immediate intervention. Otherwise, I would certainly wait as long as 3 to 4 weeks. However, I would not wait longer than that because of the danger of opacification of the lens due to hypotony. I have always done the procedure described by Chandler of opening the area over the ciliary body and placing saline or air into the anterior chamber.

In late cases, in which there is a flat chamber due to a leak caused by rupture of the bleb, I bring down a conjunctival flap without Tenon's capsule and suture it to the denuded upper 2 mm. of the cornea, after

applying 3.5% tincture of iodine to the sur-face of the bleb and making sure that the conjunctival flap that I just prepared has no tension whatever on it with the eye in the straight-ahead position. I have found that this is the most satisfactory method. When other methods are used, such as Tenon's capsule grafts or pedicle grafts into the bleb aiming at closure of the hole (the classical flap with Tenon's capsule included), there is usually no filtration because of scarring associated with previous surgery.

Dr. Gorin: Thank you, Dr. Sugar. Dr. Luntz, do you have anything to add to this?

Dr. Luntz: Just one or two minor points. As far as the early cases are concerned, I like to push fluids if, after excluding a leak, one believes that the lack of re-formation of the anterior chamber is caused by suppres-sion of the ciliary body. I think it is impor-tant to differentiate between flat or complete absence of anterior chamber and shallow anterior chamber. If the anterior chamber is flat, one should intervene surgically earlier, perhaps after 1 week. If the chamber is shallow, it is safe to wait very much longer.

Dr. Gorin: Thank you, Dr. Luntz. The next question is: What is the treatment for malignant glaucoma? What is the incidence of malignant glaucoma following glaucoma procedures?

I just want to say that the incidence has been estimated to be about 2%, but when a case such as this occurs, it is a 100% headache. What is bad about it is that the surgeon seldom foresees its occurrence. If we could learn to suspect the possibility of oc-currence of malignant glaucoma after iridec-tomy or filtering operations and warn the patient that he may need a lens extraction following the glaucoma surgery, our position would be much more comfortable. I found that in certain cases of angle-closure glau-coma, especially in older people, there is a tendency for the lens to be slightly loose. These cases may be well controlled with 2% pilocarpine. However, if a patient is given 4% pilocarpine and remains under observation for 1 hour, the anterior chamber becomes extremely shallow. This does not happen in typical angle-closure glaucoma, in which the position of the iris–lens diaphragm is more or less fixed. One gets the impression that the lens has moved forward after strong miotics and this should be a warning that malignant glaucoma may occur after opening the anterior chamber for glaucoma surgery.

Dr. Sugar: You are referring to the flat chamber after surgery for angle-closure glaucoma, in which the chamber is absent, the tension very high, and the lens is displaced forward at the first dressing. The treatment for this, which is typical malignant glaucoma, is the use of Neo-Synephrine 10% and atropine. There are some cases that respond to this treatment quite well for some time. I have not had much experience with it, since I have treated only 6 cases of malignant glaucoma in 32 years of practice. These patients have all required surgery in the form of removal of the lens.

Dr. Luntz: I was surprised to hear the mention of an incidence of 2% and was relieved to hear that Dr. Sugar has seen only 6 cases in 32 years. I have seen only 2 cases. One I saw with a chief of mine, Dr. Cross. I just mention it because this case was written up in the *British Journal of Ophthalmology*. It was a patient with typical malignant glaucoma in which Dr. Cross put a needle behind the lens into the vitreous and drew out some fluid from a pocket in the vitreous and put the patient on mydriatics and Diamox. This relieved the condition without recourse to removal of the lens. I mention this because I think this is a procedure that should be tried before attempting to remove the lens.

Dr. Gorin: I would like to stress the fact that if the condition is not relieved by medical means, prompt extraction of the lens is important. If one waits too long the vitreous frequently comes forward into contact with the cornea after removal of the lens. This results in a flat chamber that can be managed only by discission of the anterior face

of the condensed vitreous and releasing pockets of fluid trapped behind the vitreous.

Do you think that thick conjunctival blebs fail to filter adequately more often than thin blebs? I would like to ask Dr. Sugar for his opinion about this.

Dr. Sugar: I think that the thickness of the bleb depends on several factors. First of all, we know that in children and in juveniles we have the problem of filtration through the conjunctiva. This may be due simply to the known anatomic thickness of Tenon's capsule in younger people, to increased vascularization, or to the presence of some chemical substance, such as an increase in mucopolysaccharides. At any rate, thick blebs in children certainly have a greater tendency to nonfiltration.

In an older adult I am very pleased to have an adequate amount of Tenon's capsule, because I feel Tenon's capsule is protective and it prevents the most important complications that I have seen in years past with the corneoscleral trephination—the late infection and the tendency of the bleb to rupture. I happen to prefer as much Tenon's capsule as possible over a filtering fistula. I know that there are people who prefer to make the blebs thin. I am directly in conflict with them.

Dr. Gorin: I would like to make a few remarks about some work that we have been doing in the glaucoma clinic at Manhattan Eye, Ear and Throat Hospital. We have noted, while studying blebs over the years, that all well-functioning blebs are thin blebs that are not vascularized. The blood vessels come up to the edge of the bleb but do not enter the area of the bleb. Occasionally, a large blood vessel follows the contour of the bleb from 180 to 270 degrees of the circumference, but does not enter the bleb proper. On the other hand, blebs which fail to filter become vascularized early, especially in the presence of a thick-walled bleb containing Tenon's capsule or a large hard-walled bleb containing organized fibrotic tissue. We have the impression that disposal of aqueous that comes out from the anterior chamber into the filtering area may not necessarily be through the bloodstream, but may just take place by evaporation and/or percolation through the wall of a thin bleb.

It is true that a very thin bleb entails greater danger of late infection and it is best to have an anemic spongy bleb. On the other hand, a thick bleb often causes failure of the operation. I believe that Tenon's capsule is the main culprit in failure of filtering operations because of fibroblastic proliferation which takes place in the presence of Tenon's capsule, and this ultimately blocks aqueous flow through the wall of the bleb.

For the past 2 or 3 years we have tried thin conjunctival flaps. We do not even incise Tenon's capsule. We make the same incision as usual but only in the conjunctiva. We go all the way down to the limbus, partially split the limbus, and do a limbectomy. I like to call it a limbectomy instead of posterior sclerectomy. I like the opening to be anterior in order to prevent loss of communication between the anterior chamber and the filtering bed. When the opening is posterior, this communication may be lost resulting in early failure of the operation. Our results with filtering limbectomies have improved from 50% to 90% successful permanent filtration. This includes a high percentage of Negro patients who seem to filter just as well as the Caucasian patients because we have eliminated the problem of Tenon's capsule.

Dr. Sugar: Actually, I think we are talking about different things in a way, because the vascularization that you are referring to does not have anything to do with the thickness or thinness of Tenon's capsule. In either a thick or a thin functioning bleb, you have relative avascularity of the bleb. If the bleb is a failure, whether it is thick or thin, you get vascularization. This is one of the more obvious evidences of failure of function of the bleb and it has very little to do with the thickness, in my opinion.

Dr. Gorin: I would like to ask Dr. Luntz about his experience with filtering opera-

tions on Negro patients in South Africa.

Dr. Luntz: Thank you, Dr. Gorin. Perhaps I could refer to our retrospective study of surgery for open-angle glaucoma in Bantu (South African Negroes) and Caucasian patients. There were 16 failures out of 55 in Negro patients, while the rate of failure in white patients was 9 out of 51. In other words, the failure rate in open-angle glaucoma in Negro patients seems to have been rather higher than in white patients. We have the impression that the reason for the greater rate of failure in Negro patients is predominantly fibrosis of the bleb rather than fibrosis or obstruction of the fistula through the sclera.

In an attempt to overcome fibrosis of the bleb, especially in repeated operations, we have turned to the use of a plastic implant that is designed with a very large scleral flange. There have been many other attempts in the past at plastic implants. The only modification of the procedure is to concentrate more on maintaining a large bleb through the implant, rather than worrying about maintaining a fistula. We do not use thin conjunctival flaps for our fistulas; we do go through Tenon's capsule.

We use a wide prosthesis shaped to the sclera and a very small tunnel fitting into a trephine hole in the sclera. At the present time we have done the operation on 60 rabbits, which we have followed for 2 years. There have been no complications and we had reasonably good blebs. We have done this procedure in 30 patients; there were a certain number of buphthalmus cases and the rest were repeated operations in Negro patients. Analysis of the results at present shows that we achieved control of the disease (with or without the use of miotics postoperatively) in 75 to 80% of the patients we have treated. Follow-up has been from 1 to 2½ years. We removed the prosthesis after 3 months, because we were worried about the effect of the acrylic exposed to aqueous for a long time and also because we wanted to see what would happen after removal of the implant.

Dr. Gorin: Since we have been using thin flaps in our hospital, the results of filtering operations in Caucasians and Negroes do not seem to be much different. A large percentage of our patients are Negroes and we have been getting much better results. I believe that the elimination of the thick Tenon's capsule, characteristic of Negro eyes, has played an important role in the improvement of our results.

I have been asked by a number of people to comment on Dr. Posner's paper concerning the role of a cataractous lens in chronic simple glaucoma. Although this does not relate to the topic of this panel, I would like to ask Dr. Sugar to give his opinion about this concept.

Dr. Sugar: I think there is no question but that there are instances in which there is a definite relationship between cataract and glaucoma. However, it should be pointed out that in the presence of a clear lens there is absolutely no evidence that the cause for glaucoma is the lens. One could argue that in patients with heterochromic iridocyclitis there is some evidence that removal of a cataractous lens does often lead to a lessening of the uveitic response. It is important to point out that at the present time one should not consider the lens as a cause for glaucoma under ordinary circumstances.

Dr. Gorin: What are the dangers of operating on open-angle glaucoma when the eye has been treated with the long-acting miotics before surgery?

Dr. Sugar: The danger is the tendency for iritic response in patients who have miotics of any kind right up to the time of surgery. We tend to stop any miotic the day before, and, if possible, the long-acting miotics several days, possibly even longer than a week before. I find that this is not practical in many cases, but we certainly try to stop them at least 3 days before the operation.

Dr. Luntz: One must never forget the danger of long-acting miotics with general anesthesia. Some of us, like myself, do all intraocular surgery under general anesthesia.

Dr. Gorin: There has been a great deal of talk in a previous panel about prophylactic iridectomies. It seems to me that there has been a great deal of abuse and permissiveness in the recommendation of prophylactic iridectomies. I would like to ask the members of the panel what they think of a case of angle-closure glaucoma in which the tension is controlled at all times with 1 or 2% pilocarpine and in which the angle remains open gonioscopically under miotics. Would the panel consider recommending a prophylactic iridectomy on an eye such as this?

Dr. Luntz: I assume that this is a patient who has had an acute attack in the past in one eye and the angle is very narrow in the other eye. My own practice is to do a provocative test on these patients. If the provocative test is positive, then I strongly advise the patient to have prophylactic iridectomy. If the provocative test is negative, then I again explain the situation to the patient and I advise iridectomy, but I do not push it. This is my practice.

Dr. Sugar: When I have a patient with acute glaucoma and the other eye has a chamber which is shallow or shows evidence of being the same as the eye that has had the acute attack, it has usually been my practice to try to do a prophylactic iridectomy on the other eye at the same time. If I have a patient who has been controlled for a long time with miotics, I would not operate on either eye. I think that it depends a little bit on whether the eye that had an acute attack has had a very shallow chamber or not. There are varying degrees of shallowness, and I have been surprised sometimes to have a chamber which is narrow in the angle, but the rest of the chamber is not at all shallower than I would ordinarily see. In such cases I certainly would do an iridectomy on the other eye.

Dr. Harrison: I agree with the other panelists.

Chapter 32

Cataract surgery

Moderator:
Arnold I. Turtz

Panelists:
P. Robb McDonald
Ramon Castroviejo
C. D. Binkhorst

Dr. Turtz: I'm sure that all of us have had the experience in which we open an eye and the entire contents rise to greet us. Dr. McDonald, what is your precautionary management of the situation in which there is severe bulging of the anterior segment after the initial corneoscleral incision?

Dr. McDonald: I usually try to determine whether this is a positive pressure eye. If the iris is prolapsed I will nick it with a pair of scissors. If it falls back into the anterior chamber readily, I'm not too concerned, as it is just a gush of aqueous that has brought the iris out. But if it's an indication of positive pressure, I check my block and if the patient is awake and obviously not completely sedated I will call for an anesthetist to give the patient some intravenous medication. We've recently used a new drug, Innovar, which works beautifully. The patients can be spoken to but they are relaxed. If there is still evidence of positive pressure in the eye, the best thing to do is to close the wound and operate another day. This takes some intestinal fortitude because the patient is expecting an operation, but it is much better to stop while you're ahead than to go ahead and lose a lot of vitreous. I will probably schedule the patient for general anesthesia the following day.

Dr. Turtz: Do any of the panelists feel that they would do a vitreous tap in such a case and proceed, or would they prefer to cancel surgery if all of these measures fail?

Dr. Castroviejo: I would prefer to wait rather than to disturb the vitreous. I would reschedule with general anesthesia since this bulging was perhaps caused by an intra-Tenon's capsule retrobulbar injection. I would prefer to wait.

Dr. Turtz: Dr. Binkhorst, do you have any comments?

Dr. Binkhorst: I agree about checking all prophylactic measures, but I want to make a point as to the degree of bulging. If there is a slight degree of iris bulging, it is not necessary to stop, especially if you are not sure that you can do better the next time. But, of course, the whole procedure becomes very hazardous and difficult. Often in suturing these eyes the iris must be pushed back with a repositor, stitch by stitch, and in this way we succeed in suturing in the iris without doing an iridectomy.

Dr. Castroviejo: Of course, it is correct that if bulging is not pronounced one may proceed with the operation. In postponing the operation the patient can be better prepared because one can use osmotic agents that will dry the eye and make the operation much less complicated. If there is bulging and one must proceed with the operation, I would advise either a sector iridectomy or serial peripheral iridectomies throughout the extent of the incision to make sure that the bulging will not push the iris forward and bring about very extensive anterior synechiae.

Dr. Turtz: Doctor, if osmotic agents such as glycerol or mannitol put the eye in a less hazardous state, would you advocate them for routine use?

Dr. Castroviejo: I use intravenous Diamox,

500 mg., prior to the operation in all cases. In cases that aren't routine, or if there is the slightest question of glaucoma, I use mannitol or other more active osmotic agents.

Dr. Binkhorst: I agree with Dr. Castroviejo about using intravenous Diamox. I never use osmotics, and have no experience with their effect in cataract surgery.

Dr. Turtz: Thank you. Dr. Binkhorst, some people feel that the use of a phaco-prosthetic device renders the eye more vulnerable to operative and postoperative complications; and, further, that it may complicate retinal detachment surgery at a future time should it become necessary. Would you comment on this please?

Dr. Binkhorst: This can be considered from different points of view. The procedure I do now in unilateral senile cataracts is an intracapsular extraction and immediate implantation of a pseudophakos. These eyes, therefore, are a selected group because, when I get into trouble with the cataract extraction, I never implant the pseudophakos. This may be one of the reasons why we have fewer complications in these pseudophakic eyes than in aphakic eyes, and not more. There is another reason, which is a mechanical one. When the crystalline lens is removed, the lens–iris diaphragm is lost. If a pseudophakos is inserted that situation is restored, and every complication that can result from this loss is prevented.

For instance, if there is iris bulging after the cataract extraction, the iris can be pushed back in place with a pseudophakos, and iris prolapse is avoided. There will be less vitreous touch because the pseudophakos holds the vitreous behind the pupil. There are many reasons for fewer complications.

As to retinal detachment, I summed up the complications in an article in the *American Journal of Ophthalmology* a year ago, and in 200 implantations, we had 3 retinal detachments. I wouldn't say this is a signifi-

cantly lower incidence than in ordinary cataract surgery, but it is certainly not higher.

The presence of these pseudophakoi makes things easier if there is a retinal detachment. The fear of dislocating these devices by widening the pupil for examination of the fundus is more or less exaggerated; we think it's rather harmless. When we lay the patient down the pseudophakos will rest on an intact vitreous face, and in this manner I have operated upon two of these retinal detachments, one with success and one without, but not because I couldn't view the tears.

Dr. Turtz: Thank you. Dr. Castroviejo, do you have any comments?

Dr. Castroviejo: I don't use the implants. At the beginning of the passion for the implant I used it in 11 cases and lost 6 eyes. I never had the nerve to use them again. Of course, I have not used the more sophisticated implants that Dr. Binkhorst is talking about, but I feel it is a dangerous procedure that may increase complications postoperatively, and I prefer to have those things done by somebody else.

Dr. McDonald: I've had no experience with anterior chamber or Ridley lenses except to try to get them out of the vitreous when somebody else put them in. I would like to make one comment about the younger patient, from age 40 to 50, who has a mature monocular cataract. I'm always a little wary of this type of eye. I usually tell the patient that the same conditon that caused the cataract may cause some disturbance in the back of the eye. I think the incidence of retinal detachment in a monocular cataract with no obvious cause is probably higher than it is in the average aphakic patient, and I'm surprised that there were only 3 cases of detachment in over 200 cases of monocular cataract. I would expect it to be higher. I'm always wary of these patients. I'll remove the cataracts and fit them with contact lenses, but I tell them their chances of getting into trouble are probably a little greater than if it were a binocular condition.

Dr. Turtz: Thank you. Dr. Castroviejo,

would you discuss your approach to a situation in which you've taken all the precautions and still a wee bit of vitreous is lost?

Dr. Castroviejo: We have been taught that in such a case it is advisable, when performing a peripheral iridectomy, to do a larger sector iridectomy and a sphincterotomy at the 6 o'clock position to prevent displacement of the pupil upwards. That is just the opposite of what one should do, because it increases the chance of vitreous contact with the incision, which may cause several complications. First, contact between vitreous and cornea may eventually cause the development of bullous keratopathy. Second, vitreous traction to the incision may pull upon the retina and cause a detachment. Third, it may interfere with drainage of fluid through the angle and cause glaucoma.

In such cases I would proceed with the operation, and after the lens has been removed, I would close the incision very accurately. I would try to break the adhesions of the vitreous to the incision. After the stitches have been tied, a very thin spatula, 0.5 mm. wide and 15 mm. long, is introduced into the eye on one side between the iris and the vitreous and is rotated down to break the attachment of the vitreous to the incision. The moment this is done, the pupil that was somewhat deflected in the direction of the vitreous prolapse, immediately straightens out. The procedure is duplicated on the other side to make sure that all of the fibers that may have been attached both temporally and nasally are broken. If the vitreous attachments have been successfully broken, air should be injected into the anterior chamber. The air bubble will push the iris backwards, leaving a round central pupil. A strong miotic should be used. At the time of the operation, acetylcholine, 1:100, can be used to contract the pupil immediately; in addition, a strong miotic, such as pilocarpine 4, 5, or 6% can be instilled. The postoperative course of these patients will be identical to that of those patients who

have not had vitreous loss. The pupil remains round and central throughout, and there is no evidence that there has been any vitreous prolapse.

By this maneuver the pulling of the vitreous, which might induce retinal detachment, is avoided, the displacement of the pupil upward is stopped, and contact of the vitreous with the cornea and possible development of bullous keratopathy is also avoided. There should be a normal postoperative recovery without danger of these three complications.

Dr. Turtz: Thank you. Dr. McDonald, do you agree with this technique?

Dr. McDonald: I seldom do a sphincterotomy at the 6 o'clock position, though I usually have a sector iridectomy rather than a round pupil, and it is sometimes a little more difficult to tell if the vitreous is completely out of the wound. If you have a round pupil you can see by the eccentric pupil that you probably still have some tug.

Probably the only instrument I have on my tray that doesn't have Dr. Castroviejo's name on it is a Randolph cyclodialysis irrigator, which is exactly the same as his, except the hole is on the end rather than on the top. Rather than put a spatula in and free the vitreous, I will use a needle with air in it to try to get the vitreous out of the wound. I then inject air, introducing only one instrument into the anterior chamber. I think it's very important to check at the conclusion of this procedure to make sure that there are no vitreous strands underneath the conjunctiva flap. I routinely use a limbus-based flap, and if you take an applicator and roll it you can see if there is any vitreous in the wound.

Dr. Binkhorst: I think Dr. Castroviejo's method is a very elegant one and I personally use it too. I would like to emphasize again that it is possible with a repositor, stitch by stitch, to suture the vitreous inside the eye.

Dr. Turtz: While we're talking about vitreous and its complications, I have a question.

Will the panel members comment on what might be the indications for vitreous aspiration during cataract surgery? Is it ever indicated?

Dr. McDonald: I've never done it. I know there are many good surgeons who advocate softening the eye by aspirating vitreous, but I personally don't want to do it. I've never seen any of these cases postoperatively. I have seen needles stuck into the vitreous and I've seen a fair number of retinal detachments following it, so I'd prefer to take my chances on something else rather than to aspirate.

Dr. Binkhorst: I have done aspiration in a few cases and I've always ended up with a very cloudy vitreous. Also, I'm not sure that evacuating vitreous from the anterior chamber helps to keep it out of the wound during suturing. You may have the same troubles in finishing your operation as in not aspirating.

Dr. Castroviejo: I never aspirate the vitreous. I agree with Dr. McDonald.

Dr. Turtz: Dr. McDonald, would you talk about the major factors influencing corneal edema in the immediate postoperative period, and how you treat it?

Dr. McDonald: I think there are many cases which probably show slight corneal edema in the immediate postoperative period. You'll see edema above, where the suture line is, but I assume that you are talking about edema from something touching the endothelium. I think the most important factor is contact of the hyaloid face with the endothelium. This will vary, of course, depending upon the condition of the endothelium. If the hyaloid face is in contact with the endothelium and there is edema, I don't like it, but I don't do anything about it right away, because, as the chamber forms, this will disappear.

However, if there is localized edema from vitreous touch or iris touch, I think it is almost a surgical emergency. You should bring the patient to the hospital and relieve this adhesion early, because, in my experience, once there is corneal edema from something touching the endothelium, it progresses. Whether it's cotton, vitreous, iris, or a piece of glass in the angle, this should be relieved.

Dr. Binkhorst: If there is no visible reason for the edema I would rather tranquilize my nerves and the patient and simply wait, because it will clarify itself. But I would emphasize one point. I think many surgeons go into the eye with instruments that are not free of particles of dust or lint, and I can tell you a little trick. I sweep my instruments with a fine brush every time I start an operation. When I check the instruments under the microscope before and after having done this, there is a most delightful difference.

Dr. Castroviejo: If the edema is caused by vitreous contact, it must be freed right away as Dr. McDonald has suggested, instead of waiting to see the eye get worse. A case of chronic edema, if it's not too pronounced, may be reversed by removing the contact from the cornea, and this can be done in two different ways.

Using hypotensive agents and a miotic, make a very small incision at the limbus or a slanting corneal incision large enough to admit a needle. Aspirate the vitreous in the anterior chamber until you actually see collapse of the cornea when the aqueous and the vitreous that were pushing through the pupil have been withdrawn. Then resuture the incision very adequately, and with a 30 gauge needle inject air into the anterior chamber to separate the vitreous from the cornea. This may be sufficient to reverse the trend and the edema will clear up.

Another approach is to withdraw vitreous through an incision in the pars plana. A stab incision in the ciliary body may bring about hemorrhage and complicate matters, so the anterior approach is always best.

If the edema is very pronounced and has developed into bullous keratopathy, then, of course, the edematous cornea must be removed. This can be done in several ways.

One is by partial penetrating keratoplasty with tightly fitting graft and slightly beveled edges, as emphasized by Max Fine in San Francisco. In 50% of cases a surprisingly clear graft results.

A different approach can be used if the bullous keratopathy extends to the limbus. You may attempt to improve the cornea structurally and the eye functionally by a total, full-thickness lamellar graft. That means a full-thickness graft, with endothelium, placed in a lamellar bed dissected as deeply as possible without penetrating into the anterior chamber. If you use this type of graft and go as far as the limbus to get the limbic nutrition for the graft, you may find in a very high percentage of cases that the graft remains transparent, the bullous keratopathy does not recur, and vision improves.

Sometimes the keratopathy does not recur, but the interface and recipient cornea remain cloudy so that vision is not improved. Then the total lamellar full-thickness graft is used as a foundation for a partial penetrating keratoplasty.

There is another approach that entails the use of artificial endothelium with which I have no experience. The operation has been advocated by Dohlman from Boston, and I have seen some of his cases that show very promising results.

Dr. Turtz: Thank you, Dr. Castroviejo. I would like to add that we have seen successful penetrating grafts in corneas that were totally bullous in which you would not expect success. This is one area where perhaps I differ with the panel. In doing aphakic grafts on bullous corneas in which I expect vitreous corneal adhesions, I always aspirate vitreous at the beginning of the procedure. Would you consider this an indication, Dr. Castroviejo?

Dr. Castroviejo: These aphakic eyes are first prepared with osmotic agents. Second, I do aspirate vitreous if there is a vitreous tendency to prolapse. I do not aspirate through the pars plana, but through the opening made in the opaque cornea. Vitre-ous is evacuated either by sucking it out or by inserting a sponge which becomes adherent to the vitreous. You must continue to pull out and keep cutting until the vitreous forms a concavity and remains away from the cornea. Then you can put in the graft and replace this missing fluid with saline and an air bubble. In these cases it is almost essential to remove vitreous.

Dr. Turtz: I think you would agree that at the completion of these cases it is very important that you have a deep anterior chamber.

Dr. Castroviejo: Absolutely. If you do not, you will have a recurrence of the bullous keratopathy in the graft.

Dr. Turtz: Are there any other comments from the panel on this?

Dr. McDonald: I would agree with you that this is an indication, but since I do no corneal surgery I still don't have to aspirate vitreous.

Dr. Binkhorst: I think these cases may be an indication for the use of a pupil-blocking device such as the pseudophakos.

Dr. Turtz: One other question on this. I have not been able to duplicate the reported results that by using cryotherapy along with osmotic agents, the adhesion between vitreous and cornea can be broken. Have you had any experience with this?

Dr. Castroviejo: I have had no experience with cryotherapy in these cases. I have heard that they tried it at the Columbia Presbyterian Medical Center, and never had any success with it.

Dr. McDonald: I've had no experience.

Dr. Binkhorst: I've had no experience.

Dr. Turtz: I'd like to ask the panelists for their opinions as to whether the glaucoma that occasionally results from the use of alpha-chymotrypsin is a clinical problem or merely of academic interest. Is there any difference between 1:5,000 and 1:10,000 as regards effectiveness and its influence on resulting complications?

Dr. McDonald: I seldom use alpha-chymotrypsin. When it was first introduced I probably had 2 cases of unrecognized glaucoma that developed slight dehiscence of the wound. At that time I was flushing the anterior chamber with approximately 2 ml. of alpha-chymotrypsin. If I have occasion to use it now, I never take up more than .25 ml. in the syringe and use only 2 or 3 drops at the 6 o'clock and 12 o'clock positions. I don't take tensions on my patients postoperatively, but I haven't had any difficulty using this small amount. From my experience and from listening to others who have used it at Wills, I don't think there is much difference between 1:5,000 and 1:10,000 as far as the incidence of glaucoma is concerned.

Dr. Castroviejo: I used alpha-chymotrypsin in 150 cases when it first came out and didn't think that it gave better results; I have never used it since.

Dr. Turtz: Thank you. For our final topic I would like to poll the panel on their preference for sector as against peripheral iridectomy. I'd like to find out whether they feel that the use of one as against the other influences the type and number of complications which may follow, such as prolapse, hyphema, vitreous loss, vitreous-corneal adhesions, and so on.

Dr. McDonald: I'm pretty old-fashioned. I do 90% sector iridectomies in my cataract extractions. I do it for several reasons. First, it is easier to get the lens out. Second, I'm firmly convinced that if you get a retinal detachment it is easier to find the hole if you have a sector iridectomy, because many of these round pupils do not dilate fully. Third, I think if you've lost vitreous in one eye for an unexplained reason, then you should do a sector iridectomy on the other eye and slide the lens rather than to tumble it. If I do a round pupil I usually do two small iridectomies at the 11 o'clock and 1

o'clock positions, but I am known as a sector iridectomy man.

Dr. Binkhorst: Needless to say, I disagree with Dr. McDonald. I think in uncomplicated cases everything speaks against sector iridectomy and for peripheral iridectomy. I think it is much easier to deepen the anterior chamber immediately postoperatively with a round pupil than with a sector iridectomy and thereby prevent complications due to loss of chamber.

Dr. Castroviejo: Well, this is probably one of the very few disagreements that I have with Dr. McDonald. I feel that the iris should not be mutilated and I go to extremes to preserve the iris intact. I do one or two peripherals and in glaucomatous eyes controlled with miotics I even perform three peripheral iridectomies to minimize the possibility of anterior synechiae, which might complicate the postoperative recovery of these patients. I like to keep the iris, to separate the vitreous from the cornea.

Most cases of bullous keratopathy that I have seen have been with large sector iridectomies. Contact of the vitreous with the cornea is much more likely to take place with a large sector iridectomy than when the iris remains intact. I don't see any need to punish 98 patients because 1 or 2% may develop a retinal detachment. If they do develop a detachment and if the pupil doesn't dilate, then one can perform an iridectomy prior to the detachment operation.

I am convinced that the patient with a round pupil feels more comfortable than the patient with a large pupil. This can be verified by the patient who has a large sector iridectomy in one eye, and in the second eye a round pupil. He is infinitely more comfortable with the round pupil, while the eye with the large pupil suffers much glare and discomfort in the light.

Name index

A

Adams, S. T., 101, 111
Adest, 231
Ahmad, B., 16-17
Akiyama, K., 99
Allen, J. H., 129, 201
Allen, L., 201
Allt, W. E., 172
Allyn, B., 172
Alvis, 254
Amoils, S. P., 239
Anderson, J. R., 203
Andrade, R., 172
Apers, R., 83, 86
Apt, L., 7
Ashton, N. C., 27, 154
Astill, B. D., 142

B

Bagshaw, M. A., 52
Bailey, R. J., 283, 289
Bain, W. E. S., 111
Ballen, P., 192, 194
Ballintine, E. J., 259
Bannon, R. E., 85
Bänziger, T., 101, 111
Barger, G., 3, 7
Barkan, O., 103, 111, 125-126
Barraquer, J. I., 57, 71, 236, 239, 253
Baum, G., 212
Beard, C., 176, 192
Becker, B., 96, 107-108, 111
Bedford, M. A., 52, 53, 166, 193-194
Bellows, J. G., 225, 231, 235, 240-241
Benjamin, B., 221
Berger, P., 182
Berke, R. N., 127, 129
Besnainou, R., 176
Bietti, 228
Bill, A., 259
Binkhorst, C. D., 85, 309-314
Blau, R. J., 85
Blaxter, P. L., 85
Blodi, F. C., 166, 253
Bodian, 167
Boechmann, E. J., 129
Bogardus, C. R., 172

Bojano, 182
Boniuk, M., 27, 49, 52, 166
Bonnet, R., 81, 85
Borley, W. E., 27
Boruchoff, A., 134
Bourel, M., 85
Bradley, A. E., 201
Branca, 182
Brandt, E. N., 172
Branwood, A. W., 17
Breed, J. E., 172
Breinin, 282
Bronner, A., 72, 81, 83, 85
Bronsky, D., 7
Brown, D. H., 52, 235
Brown, H. W., 128-129, 297-303
Brown, S. I., 16, 17, 289
Brubaker, R. F., 236, 239
Budinger, 183
Burch, P. G., 18, 27
Burian, H. M., 85

C

Callahan, A., 129, 188, 191-192, 194
Canaan, S., 96
Capella, J. A., 289
Carlin, B., 221
Carroll, J. M., 142
Casey, W., 283
Cassady, J. R., 85
Castroviejo, R., 309-314
Celsus, 182
Chandler, P. A., 102-103, 107, 109-111, 125-126
Chavan, S. B., 289
Chi, H. H., 13, 17
Choy, M., 283
Cibis, P. A., 87-91, 94, 96
Cleasby, G. W., 26-27
Cobb, G. M., 171-172
Cogan, D. G., 131, 134
Cole, H. G., 129
Cole, J. G., 129
Coleman, D. J., 221
Coles, R. S., 160-162
Constantine, E. F., 85
Constantine, F. H., 52-54, 85
Converse, J. M., 172, 176, 181
Cooper, I. S., 225

315

Hugonnier, R., 85
Hugonnier-Clayette, J. R., 85
Hulquist, R., 239
Hysern y Molleras, 183

I

Iliff, C. E., 167, 172, 255, 257
Innes, G. S., 52
Irvine, S. R., 255, 257

J

Jansson, F., 221
Jones, I. S., 27, 166, 277-279
Juler, F. A., 85

K

Kaplan, H. S., 52
Kaplan, M., 57, 289
Katzin, H. M., 17, 114
Kaufman, H. E., 142, 160-161, 235, 239, 289
Keiker, 183
Kelman, C. D., 225, 228, 240-241, 282
Kent, R. B., 125
Kertesz, E. D., 126
Kestenbaum, A., 203
Kimura, S. J., 145, 150-151, 153-154, 161-162, 261, 266
King, J. H., Jr., 253, 260, 266, 289
Kirsch, R. E., 101, 111
Kleefeld, G., 261, 266
Knapp, H., 183
Knapp, P., 129, 297-303
Kopf, A. W., 172
Krayenbuhl, H., 279
Krill, A. E., 256-257
Kronfeld, P. C., 101, 111
Krwawicz, T., 225, 231, 235-236, 239-241
Kurose, Y., 7

L

Lake, L. H., 85
Langford, W. S., 134
Langham, M. E., 4, 7
Lederman, M., 166
Lee, W. Y., 7
Leonard, P. A. M., 85
Leopold, I. H. 7
Levitt, S. H., 171-172
Levy, P. M., 7
Leydhecker, W., 97, 99
Lieberman, T. W., 7
Lincoff, H., 35, 52, 228
Littmann, H., 253
Lombardi, G., 279
Long, R., 35
Lowe, R. F., 111
Lund, O. E., 20, 27
Luntz, M. H., 111, 118-120, 305-308
Lyle, K. T., 82, 85

M

MacDonald, I., 171-172
Mackensen, G., 253
MacLean, A., 257
Magnard, P., 72, 82, 85
Manson, N., 85
Martinez, M., 239, 289
Martola, E. L., 17, 289
Massin, M., 85
Maumenee, A. E., 18, 27, 134, 257
Maurer, 82, 85
McAuley, F. D., 171-172
McDonald, P. R., 309-314
McKenna, R. J., 171-172
McKinna, A. J., 85
McLean, J. M., 35, 85, 128-129
McPherson, S. D., 5, 7
McTighe, J. W., 253
Merriman, G., 167-168, 172
Meryman, H. T., 235
Meyer, Karl, 7, 283
Meyer-Schwickerath, G., 36
Milauskas, A. T., 202
Miller, S. J. H., 7
Miller, W. W., 27
Minsky, H., 189, 266
Mirault, 183
Mishima, S., 16-17
Montigore, 182
Moore, C. D., 85
Moore, T., 235
Moran, N. C., 7
Morimoto, P. K., 7
Mueller, F. O., 289
Mules, P. H., 201
Müller, H. K., 18, 20, 27
Mullison, E. G., 197
Mustardé, 167, 186, 188

N

Nesburn, A. B., 232, 235
Neumann, H. G., 99
Newell, F. W., 111
Newhouse, R., 112
Nichols, A., 7
Nishihara, T., 17
Norn, M. S., 259, 262, 266
Norton, E. W. D., 257
Novotny, 254

O

Obear, M. F., 181
Oelis, 231
Offret, G., 72, 81, 85
Ogle, K. N., 84-85
Okun, E., 96
Ollier, 183
O'Neill, P., 72, 85

Subject index